Inverse Problems, Tomography, and Image Processing

Inverse Problems, Tomography, and Image Processing

Edited by

Alexander G. Ramm

Kansas State University
Manhattan, Kansas

Plenum Press • New York and London

Library of Congress Cataloging-in-Publication Data

On file

Proceedings of sessions from the First Congress of the International Society for Analysis, Applications, and Computing, held June 2 – 6, 1997, at the University of Delaware, Newark, Delaware

ISBN 0-306-45828-4

A Division of Plenum Publishing Corporation
233 Spring Street, New York, N.Y. 10013

http://www.plenum.com

10 9 8 7 6 5 4 3 2 1

Printed in the United States of America

PREFACE

In this volume selected papers delivered at the special sessions on "Inverse problems" and "Tomography and image processing" are published. These sessions were organized by A. G. Ramm at the first international congress of ISAAC (International Society for Analysis, Applications and Computing) which was held at the University of Delaware, June 3–7, 1997. The papers in this volume deal with a wide variety of problems including some theoretical and numerical problems arising in various inverse problems of interest in applications (Athanasiadis, Ramm and Stratis, Crosta, Gutman, Kamimura, Kochikov, Kuramshina and Yagola, Ramm, Yakhno, Yamamoto), in tomography (Faridani, Katsevich, Sharafutdinov), and in image processing (Lina, Schempp, Lobel, Pichot, Feraud and Barlaud, Weaver) These papers will be of interest to a wide audience including mathematicians, physicists, persons working in medical imaging, and theoretically oriented engineers.

A. G. Ramm
Manhattan, KS

CONTENTS

Inverse Problems, Tomography, and Image Processing

1

INVERSE ACOUSTIC SCATTERING BY A LAYERED OBSTACLE

C. Athanasiadis,[1] A. G. Ramm,[2] and I. G. Stratis[1]

[1]University of Athens
Department of Mathematics
Panepistimiopolis, GR 157 84 Athens, Greece
E-mail: istratis@atlas.uoa.gr
[2]Department of Mathematics
Kansas State University
Manhattan, KS 66506-2602, USA
E-mail: ramm@math.ksu.edu

ABSTRACT

A uniqueness theorem is proved for the inverse acoustic scattering problem for a piecewise-homogeneous obstacle under the assumption that the scattering amplitude is known for all directions of the incident and the scattered field at a fixed frequency.

1. INTRODUCTION

The inverse problem of the scattering of a plane acoustic wave by a multilayered scatterer is studied in this work. Such a scatterer consists of a finite number of homogeneous layers, and is described in detail in Section 2. The corresponding direct scattering problem has been studied by Athanasiadis and Stratis, who have shown existence and uniqueness of its solution in [2], and have implemented the low frequency theory for the determination of the solution in [1]. Alternative formulation of a similar problem for the impedance equation has been studied in [18] and references therein. In the present work uniqueness of the solution to inverse scattering problem is established provided that the scattering amplitude is known for all directions of incident and scattered fields at a fixed frequency. The proof is based on an orthogonality result and is similar to the proofs in [7–12]. Similar ideas have been applied in [12] to some inverse scattering problems, inverse spectral problems, inverse geophysical problems, and some other inverse problems. The actual reconstruction of the scatterer is still an open problem. There is a number of papers in which the surface of an acoustically soft

Inverse Problems, Tomography, and Image Processing, edited by Ramm,
Plenum Press, New York, 1998

obstacle is found numerically from the scattering data, but these contain parameter-fitting schemes, rather than a reconstruction procedure based on an analytical or numerical inversion method, and they give no error estimate for the solution. Stability estimates for the recovered obstacle are not given in the present work. They were given in the papers [13, 14] for the case of a non-stratified soft scatterer.

2. THE DIRECT PROBLEM

Let D be a bounded closed subset of $\mathbb{R}^3$ with boundary S_0. The set D is divided into annuli-like regions D_m by surfaces S_m, where S_{m-1} surrounds S_m, and $S_{m-1} \cap S_m = \emptyset$, $m = 1,2,\dots,M$. The S_m, $m = 0,1,\dots,M$ are assumed to be $C^{1,\lambda}$-surfaces, $\lambda \in (0,1]$. Moreover we assume that the origin is contained in D_{M+1}, the "last" region. The exterior D_0 of D, as well as each of D_m, are homogeneous isotropic media of mass density ρ_m and compressibility γ_m. The wave number k_m in each region D_m is expressed in terms of the free space (D_0) wave number $k_0 > 0$, by the relation

$$k_m^2 = \frac{\gamma_0}{\gamma_m}\frac{\rho_m}{\rho_0}k_0^2. \tag{2.1}$$

We assume that a plane acoustic wave u^{inc} is incident upon D; suppressing the harmonic time dependence $\exp(-i\omega t)$, ω being the angular frequency, we have

$$u^{\text{inc}}(x,\alpha,k_0) = e^{ik_0 x\cdot\alpha}, \tag{2.2}$$

where α is the unit vector in the direction of propagation.

The total exterior acoustic field u_0 is given by the formula:

$$u_0(x,\alpha,k_0) = u^{\text{inc}}(x,\alpha,k_0) + u^{\text{sc}}(x,\alpha,k_0), \tag{2.3}$$

where u^{sc} is the scattered field given by

$$u^{\text{sc}}(x,\alpha,k_0) = A(\alpha',\alpha,k_0)\frac{e^{ik_0 r}}{r} + o\left(\frac{1}{r}\right), \quad r \to \infty \tag{2.4}$$

with $r = |x|$ and $\alpha' = \frac{x}{r}$. $A(\alpha',\alpha,k_0)$ is the scattering amplitude [6]. Formula (2.4) implies the radiation condition for the scattered field.

Let u_m be the acoustic field in D_m. Then the problem of scattering of u^{inc} by the multi-layered scatterer D, is described by the following *transmission problem*:
Find $u_m \in C^2(D_m) \cap C(\overline{D_m})$, such that

$$\Delta u_m + k_m^2 u_m = 0, \qquad \text{in } D_m, \quad m = 0,1,\dots,M+1 \tag{2.5}$$

$$\left.\begin{aligned} u_{m+1} - u_m &= 0 \\ \frac{1}{\rho_{m+1}}\frac{\partial u_{m+1}}{\partial \nu} - \frac{1}{\rho_m}\frac{\partial u_m}{\partial \nu} &= 0 \end{aligned}\right\}, \quad \text{on } S_m, \quad m = 0,1,\dots,M \tag{2.6}$$

along with (2.3) and (2.4).

It has been proved in [2] that this transmission problem has a unique solution.

Remark 2.1. The fundamental solution

$$\Phi(x,y) = \frac{e^{ik|x-y|}}{4\pi \mid x-y \mid} \tag{2.7}$$

of the Helmholtz equation $\Delta u + k^2 u = 0$ satisfies

$$\operatorname*{grad}_x \Phi(x,y) = \left(ik - \frac{1}{\mid x-y \mid} \right) \Phi(x,y) \frac{x-y}{\mid x-y \mid} \tag{2.8}$$

and the asymptotic formulas

$$\Phi(x,y) = \frac{1}{4\pi \mid x-y \mid} [1 + O(\mid x-y \mid)], \quad \mid x-y \mid \to 0 \tag{2.9}$$

and

$$\operatorname*{grad}_x \Phi(x,y) = \frac{x-y}{4\pi \mid x-y \mid^3} \left[1 + O(\mid x-y \mid^2)\right], \quad \mid x-y \mid \to 0. \tag{2.10}$$

If $\Phi_m(x,y)$ is the fundamental solution of $\Delta u + k_m^2 u = 0$ in D_m, $m = 0, 1, \ldots, M+1$, then $\Phi_m(x,y)$ satisfies (2.9) and (2.10). The asymptotic behavior for elliptic operators with smooth coefficients was derived by the parametric methods in the theory of pseudodifferential operators and also by classical methods (see [5]).

We will need also the asymptotics of the principal part of the fundamental solution to elliptic equations of the second order of the divergent form (see (3.1) with $q(x) = 0$ below) for piecewise-smooth $a(x)$. We assume that $a(x)$ has a smooth surface S as a discontinuity surface, and $a(x)$ together with its derivatives is continuous up to S from inside and outside. In this case one can assume without loss of generality that S is a plane, say the plane $x_n = 0$, and the function $a(x)$ is constant a_+ if $x_n > 0$, and $a(x) = a_-$ if $x_n < 0$. The fundamental solution g is assumed continuous across S, and $a\frac{\partial g}{\partial \nu}$ is continuous across S, where ν is the normal to S, in our case ν is directed along x_n. In [17] a formula for $g(x,y)$ is obtained, where $g(x,y)$ satisfies the above transmission conditions across S and the differential equation $\operatorname{div}[a(x) \operatorname{grad} g] + k_0^2 q(x) g = -\delta(x-y)$ in $\mathbb{R}^n$. If $a(x)$ is piecewise-constant, then a global formula for g is given in [17], see formulas (2.11) and (2.12) below. In [4], it is claimed that g is of the form $c \mid x-y \mid^{-1}$ if $n = 3$, where $c = [(a_+ + a_-)(2\pi)]^{-1}$. This claim is not correct and we give below the correct formula. However, if y, the pole of $g(x,y)$, belongs to the interface S, then, as $|x-y| \to 0$, one obtains $g \sim c|x-y|^{-1}$, with c defined above as in [4].

Let $\gamma := (a_+ - a_-)/(a_+ + a_-)$, $\rho := \mid \hat{x} - \hat{y} \mid$, $\hat{x} := (x_1, \ldots, x_{n-1})$, $A_\pm := (4\pi a_\pm)^{-1}$, $r := \mid x-y \mid$. We claim that the following global formula holds

$$g = A_+ \left[\frac{1}{r} + \frac{\gamma}{(\rho^2 + [\mid x_3 \mid + \mid y_3 \mid]^2)^{1/2}} \right], \; y_3 > 0, \tag{2.11}$$

$$g = A_- \left[\frac{1}{r} - \frac{\gamma}{(\rho^2 + [\mid x_3 \mid + \mid y_3 \mid]^2)^{1/2}} \right], \; y_3 < 0. \tag{2.12}$$

The idea of the proof of formulas (2.11)–(2.12) is simple: one Fourier-transforms the equation for g with respect to transversal variables $\hat{x}$ and gets an ordinary differential equation for the function $\widetilde{g}$, the Fourier transform of the above g. The solution to this equation with the transmission conditions at $x_3 = 0$ leads to the formula:

$$\widetilde{g} = \frac{\exp(-\xi \mid x_3 - y_3 \mid)}{2\xi a_+} + \gamma \frac{\exp(-\xi[\mid x_3 \mid + \mid y_3 \mid])}{2\xi a_+}, \; y_3 > 0, \tag{2.13}$$

$$\widetilde{g} = \frac{\exp(-\xi \mid x_3 - y_3 \mid)}{2\xi a_-} - \gamma \frac{\exp(-\xi[\mid x_3 \mid + \mid y_3 \mid])}{2\xi a_-}, \; y_3 < 0. \tag{2.14}$$

Inverse transforming (2.14) with respect to ξ-variable, one gets (2.11), (2.12). Let us note that (2.11), (2.12) hold locally for equations with variable coefficients.

Remark 2.2. The assumption that the S_m, $m = 0, 1, \dots, M$ are of class $C^{1,\lambda}$, $\lambda \in (0, 1]$, may be weakened to S_m being Lipschitz surfaces (see [15, 16]).

3. UNIQUENESS OF SOLUTIONS TO THE INVERSE PROBLEM

We start this section by noticing that (2.5) may be written in the following unified way

$$(Lu)(x) := \operatorname{div}[a(x) \operatorname{grad} u(x)] + k_0^2 q(x) u(x) = 0, \text{ in } \bigcup_{m=0}^{M+1} D_m, \tag{3.1}$$

where

$$u_m(x) = u(x) \chi_{D_m}(x), \quad m = 0, 1, \dots, M+1 \tag{3.2}$$

$$a(x) = \begin{cases} 1 & , \quad x \in D_0 \\ \dfrac{\rho_{m-1}}{\rho_m} & , \quad x \in D_m \cup S_{m-1}, \; m = 1, 2, \dots, M+1 \end{cases} \tag{3.3}$$

$$q(x) = \begin{cases} 1 & , \quad x \in D_0 \\ \dfrac{\rho_{m-1}}{\rho_m} \dfrac{k_m^2}{k_0^2} & , \quad x \in D_m \cup S_{m-1}, \; m = 1, 2, \dots, M+1, \end{cases} \tag{3.4}$$

$\chi_{D_m}(x)$ being the characteristic function of D_m. Using the notation $[h(x)] = h^+(x) - h^-(x)$, $h^+(x)$ $(h^-(x))$ denoting the limit of h on S from the exterior (interior) of S, we may write (2.6) as

$$[u] = 0 \quad \text{and} \quad \left[q \frac{\partial u}{\partial \nu} \right] = 0, \text{ on } S_m. \tag{3.5}$$

Moreover, in view of (2.3) we have

$$u(x) = u^{\text{inc}}(x) + u^{\text{sc}}(x), \tag{3.6}$$

while u^{sc} is assumed to satisfy the Sommerfeld radiation condition

$$\lim_{r \to \infty} r \left(\frac{\partial u^{\text{sc}}}{\partial r} - i k_0 u^{\text{sc}} \right) = 0, \tag{3.7}$$

uniformly in all directions $\frac{x}{r}$.

Therefore, the direct transmission problem (2.3)–(2.6) may be written as the problem consisting of (3.1), (3.5)–(3.7), and will be denoted by (DTP).
Now, let

$$\mathcal{H} := H^1(D) \cap \{h \in H^1(\overline{D_0}_{loc}) : \ h \text{ satisfies } (3.6) \text{ and } (3.7)\}. \tag{3.8}$$

We denote by H_0 the set of h which satisfy (3.8) with the condition that h solves (3.6) dropped and (3.7) replaced for the elements of H_0 by the condition that h vanishes near infinity. For the use of such spaces we refer to [3]. We are now in a position to give

Definition 3.1. (DTP) has a weak solution $u \in \mathcal{H}$ iff

$$\int_{\mathbb{R}^3} \{-a(x)\,\mathrm{grad}\, u(x)\cdot \mathrm{grad}\, v(x) + k_0^2 q(x)u(x)v(x)\}\,dx = 0, \ \forall v \in H_0. \tag{3.9}$$

Let us note that the transmission conditions (3.5) are incorporated in (3.9).

The *inverse transmission problem* consists of finding D (i.e. the surfaces S_m, $m = 0,1,\dots,M$), given the scattering amplitude $A(\alpha',\alpha,k_0)$ for all directions of incident and scattered fields at a fixed $k_0 > 0$. In this paper we study the uniqueness of the solutions to the inverse transmission problem. The main uniqueness result is proved by an approach similar to that used in [7–12].

For the formulation of the results, we assume that there are two multi-layered scatterers $D^{(1)}$ and $D^{(2)}$. Each $D^{(j)}$ is stratified by surfaces $S_m^{(j)}$ into layers $D_m^{(j)}$, $m = 0,1,\dots,M$ and $j = 1,2$, as described in Section 2.

We start with the following orthogonality result.

Proposition 3.1. *Let us assume that*

$$A^{(1)}(\alpha',\alpha,k_0) = A^{(2)}(\alpha',\alpha,k_0), \tag{3.10}$$

for all α', α on the unit sphere, and a fixed $k_0 > 0$. Let w_j be the solution of $L^{(j)}w_j = 0$ in Ω, $j = 1,2$, where Ω is any domain containing $\overline{D^{(1)} \cup D^{(2)}}$. Then

$$\int_{D^{(1)}} \{a_1(x)\,\mathrm{grad}\, w_1(x)\cdot \mathrm{grad}\, w_2(x) + k_0^2 q_1(x)w_1(x)w_2(x)\}\,dx =$$
$$\int_{D^{(2)}} \{a_2(x)\,\mathrm{grad}\, w_1(x)\cdot \mathrm{grad}\, w_2(x) + k_0^2 q_2(x)w_1(x)w_2(x)\}\,dx \tag{3.11}$$

Proof: Let $w := w_1 - w_2$, $a := a_1 - a_2$, and $q := q_1 - q_2$. Subtract from (3.1) with $w = w_1$, $a = a_1$, $q = q_1$ this equation with $w = w_2$, $a = a_2$, $q = q_2$, to get

$$\mathrm{div}(a_1\,\mathrm{grad}\, w) + k_0^2 q_1 w = -\,\mathrm{div}(a\,\mathrm{grad}\, w_2) + k_0^2 q w_2. \tag{3.12}$$

Let $\Omega_0 := \mathbb{R}^3 \setminus (\overline{D^{(1)}} \cup \overline{D^{(2)}})$. We have

$$\Delta w + k_0^2 w = 0, \text{ in } \Omega_0. \tag{3.13}$$

From (3.10), (2.3), (2.4) we derive that

$$w(x) = O\left(\frac{1}{|x|^2}\right), \quad |x| \to \infty, \tag{3.14}$$

whereby

$$w(x) = 0 \quad \text{for } |x| \quad \text{large.} \tag{3.15}$$

Hence, by the unique continuation principle, we obtain

$$w(x) = 0, \quad x \in \Omega_0. \tag{3.16}$$

Multiplying (3.12) by $\varphi \in H_0^1(\Omega)$ and integrating over Ω we get

$$\int_\Omega \{-a_1 \operatorname{grad} w \cdot \operatorname{grad} \varphi + k_0^2 q_1 w \varphi\} \, dx = \int_\Omega \{a \operatorname{grad} w_2 \cdot \operatorname{grad} \varphi + k_0^2 q w_2 \varphi\} \, dx \tag{3.17}$$

Now, let Ω_* be any open bounded set in $\mathbb{R}^3$, containing $D^{(1)} \cup D^{(2)}$, such that $\overline{\Omega}_* \subset \Omega$. Let $\psi \in C_0^\infty(\Omega)$, $\psi = 1$ in Ω_*. Then $\varphi := \psi w_1 \in H_0^1(\Omega)$. Hence

$$\begin{aligned} &\int_\Omega \{-a_1 \operatorname{grad} w \cdot \operatorname{grad} \varphi + k_0^2 q_1 w \varphi\} \, dx = \\ &\int_\Omega \{-a_1 \operatorname{grad} w \cdot \operatorname{grad} w_1 + k_0^2 q_1 w w_1\} \, dx = \int_\Omega (L^{(1)} w_1) w \, dx = 0, \end{aligned} \tag{3.18}$$

and so

$$\int_\Omega \{a \operatorname{grad} w_2 \cdot \operatorname{grad} \varphi + k_0^2 q w_2 \varphi\} \, dx = 0. \tag{3.19}$$

But in Ω_0 we have $a = 0$, $q = 0$, while in $D^{(1)} \cup D^{(2)}$ we may take $\varphi = w_1$, whereby (3.11) follows. □

We now prove:

Theorem 3.2. *If (3.10) holds, then $D^{(1)} = D^{(2)}$.*

Proof: As mentioned in the description of the inverse transmission problem, it suffices to show that $S_m^{(1)}$ coincides with $S_m^{(2)}$, $m = 0, 1, \dots, M$. Suppose, to the contrary, that there is a $m_0 \in \{0, 1, \dots, M\}$ such that $S_{m_0}^{(1)}$ does not coincide with $S_{m_0}^{(2)}$. Let $\widetilde{D}^{(j)}$, $j = 1, 2$, denote the domain circumscribed by $S_{m_0}^{(j)}$. Assume that $\widetilde{D}^{(1)}$ is not contained in $\widetilde{D}^{(2)}$. Without loss of generality, we suppose that $m_0 = 0$ (and hence $\widetilde{D}^{(j)} = D^{(j)}$). Let z be on the part of $S_0^{(1)}$ which is not inside $D^{(2)}$. Consider a ball B_z, centered at z, having no common points with $\overline{D^{(2)}}$, while its part inside $D^{(1)}$ lies in the first layer $D_1^{(1)}$, without touching $S_1^{(1)}$. Let $w_j(x,y)$ be the Green function of $L^{(j)}$, and $y \in \Omega_0$. Write (3.11) as

$$\begin{aligned} &\int_{D^{(1)} \cap B_z} \{a_1(x) \operatorname{grad} w_1(x,y) \cdot \operatorname{grad} w_2(x,y) + k_0^2 q_1(x) w_1(x,y) w_2(x,y)\} \, dx = \\ &= \int_{D^{(1)} \setminus B_z} \{-a_1(x) \operatorname{grad} w_1(x,y) \cdot \operatorname{grad} w_2(x,y) - k_0^2 q_1(x) w_1(x,y) w_2(x,y)\} \, dx + \\ &+ \int_{D^{(2)}} \{a_2(x) \operatorname{grad} w_1(x,y) \cdot \operatorname{grad} w_2(x,y) + k_0^2 q_2(x) w_1(x,y) w_2(x,y)\} \, dx. \end{aligned} \tag{3.20}$$

Note that the right-hand side of (3.20) is bounded as $y \to z$.

When $y \to z$, we observe that $O(|x-y|)$ is small, for $x \in D^{(1)} \cap B_z$. Hence, by formulas (2.11)–(2.12) for the principal parts of the fundamental solutions of the second-order elliptic differential equations with discontinuous coefficients we obtain

$$\left| \int_{D^{(1)} \cap B_z} k_0^2 q_1(x) w_1(x,y) w_2(x,y)\, dx \right| \leq c_1, \tag{3.21}$$

and, using formulas (2.11)–(2.12) again, we get:

$$\int_{D^{(1)} \cap B_z} a_1(x)\, \mathrm{grad}\, w_1(x,y) \cdot \mathrm{grad}\, w_2(x,y)\, dx \geq c_2 \int_{D^{(1)} \cap B_z} \frac{dx}{|x-y|^4}, \tag{3.22}$$

where c_1 and c_2 are positive constants.

The right-hand side of (3.22) tends to $+\infty$ as $y \to z$ if $z \in \mathbb{R}^3$, and therefore all the terms in (3.20), except one, are bounded. Thus, a contradiction. If the dimension of the space is greater than 3, the conclusion of Theorem 3.2 remains valid and the argument needs only a slight modification.

Hence $D^{(1)}$ must be contained in $D^{(2)}$. Arguing similarly we obtain that $D^{(2)}$ must be contained in $D^{(1)}$, and therefore that $D^{(1)} = D^{(2)}$. Hence $S_0^{(1)}$ coincides with $S_0^{(2)}$. Now, we follow the above procedure stepwise; repeating it, we conclude that $S_m^{(1)}$ coincides with $S_m^{(2)}$ for all $m = 0, 1, \ldots, M$, □

Remark 3.1. The previous result and proof remain valid for variable coefficients a, q belonging to the class of piecewise continuous functions with a non-zero jump at S_m.

REFERENCES

1. C. Athanasiadis and I. G. Stratis: Low frequency acoustic scattering by an infinitely stratified scatterer, *Rend. Mat. Appl.* **15**, 133–152 (1995).
2. C. Athanasiadis and I. G. Stratis: On some elliptic transmission problems, *Ann. Polon. Math.* **63**, 137–154 (1996).
3. R. Dautray and J.-L. Lions: *Mathematical Analysis and Numerical Methods for Science and Technology*, Vol. 4: *Integral Equations and Numerical Methods*, Springer, Berlin (1990).
4. S. M. Kozlov: Asymptotics of fundamental solutions of divergent-type second order differential equations, Matem. Sbornik, 113 (155), N2, (1980), 302-323; English transl. in *Math. USSR Sb.*, **41**, 249–267 (1982).
5. C. Miranda: *Partial Differential Equations of Elliptic Type*, Springer, New York (1970).
6. A. G. Ramm: *Scattering by Obstacles*, Reidel, Dordrecht (1986).
7. A. G. Ramm: Completeness of the products of solutions to PDE and uniqueness theorems in inverse scattering, *Inverse Problems*, **3**, 77–82 (1987).
8. A. G. Ramm: A uniqueness theorem for a boundary inverse problem, *Inverse Problems* **4**, 1–5 (1988).
9. A. G. Ramm: Multidimensional inverse problems and completeness of the products of solutions to PDE, *J. Math. Anal. Appl.* **134**, 211–253 (1988).
10. A. G. Ramm: Multidimensional inverse problems: uniqueness theorems, *Appl. Math. Lett.* **1**, 377–380 (1988).
11. A. G. Ramm: Completeness of the products of solutions of PDE and inverse problems, *Inverse Problems* **6**, 643–664 (1990).
12. A. G. Ramm: *Multidimensional Inverse Scattering Problems*, Longman Scientific & Wiley, New York (1992).
13. A. G. Ramm: Stability of the solution to inverse obstacle scattering problem, *J. Inverse and Ill-Posed Problems* **2**, 269–275 (1994).
14. A. G. Ramm: Stability estimates for obstacle scattering, *J. Math. Anal. Appl.* **188**, 743–751 (1994).
15. A. G. Ramm: Uniqueness theorems for inverse obstacle scattering problems in Lipschitz domains, *Applicable Analysis* **59**, 377–383 (1995).
16. A. G. Ramm: Existence and uniqueness of scattering solutions in non-smooth domains, *J. Math. Anal. Appl.* **201**, 329–338 (1996).

17. A. G. Ramm: Fundamental solutions to some elliptic equations with discontinuous senior coefficients and an inequality for these solutions, *Math. Inequalities and Applic.* **1**, N1, 99–104 (1998).
18. P. C. Sabatier: On the scattering by discontinuous media, in *Inverse Problems in Partial Differential Equations*, (D. Colton, R. Ewing, W. Rundell eds.), SIAM, Philadelphia, 85–100 (1990).

2

SCALAR AND VECTOR BACKPROPAGATION APPLIED TO SHAPE IDENTIFICATION FROM EXPERIMENTAL DATA: RECENT RESULTS AND OPEN PROBLEMS

Giovanni F. Crosta

DISAT, Università degli Studi di Milano
15, via Emanueli; I 20126 Milano, Italy
E-mail: giovanni@alpha.disat.unimi.it

ABSTRACT

The inverse problem considered herewith consists of determining the shape of a two dimensional, perfectly conducting obstacle from knowledge of the incident monochromatic plane electromagnetic wave and of a set of laboratory measurements related to the scattered wave: the Ipswich data. The solution algorithm and its numerical implementation rely on approximate back propagation (ABP). The latter is an algebraic transformation, which is deduced from the properties of complete families of base functions and relates the far field scattering coefficients to those on the obstacle boundary. The features presented herewith for the first time are: **a**) a consistency result for a forward propagator, which transforms least squares boundary coefficients into far field scattering coefficients; **b**) the development and testing of a scalar ABP method for two dimensional electromagnetic problems, where polarization is vertical; **c**) the outline and the implementation of a vector ABP method for horizontal polarization; **d**) the application of both methods to the inversion of experimental data. Since general conditions for the well posedness of ABP methods are still unknown, the main related open problems are also stated.

1. INTRODUCTION

The reconstruction of the shape of an obstacle from knowledge of the incident plane wave of fixed wavevector and of the scattering amplitude, given on the surface of the unit sphere, S^2, or respectively, the unit disk, S^1, is an inverse problem of class *IP31* according to [10, Section II.3].

Inverse Problems, Tomography, and Image Processing, edited by Ramm,
Plenum Press, New York, 1998

Approximate back propagation (ABP) methods have been developed during the past few years and applied to the numerical solution of said inverse problem in the acoustic (scalar) case, where the scatterer is three dimensional, star shaped, axially symmetric, smooth and non penetrable. Only simulated data were used: the values of the scattering amplitude were supplied at regularly spaced grid points on S^2. Detailed accounts are provided in [4–7]. The satisfactory performance of these methods on a wide class of examples, even when noise is added to the data, has motivated this author to extend the ABP scheme to the reconstruction of an impenetrable electromagnetic scatterer both in the scalar and vector cases. This task has been undertaken in the past few months. The development, testing and validation of the corresponding ABP algorithms is made more attractive by the availability of laboratory measurements, the Ipswich data sets [8].

The reconstruction algorithms are based on a relation i.e., ABP, between the scattering coefficients, which appear in the approximate representations of the far and, respectively, the boundary scattered waves.

To date ABP is the result of heuristics, which draws its motivation from a solution procedure for the direct problem, named the affine least squares (ALS) scheme.

Section 2 is devoted to the forward problem and to the ALS scheme in particular, where the finite dimensional subspace spanned by outgoing spherical (cylindrical) wave functions, named $X_1^{(L)}$, plays a basic role. The properties of the coefficients $c_\lambda^{(L)}$, by which the scattered field on the obstacle boundary, Γ, is represented as a linear combination of base functions, have been known for a long time [1,4,9]. On the other hand, the ALS scheme still deserves attention: the scheme is shown herewith to be consistent for spheres (disks): see Theorem 2.2. Nonetheless, the "effectiveness" of the scheme is an open problem: Problems 2.2 and 2.3.

Section 3 deals with the scalar inverse problem, where the unknown is a (finite dimensional) vector, ψ, of shape parameters, subject to constraints. Shape reconstruction is restated in the least squares sense. The $L^2(\Gamma)$-norm of the boundary defect, i.e., incident + scattered wave on Γ, is minimized by a conjugate directions algorithm. The latter is adapted to process a set of the Ipswich data, where geometry is 2-dimensional, polarization is vertical and the argument of the scattering amplitude has been measured up to an additive, unknown constant. The computational results obtained so far and described below for the first time, are satisfactory. Since an iterative algorithm is a discrete time dynamical system, a picture of the phase flow is derived from the minimization runs, with the aim of providing further insight into the properties of ABP.

Section 4 attacks a 2-dimensional shape reconstruction problem in the vector case, where polarization of the incident electromagnetic wave is horizontal. The vector ALS scheme is outlined (Proposition 4.2, Theorem 4.3 and Proposition 4.4), then the $X_1^{(L)}$-ABP method is derived (Proposition 4.5). The properties of all of these methods still have to be determined. Nonetheless, numerical implementation is attempted on another set of Ipswich data and the preliminary computational results are shown. Although performance of the vector ABP is poorer than in the scalar case, the subject is worth further, much deeper investigation.

2. THE AFFINE LEAST SQUARES SCHEME IN $X_1^{(L)}[\Gamma]$ (ALS-$X_1^{(L)}$)

2.1. Outline of the Direct Problem

In order to justify the ABP method one must start from a scheme, which approximately solves the boundary integral equations of forward scattering.

With reference to the three dimensional acoustic scattering problem, let $u := e^{i\mathbf{k}\cdot\mathbf{r}}$ denote the unit amplitude incident plane wave, the incident wavevector, $\mathbf{k}$, of which is given; the wavenumber is $k := |\mathbf{k}|$. Let $\Omega \subset \mathbb{R}^3$ denote the obstacle, which is star shaped with respect to the origin, $\mathbf{O}$, and the boundary of which, $\partial\Omega := \Gamma$, is sufficiently smooth. Then the scattered wave v is a solution to the exterior boundary value (BV) problem for the scalar Helmholtz equation (HE)

$$(\Delta^2 + k^2)v = 0 \;\text{ in } \mathbb{R}^3 \backslash \bar{\Omega} \tag{2.1}$$

subject to the Sommerfeld radiation condition at infinity and to the following Dirichlet BC, which characterizes an acoustically soft scatterer

$$(u+v)|_\Gamma = 0. \tag{2.2}$$

Let λ be the triple of indices $\lambda := \{p,m,l\}$ such that $p = 0,1; p \leq m \leq l(\leq \infty)$ and let $\{v_\lambda\}$ be the family of outgoing spherical wave functions

$$v_\lambda[\mathbf{x}] = g_{ml} P_l^m[\cos\theta] h_l^{(1)}[kr]((1-p)\cos m\phi + p\sin m\phi), \tag{2.3}$$

where $\{r, \theta, \phi\}$ are the spherical coordinates of $\mathbf{x}$, $P_l^m[\cdot]$ is the associate Legendre function, g_{ml} is the normalization factor of the surface harmonics and $h_l^{(1)}$ is the spherical Hankel function of the 1st kind.

It is well known that on or outside S_R^2, the surface of the sphere of radius R circumscribed to Ω, the scattered wave is represented by the converging series

$$v := \sum_\lambda f_\lambda v_\lambda, \tag{2.4}$$

where f_λ is the far field scattering coefficient.

A standard result, which can be deduced from the Helmholtz formulas and the addition theorem for spherical Bessel functions is

$$f_\lambda = -\frac{ik}{4\pi}\langle u_\lambda|_\Gamma \partial_N(u+v)\rangle. \tag{2.5}$$

where $\partial_N[\cdot]$ stands for normal differentiation, with the unit vector $\hat{\mathbf{N}}$ pointing outside Ω, $\langle\cdot|_\Gamma\cdot\rangle$ is the inner product in $L^2(\Gamma)$ and

$$u_\lambda := \mathrm{Re}[v_\lambda]. \tag{2.6}$$

If $\partial_N v|_\Gamma$ were known, then all f_λ's could be determined and the forward scattering problem would be exactly solved. With the exception of the sphere (see e.g., [12]) one has to implement some procedure aimed at approximating the values of $\{f_\lambda\}$.

The ALS-$X_1^{(L)}$ scheme is one of them. It consists of three steps: projection, differentiation, forward propagation, which will be defined in the next two Subsections.

2.2. The Least Squares Boundary Coefficients

Let L be the approximation order such that, λ belongs to the set

$$\Lambda(L) := \{p,m,l|p = 0,1; p \leq m \leq l \leq L\} \tag{2.7}$$

and introduce both the finite dimensional subspace of $L^2(\Gamma)$ spanned by the corresponding outgoing wave functions

$$X_1^{(L)}(\Gamma) := \mathrm{Span} v_\lambda|_\Gamma | \lambda \in \Lambda(L) \tag{2.8}$$

and the orthogonal decomposition $L^2(\Gamma) = X_1^{(L)}(\Gamma) \bigoplus (X_1^{(L)})^\perp(\Gamma)$.

Although the series in Eq. (2.4) generally is known not to converge on Γ (if it does, one says that the Rayleigh hypothesis holds or, more briefly, that Ω is a Rayleigh obstacle), it always makes sense to consider linear combinations of $v_\lambda | \lambda \in \Lambda(L)$ on Γ and state the following Problem.

Problem 2.1. Given Γ, *u and L* **find** *the vector of least squares boundary coefficients* $[c_\lambda^{(L)}] := \mathbf{c}^{(L)}$ *i.e.,* $c_\lambda^{(L)} | \lambda \in \Lambda(L)$ *such that*

$$B_{DA}^{(L)} := \frac{1}{2} \left\| u + \sum_{\lambda \in \Lambda(L)} c_\lambda^{(L)} v_\lambda \right\|_{L^2(\Gamma)^2} = \min. \tag{2.9}$$

This problem is well posed, as it appears from the following properties, which are easy to derive.

Lemma 2.1.

I. $\exists! \mathbf{c}^{(L)}$ *given by the solution to the algebraic system* $\mathbf{P}^{(L)} \cdot \mathbf{c}^{(L)} = -\mathbf{g}^{(L)}$, *where* $\mathbf{g}^{(L)}$ *is a vector of inner products and* $\mathbf{P}^{(L)}$ *a Gramian matrix*

$$\mathbf{g}^{(L)} = [\langle v_\lambda |_\Gamma u \rangle], \quad \mathbf{P}^{(L)} = [P_{\lambda\mu}^{(L)}] = [\langle v_\lambda |_\Gamma v_\mu \rangle], \quad \lambda, \quad \mu \in \Lambda(L). \tag{2.10}$$

II.

$$\min B_{DA}^{(L)} = \frac{1}{2} \left\| (u_1^{(L)})^\perp \right\|_{L^2(\Gamma)}^2, \tag{2.11}$$

where $(u_1^{(L)})^\perp$ *is the orthogonal complement of u to* $X_1^{(L)}(\Gamma)$.

2.3. The Approximately Forward Propagated (AFP) Coefficients

Knowledge of an approximation

$$v_1^{(L)} := \sum_{\lambda \in \Lambda(L)} c_\lambda^{(L)} v_\lambda \tag{2.12}$$

to v not just in $X_1^{(L)}(\Gamma)$ but in an exterior neighborhood of Γ allows differentiation

$$\partial_N v_1^{(L)}|_\Gamma = \sum_{\lambda \in \Lambda(L)} c_\lambda^{(L)} \partial_N v_\lambda |_\Gamma. \tag{2.13}$$

Forward propagation is finally defined by the following affine transformation of $\mathbf{c}^{(L)}$ (hence the name of the method)

$$\mathbf{p}^{(L)} := \mathcal{R}\mathbf{L}^{(L)} \cdot \mathbf{c}^{(L)} + \mathbf{b}^{(L)}, \tag{2.14}$$

where $\mathcal{R}\mathbf{L}^{(L)}$ is a matrix of inner products and $\mathbf{b}^{(L)}$ a vector, both obtained from known quantities

$$\mathcal{R}\mathbf{L}^{(L)} := -\frac{ik}{4\pi}[\langle u_\lambda|_\Gamma \partial_N v_\mu\rangle],$$
$$\mathbf{b}^{(L)} := -\frac{ik}{4\pi}[\langle u_\lambda|_\Gamma \partial_N u\rangle]; \quad \lambda, \quad \mu \in \Lambda(L). \tag{2.15}$$

Not only the sizes, but also the entries of $\mathbf{c}^{(L)}$ and $\mathbf{p}^{(L)}$ depend on L. Namely, the functions v_λ are generally not orthogonal in $L^2(\Gamma)$.

The numerical implementation of the ALS-$X_1^{(L)}$ scheme on a wide class of shapes in the resonance region, where e.g., diam$[\Omega] \sim \frac{2\pi}{k}$, has yielded coefficients $\mathbf{p}^{(L)}$, the values of which are close to those obtained from the Waterman [13] **T** matrix method. This notwithstanding, the following Problem remains open.

Problem 2.2. *Show there $\exists$ a class of obstacles such that, given u and L, the ALS-$X_1^{(L)}$ scheme is "effective," i.e.,*

$$|f_\lambda - p_\lambda^{(L)}| \leq |f_\lambda - c_\lambda^{(L)}|, \quad \forall\lambda \in \Lambda(L). \tag{2.16}$$

The next statement, which holds for $n = 2$ and $n = 3$, is related to inequality (2.16) and to the consistency of the AFP scheme.

A few definitions about the two dimensional case are needed at this point. Polar coordinates are used such that, $\mathbf{x} = \{r, \phi\}$ and the base functions, still denoted by $\{v_\lambda\}$, are the outgoing cylindrical waves

$$v_\lambda[\mathbf{x}] = \sqrt{\epsilon_m} H_m^{(1)}[kr]((1-p)\cos m\phi + p\sin m\phi), \tag{2.17}$$

where $\lambda = \{p, m\}$. Indices range in $\{p = 0, 1; p \leq m\}$ and $H_m^{(1)}[\cdot]$ are Hankel's functions of the first kind. The entries of $\mathcal{R}\mathbf{L}^{(L)}$ and $\mathbf{b}^{(L)}$ are then determined by choosing v_λ of Eq. (2.17) and the corresponding u_λ; also the factor $\frac{ik}{4\pi}$ must be replaced by $\frac{i}{4}$.

Theorem 2.2. *Let $n = 2$ or 3 and Ω be a disk or, respectively a sphere of radius R, i.e., $\Gamma = S_R^{n-1}$. Then, $\forall L \geq 0$ the equality sign holds in inequality (2.16) and*

$$c_\lambda^{(L)} \overset{a)}{=} f_\lambda \overset{b)}{=} p_\lambda^{(L)}, \quad \forall\lambda \in \Lambda(L) \tag{2.18}$$

i.e., the AFP scheme is consistent.

Proof:

a) The argument is the same for both values of n. The series on the right side of Eq. (2.4) converges uniformly on and outside S_R^{n-1}; moreover the functions v_λ are orthogonal in $L^2(S_R^{n-1})$. The latter property implies that each of the least squares coefficients $c_\lambda^{(L)}$ is independent of L, being a Fourier coefficient, and coincides with f_λ.

Namely, the equations in the system $\mathbf{P}^{(L)} \cdot \mathbf{c}^{(L)} = -\mathbf{g}^{(L)}$ decouple to

$$\langle v_\lambda|_\Gamma v_\lambda\rangle c_\lambda = -\langle v_\lambda|_\Gamma u\rangle, \quad \lambda \in \Lambda(L). \tag{2.19}$$

Since $u|_\Gamma = -v|_\Gamma = -\Sigma_\lambda f_\lambda v_\lambda$, there follows $c_\lambda^{(L)} = f_\lambda$, $\forall\lambda \in \Lambda(L)$, independent of L.

b) The entries of $\mathcal{R}\mathbf{L}^{(L)}$ in Eq. (2.14) have simple expressions, because of orthogonality of the base functions. To begin with, let $n = 2$. By taking the result **a)** into account one writes

$$p_\lambda^{(L)} = -\frac{\mathrm{i}}{4}\langle u_\lambda|_\Gamma \partial_N u\rangle - \frac{\mathrm{i}}{4} J_m[Z]\partial_r H_m^{(1)}|_{r=R} f_\lambda, \tag{2.20}$$

where $Z := kR$ and J_m is the ordinary Bessel function. Before replacing f_λ by the right side of Eq. (2.23) one needs to prove the uniform convergence of the series of normal derivatives at least in the annulus $R \le r \le R_1$. The summand to be estimated is $f_\lambda \partial_r v_\lambda$. Its dependence on R and r is represented by $f_\lambda \sim \frac{J_m[Z]}{H_m^{(1)}[Z]}$ and $\partial_r v_\lambda \sim \mathrm{d}_z H_m^{(1)}[z]$, with $z := kr$. The recurrent formulas for Bessel functions and their asymptotic properties for large m yield

$$\mathrm{d}_z H_m^{(1)}[z] \sim -\frac{1}{z}\sqrt{\frac{2m}{\pi}}\left(\frac{2m}{\mathrm{e}z}\right)^m \tag{2.21}$$

and therefore

$$|f_\lambda \mathrm{d}_z v_\lambda| \sim \frac{1}{z}\sqrt{\frac{m}{2\pi}}\left(\frac{\mathrm{e}Z}{2m}\right)^m\left(\frac{Z}{z}\right)^m, \quad z = kr, \quad Z = kR. \tag{2.22}$$

From Eq. (2.17), the dependence of $|f_\lambda \mathrm{d}_z v_\lambda|$ on ϕ is uniformly bounded in $[0, 2\pi]$. Moreover the summands of Eq. (2.22) give rise to a series, which converges on S_R^1 and to a greater extent for $r > R$ i.e., $z > Z$. In other words, convergence in the region of interest is uniform. As a consequence one has

$$f_\lambda = -\frac{\mathrm{i}}{4}\langle u_\lambda|_\Gamma \partial_N u + \sum_\mu f_\mu \partial_N v_\mu\rangle. \tag{2.23}$$

The right side of Eq. (2.23) coincides with that of Eq. (2.20) i.e., $p_\lambda^{(L)} = f_\lambda$, $\forall\lambda \in \Lambda(L)$, independently of L: Eq. (2.20) corresponds to the forward propagation of f_λ itself.

Next assume $n = 3$ and, without loss of generality, let $\phi_{\text{inc}} = 0$, $\theta_{\text{inc}} = \pi$. The normal derivative of the scattered field is given by (see e.g., [12])

$$\partial_N v|_{r=R} = -\partial_N u|_{r=R} - \frac{ik}{Z^2}\sum_{m=0}^{\infty}(-i)l(2l+1)\frac{P_l[\cos\theta]}{h_l^{(1)}[Z]}, \tag{2.24}$$

where $P_l[\cdot]$ is the Legendre polynomial of degree l. Obviously $|\partial_N u|$ is bounded. The uniform bound $|P_l[\cos\theta]| \le 1$, $\theta \in [0, \pi]$, $\forall l$, and the asymptotic estimate of $h_l^{(1)}$ for large l

$$|h_l^{(1)}[Z]| \sim \frac{\sqrt{2}}{Z}\frac{2l}{\mathrm{e}Z}\left(\frac{1l}{\mathrm{e}Z}\right)l, \tag{2.25}$$

together imply the uniform convergence of the series on the right side of Eq. (2.24). The required comparison between the right sides of Eqs. (2.23) and 2.20 is now possible and the conclusion is the same as with $n = 2$. With a different incidence angle, nothing changes, because of spherical symmetry. □

Theorem 2.2 presents a situation, where the fixed point of the affine map Eq. (2.14) is explicitly determined. Theorem 2.2 is also of practical relevance in the verification of computer codes during the early development stages.

In dealing with the left side of inequality (2.16), with L finite, and regardless of the Rayleigh hypothesis, one derives the estimate for the far field defect

$$\left\| \sum_{\lambda\in\Lambda(L)} (f_\lambda - p_\lambda^{(L)}) v_\lambda \right\|_{L^2(S_R^2)^2}$$

$$\leq \left(\frac{k^2}{4\pi}\right)^2 \left\| [\partial_N (v_1^{(L)})^\perp]_3^{(L)} \right\|_{L^2(\Gamma)^2} \sum_{\lambda\in\Lambda(L)} \left(|h_l^{(1)}| \|u_\lambda\|^2_{L^2(\Gamma)} \right), \tag{2.26}$$

where $[\cdot]^{(L)_3}$ denotes the orthogonal projection of a function in $L^2(\Gamma)$ onto

$$X_3^{(L)}(\Gamma) := \mathrm{Span}\{u_\mu|_\Gamma | \mu \in \Lambda(L)\}.$$

Inequality (2.26) brings about another question, which has no satisfactory answer yet i.e.,

Problem 2.3. *Provide best estimates for orthogonal complements of arbitrary $L^2(\Gamma)$ functions to e.g., the subspaces $X_1^{(L)}(\Gamma)$ and $X_3^{(L)}(\Gamma)$.*

With star shaped and smooth, but otherwise arbitrary obstacles, one may consider to check inequality (2.16) by a numerical procedure. Strictly speaking, this is contradictory. Namely, the exact values of f_λ cannot be determined numerically. At most, f_λ can be computed with reasonably high precision only for the sphere. On the other hand $c_\lambda^{(L)}$ and $p_\lambda^{(L)}$, which by definition are the solutions to approximation problems, are easily obtained from suitable computer codes and one is faced with a relation (inequality (2.16)), where the third ingredient, f_λ, is unknown.

An attempt at overcoming this difficulty relies on the "trusted method" introduced and implemented in [7] and which will not be described here.

3. SHAPE IDENTIFICATION BY THE SCALAR $X_1^{(L)}$-ABP

3.1. The Basic Minimization Algorithm

Since the obstacle shape is unknown in the inverse problem, a few pieces of prior information are useful. In the 3-dimensional acoustic case one may choose to describe the surface of the obstacle by the function $r_\Gamma \in \mathcal{C}^2[0,\pi]$ of colatitude θ alone and to parameterize it according to

$$\frac{1}{r_\Gamma^2(\theta)} = \psi_1 + \psi_2 \cos\theta + \psi_3 \sin\theta + \psi_4 \cos 2\theta + \dots \tag{3.1}$$

i.e, by a linear combination of the first I trigonometric functions. Here $\{\psi_1, \psi_2, \dots, \psi_I\}$ are the shape parameters, which form the entries of the shape parameter vector $\psi \in \mathbb{R}^I$. Representing $\frac{1}{r_\Gamma^2}$ instead of e.g., r_Γ is convenient when dealing with spheroids (or ellipses, when $n = 2$), which are exactly parameterized by the pair $\{\psi_1, \psi_4\}$. When smoothness and two sided constraints

$$(0 <) r_{\min} \leq r_\Gamma[\theta] \leq r_{\max} \quad \forall \theta \in [0,\pi] \tag{3.2}$$

are taken into account, one must select

$$\vec{\psi} \in \Psi_{\text{ad}} \subset \mathbb{R}^I \tag{3.3}$$

where Ψ_{ad} is the corresponding bounded set of admissible parameters.

In addition to u, the inverse problem data are the complex values of the scattering amplitude $S_A[\hat{\mathbf{x}}, \mathbf{k}]$, ideally provided $\forall \hat{\mathbf{x}} \in S^2$; in practice they are given at uniformly or otherwise regularly spaced grid points on S^2. From $S_A[\hat{\mathbf{x}}, \mathbf{k}]$ one obtains the estimates of order L, $\varphi^{(L)}$, of the far field scattering coefficients $\{f_\lambda | \lambda \in \Lambda(L)\}$ by carrying out the inner products

$$\varphi_\lambda^{(L)} = \langle v_\lambda^{\text{asympt}} |_{S^2} S_A \rangle, \quad \lambda \in \Lambda(L) \tag{3.4}$$

where $v_\lambda^{\text{asympt}}$ is the asymptotic counterpart of the base function v_λ as $r \to \infty$. Due to the orthogonality of $\{v_\lambda^{\text{asympt}}\}$ in $L^2(S^2)$, the values of $\varphi_\lambda^{(L)}$ are independent of L.

The following characterizes the $X_1^{(L)}$-ABP method.

Definition 3.1. Assume

$$\exists [\mathcal{R}\mathbf{L}^{(L)}]^{-1} \tag{3.5}$$

for the given L and for the involved class of obstacles. Then the affine map

$$\mathbf{M}^{(L)}[\cdot] := [\mathcal{R}\mathbf{L}^{(L)}]^{-1} \left([\cdot] + \frac{ik}{4\pi} \mathbf{b}^{(L)} \right) \tag{3.6}$$

is the scalar $X_1^{(L)}$-approximate backpropagator of order L.

Eq. (3.6) is derived from Eq. (2.14) and is intended to transform far field coefficients, or estimates thereof, into boundary coefficients, which are "close" to the $\mathbf{c}^{(L)}$ introduced by Lemma 2.1.

From Definition 3.1 one reformulates the obstacle reconstruction problem in the least squares sense.

Problem 3.1. Given *u, L, Ψ_{ad} and a vector $\vec{\varphi}^{(L)}$ of far field coefficients,* **find** *$\vec{\psi}^* \in \Psi_{\text{ad}}$ such that*

$$B_{DA}^{(L)}[\vec{\psi}^*] := \frac{1}{2} \left\| u + \sum_{\lambda \in \Lambda(L)} \xi_\lambda^{(L)} v_\lambda \right\|^2_{L^2(\Gamma[\vec{\psi}^*])} = \min, \tag{3.7}$$

where

$$\vec{\xi}^{(L)} = \mathbf{M}^{(L)}[\varphi^{(L)}]. \tag{3.8}$$

The only unknown in Eq. (3.7) is $\vec{\psi}$, on which everything depends, except $\vec{\varphi}^{(L)}$. Namely, v_λ and u are evaluated on Γ, which is parameterized by $\vec{\psi}$; the entries of $\mathcal{R}\mathbf{L}^{(L)}$ and of $\mathbf{b}^{(L)}$ in $\mathbf{M}^{(L)}$ of Eq. (3.6) are also functions of $\vec{\psi}$.

One possible algorithm aimed at minimizing $B_{DA}^{(L)}$ of Eq. (3.7) by the scalar $X_1^{(L)}$-ABP method consists of the following steps.

Algorithm 1.

1. Fix L, Ψ_{ad}, hence I, and the stopping values $B_{\min}$ and $G_{\min}$ of, respectively, the objective function $B_{DA}^{(L)}$ and the $\mathbb{R}^I$-norm of its gradient, $\nabla_{\vec{\psi}} B_{DA}^{(L)}$.
   Also, let $u = e^{i\mathbf{k}\cdot\mathbf{r}}$ and $S_A[\hat{\mathbf{x}}, \mathbf{k}], \hat{\mathbf{x}} \in S^{n-1}$ be known.
2. Estimate $\vec{\varphi}^{(L)}$ once for all by means of Eq. (3.4).
3. Supply the initial shape guess $\psi^{(0)}$.
4. Compute $\mathbf{M}^{(L)}[\cdot]$ of Eq. (3.6)
5. Solve for $\xi_\lambda^{(L)}$ of Eq. (3.8).
6. On error (e.g., $\neg\exists[\mathcal{R}\mathbf{L}^{(L)}]^{-1}$), stop; else, continue.
7. Compute $B_{DA}^{(L)}$. If $B_{DA}^{(L)} < B_{\min}$, stop; else continue.
8. Solve for the gradient of $\xi_\lambda^{(L)}$ with respect to ψ, $\nabla_{\vec{\psi}} \xi_\lambda^{(L)}$.
9. On error, stop ; else, continue.
10. Compute $\nabla_{\vec{\psi}} B_{DA}^{(L)}$. If $\| \nabla_{\vec{\psi}} B_{DA}^{(L)} \|_{\mathbb{R}^I} < G_{\min}$, then stop; else continue.
11. If a max # of iterations either main (N_{main}) or line search or step divide is reached, then stop; else update $\vec{\psi}$ by a constrained conjugate gradient rule.
12. Go to step 4.

By denoting the boundary defect by $w[\vec{\psi}] := u + \sum_{\lambda\in\Lambda(L)} \xi_\lambda^{(L)} v_\lambda$, one can easily verify that the above mentioned gradient of $B_{DA}^{(L)}$ is given by

$$\begin{aligned}
&\nabla_{\vec{\psi}} B_{DA}^{(L)} \\
&= \int \oint \operatorname{Re}\left[w^* \left(\sum_{\lambda\in\Lambda(L)} \xi_\lambda^{(L)} \nabla_{\vec{\psi}} v_\lambda + \sum_{\lambda\in\Lambda(L)} \nabla_{\vec{\psi}} \xi_\lambda^{(L)} v_\lambda + \nabla_{\vec{\psi}} u \right)\right] J[\vec{\psi}] d\omega \\
&+ \left(\frac{1}{2}\right) \int \oint |w|^2 \nabla_{\vec{\psi}} J[\vec{\psi}] d\omega
\end{aligned} \tag{3.9}$$

where $J[\psi]$ is the Jacobian and $\nabla_{\vec{\psi}} \xi_\lambda^{(L)}$ solves the algebraic system

$$\mathcal{R}\mathbf{L}^{(L)} \cdot \nabla_{\vec{\psi}} \xi_\lambda^{(L)} = -\nabla_{\vec{\psi}} \mathcal{R}\mathbf{L}^{(L)} \cdot \xi_\lambda^{(L)} - \nabla_{\vec{\psi}} \mathbf{b}^{(L)} \tag{3.10}$$

subject to Eq. (3.5).

The numerical results in the 3 dimensional acoustic case have been described by previous papers [4–7] and will not be reported here. The relevant fact is that shape reconstruction remains satisfactory in some examples even if 30% noise is added to the estimated coefficients $\vec{\varphi}^{(L)}$.

The widely documented success in many instances does not however constitute a proof of the well posedness of Algorithm 1. Steps 2 through 12 do generate a (finite) minimizing sequence $\{\psi^{(t)} | t = 0, 1, \ldots, N_{\text{main}}\}$ but the validity of Eq. (3.5) for a class of star shaped, smooth and constrained obstacles other than spheres ($n = 3$) or disks ($n = 2$) has not yet been generally established.

3.2. Application to Scalar Electromagnetic Problems

The application of the scalar $X_1^{(L)}$-ABP method to the Ipswich data, which come from vertical polarization experiments, will now be presented.

In addition to acoustic scattering, the scalar HE is met when the obstacle is a perfectly electrical conducting (PEC) right cylinder of infinite length and star shaped cross section, illuminated by a vertically polarized electromagnetic wave: namely, the electric vector of the latter is parallel to the axis, $\hat{\mathbf{z}}$, of the cylinder.

The forward problem and its approximate solution method differ from the case of Section 2 by the spatial dimension ($n = 2$) and by the obvious implications for the base functions.

The relevant angle in obstacle parameterization, Eq. (3.1) is azimuth, ϕ. The incident wave is

$$\mathbf{E}^{(\mathrm{inc})} := \hat{\mathbf{z}} e^{\mathbf{ik}\cdot\mathbf{r}} \tag{3.11}$$

and the scalar HE Eq. (2.1) holds for $E_z^{(\mathrm{sc})}$, the z-component of the scattered $\mathbf{E}^{(\mathrm{sc})}$ wave. The boundary condition on the PEC obstacle is

$$(E_z^{(\mathrm{inc})} + E_z^{(\mathrm{sc})})|_\Gamma = 0. \tag{3.12}$$

The base functions are those of Eq. (2.17). Obviously

$$\Lambda(L) = \{p, m | p = 0, 1; p \leq m \leq L\}. \tag{3.13}$$

The entries of $\mathbf{M}^{(L)}$ of Eq. (3.6) have to be changed accordingly. The boundary defect norm is now

$$B_{DV}^{(L)}[\Psi] := \frac{1}{2} \left\| E_z^{(\mathrm{inc})} + \sum_{\lambda \in \Lambda(L)} \xi_\lambda^{(L)} \upsilon_\lambda \right\|_{L^2(\Gamma[\Psi])^2} \tag{3.14}$$

The experimental data [8] from a given 2-D scatterer correspond to

$$k = \frac{2\pi}{3} [\mathrm{cm}^{-1}], \quad |E_z^{(\mathrm{inc})}| = 1 \quad \text{and} \quad \phi_{\mathrm{inc}} = \text{known}. \tag{3.15}$$

Typical values are $\phi_{\mathrm{inc}} = 180, 200, 220, \ldots$, sexagesimal degrees (deg). Radar cross section (RCS) σ is defined by (see e.g., p. 7 of [2])

$$\sigma[\hat{\mathbf{x}}, \mathbf{k}] = \frac{4}{k} |S_A[\hat{\mathbf{x}}, \mathbf{k}]|^2. \tag{3.16}$$

For every value of ϕ_{inc} the available data pairs are $\{10\,\mathrm{Log}_{10} \frac{k\sigma}{2\pi}, \chi[\phi_j]\}$, measured every half degree in the $[0, 360°]$ interval, where $\chi[\cdot]$ is the phase angle. A few data pairs are missing in a neighborhood of $\phi_{\mathrm{inc}} + 180°$, the back scattering sector.

From the preprocessing of a few Ipswich data sets originated by the disk of radius $R = 1.59$ cm it turns out that the phase angle supplied at azimuth ϕ_j is such that

$$\angle S_A[\phi_j] = \chi[\phi_j] + \gamma_0 \cdot 180°, \tag{3.17}$$

where γ_0 is an unknown constant, from now on called the phase offset.

The shape reconstruction algorithm must therefore be modified to accommodate for the this additional unknown. The following two stage procedure is implemented.

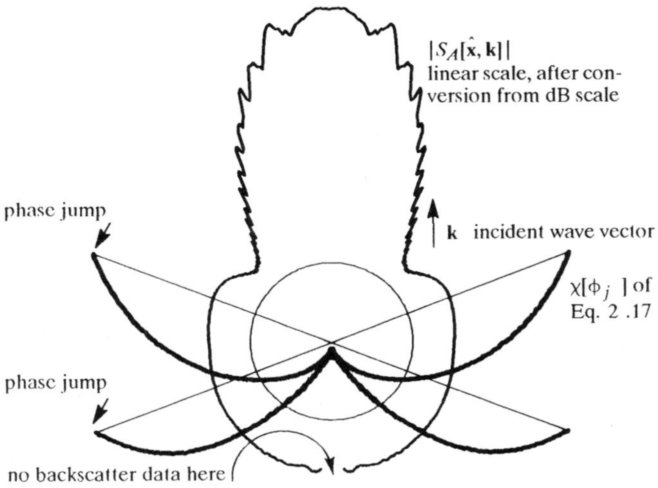

Figure 1. Polar diagrams of raw Ipswich V-polarization data from the **ips001/ips001vv.180** file.

Algorithm 2.

1. Fix L, Ψ_{ad}, $B_{\min}$ and $G_{\min}$.
2. Supply k, ϕ_{inc}, and $\vec{\psi}^{(0)}$.
3. (γ_0-stage)

   Estimate $\vec{\varphi}^{(L)}[\gamma_0^{(t)}]$ from the counterpart of Eq. (3.4), where $v_\lambda^{\text{asympt}}$ is now derived from Eq. (2.17).
4. Keep $\vec{\psi}^{(t)}$ fixed and update $\gamma_0^{(t)}$ by a conjugate gradient rule based on $\frac{\partial B_{DV}^{(L)}}{\partial \gamma_0^{(t)}}$.
5. If no $\vec{\psi}_0$-stage stopping condition is met, then go to step 3, else, continue.
6. ($\vec{\psi}$-stage)

   Keep $\gamma_0^{(t)}$ fixed, update $\vec{\psi}^{(t)}$ by a conjugate gradient rule based on $\nabla_{\vec{\psi}} B_{DV}^{(L)}$.
7. If no γ_0-stage stopping condition is met, then go to step 6, else, continue.
8. If a max # of main iterations is reached, then stop; else go to step 3.

A typical polar diagram of raw Ipswich data coming from the file **ips001/ips001vv.180** (vertical polarization, $\phi_{\text{inc}} = 180°$) is shown in Fig. 1 above. The thickest curve corresponds to $\chi[\cdot]$, exhibiting phase jumps; the backscatter sector, where data are missing, is also shown. When said data are processed by Algorithm 2 the optimal values $\vec{\psi}^*$ and $\gamma_0{}^*$ are found. Fig. 2 above shows the polar diagram of $\angle S_A{}^*$, which corresponds to $\gamma_0{}^* = -0.867$.

A set of shape reconstruction results and some of the corresponding numerical values are shown in Fig. 3 and Table 1. The raw data file is **ips001/ips001vv.240**. The reference shape is

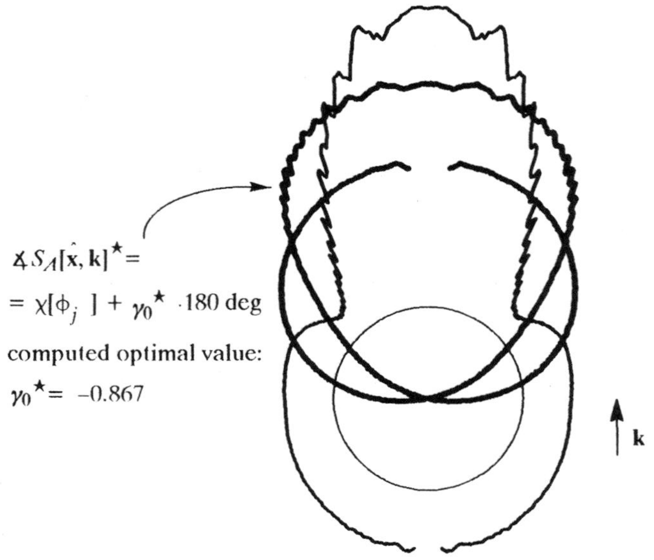

Figure 2. Polar diagrams after the optimization of γ_0.

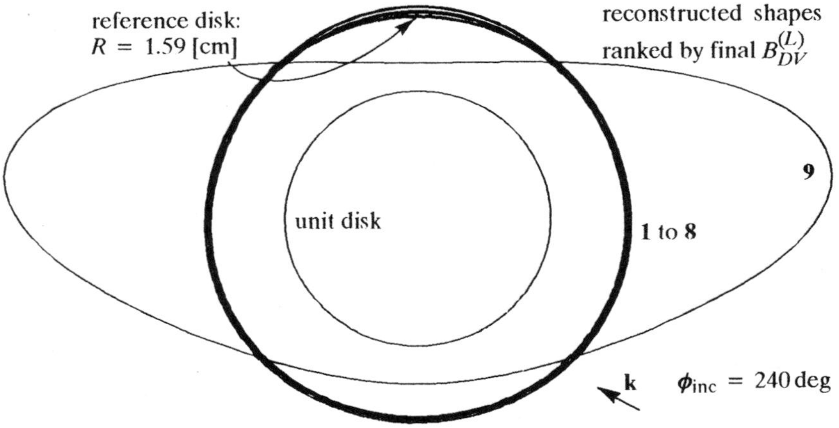

Figure 3. Shapes reconstructed from the **ips001/ips001vv.240** file. $L = 5$, $I = 6$, $n_p = 127$ and $N_{\mathrm{main}} = 15$.

Table 1. Some Numerical Values Related to Runs **1**, **2**, **8** and **9** of Fig. 3

Here r_0 denotes the radius of the initial shape at $\phi = \frac{\pi}{4}$. The best and worst results are labelled by **1** and **9** respectively.

1)	$r_0 = .571753D+00$; $N_{\mathrm{main}} = 15$; $B = .1041D+00$; $\lVert \nabla B \rVert = .8770D+00$
2)	$r_0 = .132250D+01$; $N_{\mathrm{main}} = 15$; $B = .1042D+00$; $\lVert \nabla B \rVert = .8669D+00$
8)	$r_0 = .174901D+01$; $N_{\mathrm{main}} = 15$; $B = .1066D+00$; $\lVert \nabla B \rVert = .8804D+00$
9)	$r_0 = .152087D+01$; $N_{\mathrm{main}} = 15$; $B = .7990D+02$; $\lVert \nabla B \rVert = .1881D+04$

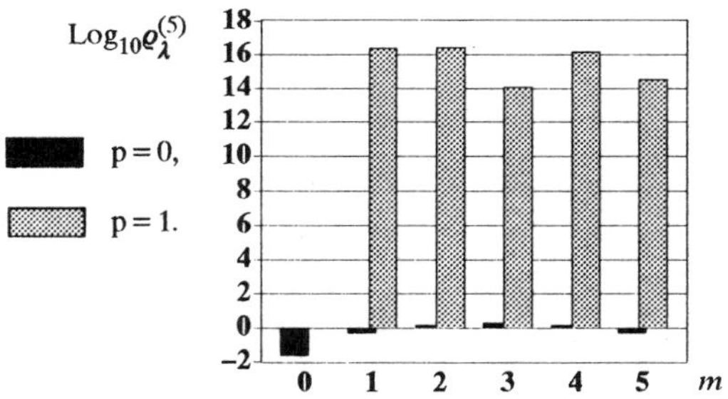

Figure 4. Bar chart of the relative estimation error affecting the far field coefficients of run **1** in Table 1.

the already mentioned disk and $\phi_{\text{inc}} = 240°$. Each of the 9 minimization runs is initialized by an ellipse such that the ratio

$$\eta := \frac{\psi_4^{(0)}}{\psi_1^{(0)}} \tag{3.18}$$

is fixed: $\eta = 0.6$. The ellipses in this set thus have the same eccentricity and differ by the half axes. The approximation order is $L = 5$, the unknown shape parameters are $I = 6$, the number of grid points on the perimeter is $n_p = 127$ and the maximum allowed number of main loop iterations is $N_{\text{main}} = 15$. The 9 reconstructed shapes are ranked by the final value of $B_{DV}^{(5)}$. The radius $r_\Gamma^{(0)}[\phi = \pi/4]$ of the initial ellipse (labelled by r_0) is also listed. Thicker lines correspond to better results. One notices that 8 out of 9 runs reconstruct the disk accurately.

Since the quality of reconstruction is affected by step 3, where $\varphi^{(L)}[\gamma_0^{(t)}]$ is estimated, it is useful to compute the following quantity, a relative estimation error

$$\rho_\lambda^{(L)} := \left| \frac{\varphi_\lambda^{(L)} - f_\lambda}{f_\lambda} \right|, \tag{3.19}$$

where f_λ comes from the known formula for the disk. A bar chart of $\text{Log}_{10}\,\rho_\lambda^{(L)}$ for $L = 5$ is shown in Fig. 4. Estimation errors for $p = 0$ are small, whereas those for $p = 1$ are extremely large. This should not mislead: the exact values of $|f_{1,m}|$ are 0, the computed ones are close to machine zero. Even if $|\varphi_{1,m}^{(L)}|$ is large in relative terms, it remains small in absolute terms and has no repercussion on the identified shape.

In order to gain insight into the properties of minimization algorithms in general and of those based on ABP in particular, it is useful to regard the sequence of shape parameters generated by the iterative procedure of e.g., Algorithm 2 as the trajectory in state space of a discrete time dynamical system

$$\mathcal{S} : \begin{cases} \vec{\psi}[t+1] = \vec{F}[t, \psi[t]] \\ \vec{\psi}[t=0] = \vec{\psi}^{(0)} \end{cases}, \tag{3.20}$$

where the generating function $\vec{F}[\cdot,\cdot]$ makes the energy $B_{DV}^{(L)}$ strictly decay in time: $B_{DV}^{(L)}[t+1] < B_{DV}^{(L)}[t]$.

Open problems related to Eq. (3.20) are:

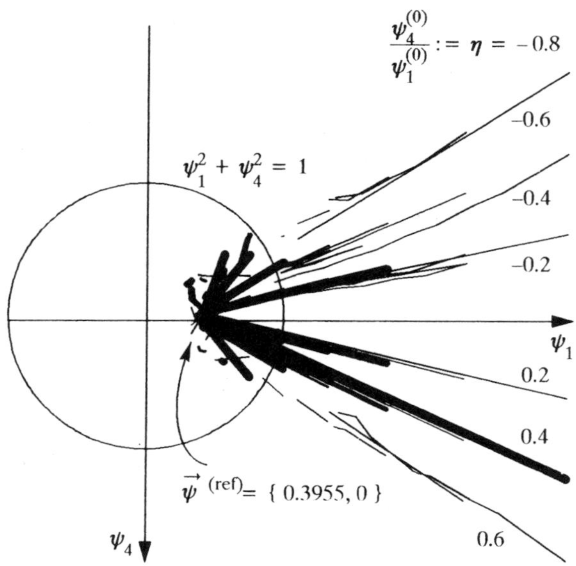

Figure 5. Collection of the trajectories of $\mathcal{S}$, where $\Psi_{ad} \subset \Omega\mathbb{R}^6$ is projected onto $\{\psi_1, \psi_4\}$, the initial states lie on the rays of Eq. (3.18) and the raw data are the same as in Fig. 3.

a. to determine the equilibrium states of $\mathcal{S}$;

b. to determine the corresponding attraction domains.

The qualitative properties of $\mathcal{S}$ can be outlined by

I. selecting two relevant components of the state vector $\vec{\psi}$ e.g., ψ_1 and ψ_4;

II. projecting Ψ_{ad} onto the $\{\psi_1, \psi_4\}$ plane ;

III. if the reference shape is known, representing $\vec{\psi}^{(ref)}$ in said plane and recalling that $\vec{\psi}^{(ref)}$ shall correspond to an equilibrium state of $\mathcal{S}$;

IV. drawing the trajectories generated by each minimization run and collecting the results.

Figure 5 depicts the implementation of rules I) to IV) to the same data set as Fig. 3, where several initial value problems for $\mathcal{S}$ have been solved. There $\{\psi_1{}^{(ref)}, \psi_4{}^{(ref)}\} = \{0.3955, 0\}$ and the loci of initial shapes lie on rays such that $-0.8 \leq \eta \leq 0.6$.

A remark about uniqueness. Fig. 5 provides no evidence of any attractor other than $\vec{\psi}^{(ref)}$, at least in the numerically explored η-sector. In fact, the attraction domain seems to include the strip $\psi_1{}^{(ref)} \leq \psi_1 \leq 3.1$. The reference disk in this and in the next Section is such that, $kR = \frac{2\pi}{3} \cdot 1.59$. In the algorithm one deliberately ignores that the obstacle is a disk, otherwise the only unknown were ψ_1. Therefore, even if single wavevector $S_A[\cdot,\cdot]$ data were exact and available $\forall \hat{\mathbf{x}} \in S^1$, one could not apply the uniqueness result for the small obstacle: Cor. 5.3 on p. 107 of [3] and Section III.8 of [10], because $kR > j_{0,0} \simeq 2.4048$ the first zero of J_0. One could overcome this limitation on kR and uniquely reconstruct disks (and spheres) of arbitrary radius by an algorithm, which determines the symmetry properties of $S_A[\cdot,\cdot]$ and implements the results of Section IV.4 of [10]. This is a subject of investigation.

4. THE VECTOR $X_1^{(L)}$-ABP APPLIED TO HORIZONTAL POLARIZATION DATA

4.1. The Approximate Forward Propagator

Let the cylinder of Section 3 be now illuminated by the horizontally polarized monochromatic plane wave

$$\mathbf{H}^{(\mathrm{inc})} := \hat{\mathbf{z}} e^{i\mathbf{k}\cdot\mathbf{r}}, \tag{4.1}$$

where $\mathbf{H}^{(\mathrm{inc})}$ is the incident magnetic field. Outside the obstacle, the z-component $H_z^{(\mathrm{sc})}$ of the scattered magnetic field $\mathbf{H}^{(\mathrm{sc})}$ complies with

$$(\Delta^2 + k^2) H_z^{(\mathrm{sc})} = 0 \ \text{ in } \mathbb{R}^3 \backslash \bar{\Omega} \tag{4.2}$$

and a suitable radiation condition. Since the surface of the obstacle is PEC, then the boundary condition involves the tangential ($\vec{\tau}$) components of the incident and scattered electric fields

$$(E_\tau^{(\mathrm{inc})} + E_\tau^{(\mathrm{sc})})|_\Gamma = 0. \tag{4.3}$$

Moreover, $\mathbf{E}^{(\mathrm{inc}),(\mathrm{sc})}\mathbf{H}^{(\mathrm{inc}),(\mathrm{sc})}$ are related by the Maxwell equations in time harmonic regime i.e.,

$$ikZ_0 \mathbf{H}^{(\mathrm{inc}),(\mathrm{sc})} = \nabla \times \mathbf{E}^{(\mathrm{inc}),(\mathrm{sc})}, \quad -ikY_0 \mathbf{E}^{(\mathrm{inc}),(\mathrm{sc})} = \nabla \times \mathbf{H}^{(\mathrm{inc}),(\mathrm{sc})} \tag{4.4}$$

$$\nabla \cdot \mathbf{H}^{(\mathrm{inc}),(\mathrm{sc})} = 0, \quad \nabla \cdot \mathbf{E}^{(\mathrm{inc}),(\mathrm{sc})} = 0, \tag{4.5}$$

where $Z_0 := \sqrt{\frac{\mu_0}{\epsilon_0}}$ is the free space impedance and $Y_0 := \frac{1}{Z_0}$.

In the inverse problem, prior knowledge about the obstacle is the same as in Subsection 3.2. In particular the unknown cross section is parameterized according to the counterpart of Eq. (3.1) and subject to the same type of two sided constraints. The data, in addition to Eq. (4.1), consist of {RCS, phase angle} pairs collected and organized as already described in Subsection 3.2 such that, once again, the unknowns are $\{\vec{\psi}, \gamma_0\}$.

Since the obstacle geometry is essentially two dimensional, work is needed to scalarize the BV problem for the vector HE, Eqs. (4.2) and (4.3), subject to Eqs. (4.4) and (4.5). Furthermore, in order to eventually apply the ABP method, the BC Eq. (4.3) has to be restated in the least squares sense.

The purpose of this Subsection is to describe the solution to the following two problems.

Problem 4.1. Given $\vec{\psi}, \mathbf{H}^{(\mathrm{inc})}$ *and* L, *assume that the approximate scattered field on* Γ, $H_{z,\Gamma}^{(\mathrm{sc},L)}$, *is represented by the linear combination*

$$H_{z,\Gamma}^{(\mathrm{sc},L)} := \sum_{\lambda \in \Lambda(L)} c_{z,\lambda}^{(L)} v_\lambda \tag{4.6}$$

where $\Lambda(L)$ *has been defined by Eq. (3.13) and* $\{v_\lambda\}$ *is the same as in Eq. (2.17),* **find** *the vector* $\mathbf{c}_z^{(L)}$ *in such a way that the boundary defect norm*

$$B_{DH}^{(L)}[\vec{\psi}] := \frac{1}{2} \| E_\tau^{(\mathrm{inc})} + E_\tau^{(\mathrm{sc},L)} \|_{L^2(\Gamma[\vec{\psi}])}^2 \tag{4.7}$$

is minimized.

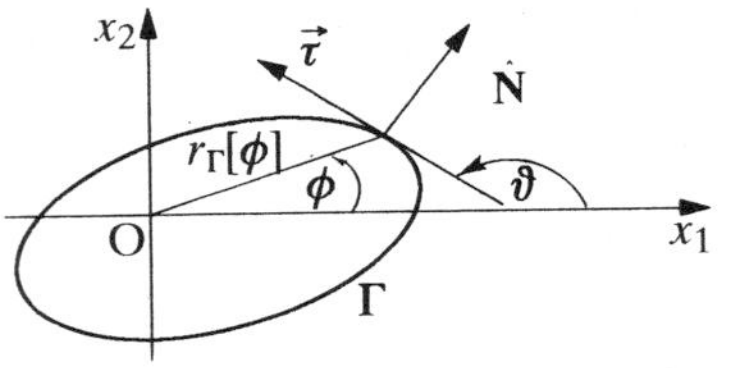

Figure 6. Geometry of the obstacle cross section.

Problem 4.2. Given $\mathbf{c}_z^{(L)}$, *which solves Problem 4.1,* **find** *the counterpart of Eq. (2.14) such that, the far scattered field, $H_{z,F}^{(\mathrm{sc},L)}$, can be approximated by*

$$H_{z,F}^{(\mathrm{sc},L)} := \sum_{\lambda\in\Lambda(L)} p_{z,\lambda}^{(L)} v_\lambda. \tag{4.8}$$

The geometry of the obstacle cross section in the $\{x_1,x_2\}$ plane and a few related quantities have to be introduced. With reference to Fig. 6, $r_\Gamma{}' := \frac{\mathrm{d}r_\Gamma}{\mathrm{d}\phi}$; the angle ϑ (not to be confused with colatitude, θ, of Section 2) complies with

$$\cos\vartheta = \frac{r_\Gamma'\cos\phi - r_\Gamma\sin\phi}{\sqrt{(r_\Gamma')^2 + r_\Gamma^2 - 4r_\Gamma r_\Gamma'\sin\phi\cos\phi}} \tag{4.9}$$

$$\sin\vartheta = \frac{r_\Gamma'\sin\phi + r_\Gamma\cos\phi}{\sqrt{(r_\Gamma')^2 + r_\Gamma^2 - 4r_\Gamma r_\Gamma'\sin\phi\cos\phi}} \tag{4.10}$$

One can easily prove the following Helmholtz formula for the magnetic field scattered by the class of PEC obstacles considered herewith.

Lemma 4.1. *Let*

$$(\hat{\mathbf{N}}\times\mathbf{E})|_\Gamma = \mathbf{0} \tag{4.11}$$

then

$$\begin{aligned} H_z^{\mathrm{sc}} =& -\partial_1\left[\int_\Gamma H_z^{\mathrm{Tot}}[\mathbf{x}']\Phi[\mathbf{x}-\mathbf{x}']\sin\vartheta \mathrm{d}\mathbf{x}'\right] \\ &+ \partial_2\left[\int_\Gamma H_z^{\mathrm{Tot}}[\mathbf{x}']\Phi[\mathbf{x}-\mathbf{x}']\cos\vartheta \mathrm{d}\mathbf{x}'\right] \end{aligned} \tag{4.12}$$

where $\mathbf{x} := x_1, x_2, z$, $H_z^{\mathrm{Tot}}|_\Gamma := (H_z^{\mathrm{sc}} + H_z^{\mathrm{inc}})|_\Gamma$ *and* $\Phi[\cdot]$ *is the fundamental solution*

$$\Phi[\mathbf{x}-\mathbf{x}'] := \frac{\mathrm{i}}{4}H_0^{(1)}[k|\mathbf{x}-\mathbf{x}'|]. \tag{4.13}$$

By letting m of Eq. (3.13) range in $p \le m \le \infty$, *the far scattered field, on or outside the circumference enclosing the obstacle, is represented by*

$$\begin{aligned} &H_{z,F}^{(\mathrm{sc})}[\mathbf{x}] \\ &= -\frac{\mathrm{i}}{4}\sum_\lambda(\partial_1 v_{0m}\langle u_{0m}|_\Gamma H_z^{\mathrm{Tot}}\sin\vartheta\rangle + \partial_2 v_{1m}\langle u_{1m}|_\Gamma H_z^{\mathrm{Tot}}\sin\vartheta\rangle) \\ &\quad+\frac{\mathrm{i}}{4}\sum_\lambda(\partial_2 v_{0m}\langle u_{0m}|_\Gamma H_z^{\mathrm{Tot}}\cos\vartheta\rangle + \partial_1 v_{1m}\langle u_{1m}|_\Gamma H_z^{\mathrm{Tot}}\cos\vartheta\rangle). \end{aligned} \tag{4.14}$$

One goes over from Eq. (4.12) to Eq. (4.14) by applying the addition theorem for $H_0^{(1)}[k|\mathbf{x}-\mathbf{x}'|]$.

The solution to Problem 4.1 can be easily obtained and reads as follows.

Proposition 4.2. *Let*

$$\begin{aligned}\mathbf{P}^{(L)} &= \frac{\mathrm{i}}{k} Z_0 [\langle v_{pm} |_\Gamma \partial_2 v_{ql} \cos\vartheta - \partial_1 v_{ql} \sin\vartheta\rangle],\\ \mathbf{g}^{(L)} &:= [\langle v_{pm} |_\Gamma E_1^{(\mathrm{inc})} \cos\vartheta + E_2^{(\mathrm{inc})} \sin\vartheta\rangle],\\ p,q &= 0,1; \quad p \le m \le L; \quad q \le l \le L\end{aligned} \tag{4.15}$$

where $E_1^{(\mathrm{inc})} = -Z_0 \mathrm{e}^{i\mathbf{k}\cdot\mathbf{r}} \sin\phi_{\mathrm{inc}}$, $E_2^{(\mathrm{inc})} = Z_0 \mathrm{e}^{i\mathbf{k}\cdot\mathbf{r}} \cos\phi_{\mathrm{inc}}$ *and* **assume** $\exists[\mathbf{P}^{(L)}]^{-1}$. *Then the vector* $\mathbf{c}_z^{(L)}$ *is obtained from solving the algebraic system* $\mathbf{P}^{(L)} \cdot \mathbf{c}_z^{(L)} = -\mathbf{g}^{(L)}$.

The main result in this Subsection consists of the solution to Problem 4.2.

Theorem 4.3. *Consider the approximate boundary scattered magnetic field of Eq. (4.6). For* $0 \le m \le L+1$ *define the sequences*

$$\{\sigma_{0,m}^-\} := \{0, \sqrt{2}, 1, \dots, 1\}, \tag{4.16}$$

$$\{\sigma_{0,m}^+\} := \{\sqrt{2}, 1, \dots, 1, 0, 0\} \tag{4.17}$$

$$\{\sigma_{1,m}^-\} := \{0, 0, 1, \dots, 1\}, \tag{4.18}$$

$$\{\sigma_{1,m}^+\} = \{\sigma_{0,m}^+\} := \{\sigma_m^+\}. \tag{4.19}$$

With reference to $\mathbf{c}_z^{(L)}$ *of Proposition 4.2, let p, q, m and l vary as in Eq. (4.15) and define the vectors*

$$[C_{p,m}^{(L)}] := [\langle u_{pm} |_\Gamma H_z^{\mathrm{inc}} \cos\vartheta\rangle] + [\langle u_{pm} |_\Gamma v_{ql} \cos\vartheta\rangle] \cdot \mathbf{c}_z^{(L)} \tag{4.20}$$

$$[S_{p,m}^{(L)}] := [\langle u_{pm} |_\Gamma H_z^{\mathrm{inc}} \sin\vartheta\rangle] + [\langle u_{pm} |_\Gamma v_{ql} \sin\vartheta\rangle] \cdot \mathbf{c}_z^{(L)}. \tag{4.21}$$

Then the entries of $\mathbf{p}_z^{(L)}$ *are given by*

$$\begin{aligned}p_{z,l,m}^{(L)} = &-\frac{ik}{8}\{-\sigma_{p,m}^- S_{p,m-1}^{(L)} + \sigma_m^+ S_{p,m+1}^{(L)}\\ &+ (2p-1)(\sigma_{1-p,m}^- C_{1-p,m-1}^{(L)} + \sigma_m^+ C_{1-p,m+1}^{(L)})\}\end{aligned} \tag{4.22}$$

The proof, which is not worked out herewith, relies on the following expressions for the tangential electric fields

$$E_\tau^{(\mathrm{inc})} = E_1^{(\mathrm{inc})} \cos\vartheta + E_2^{(\mathrm{inc})} \sin\vartheta \tag{4.23}$$

$$E_\tau^{(\mathrm{sc},L)} = \frac{\mathrm{i}}{k} Z_0 \sum_{\lambda \in \Lambda(L)} (\partial_2 v_\lambda \cos\vartheta - \partial_1 v_\lambda \sin\vartheta) c_{z,\lambda}^{(L)} \tag{4.24}$$

and on the properties of the Bessel functions. At some stage, termwise differentiation of a linear combination like that of Eq. (2.13) is carried out and the result is inserted into Eq. (4.14).

As in the scalar case, work towards the AFP of Theorem 4.3 has been heuristically guided, because there is still no proof of its general "effectiveness": in other words also the vector counterpart of Problem 2.2 is open.

In order to simplify further implementation, Eq. (4.24) must be recast in matrix form.

Proposition 4.4. *From the sequences of Eqs. (4.16) through (4.19) form the matrices $\mathbf{F}_C^{(L)}$ and $\mathbf{F}_S^{(L)}$, which e.g., for $L = 4$ read*

$$\mathbf{F}_S^{(4)} := \begin{bmatrix} \begin{matrix} 0 & \sqrt{2} & 0 & 0 & 0 \\ -\sqrt{2} & 0 & 1 & 0 & 0 \\ 0 & -1 & 0 & 1 & 0 \\ 0 & 0 & -1 & 0 & 1 \\ 0 & 0 & 0 & -1 & 0 \\ 0 & 0 & 0 & 0 & -1 \end{matrix} & \mathbf{0} \\ \mathbf{0} & \begin{matrix} 0 & 1 & 0 & 0 \\ -1 & 0 & 1 & 0 \\ 0 & 0 & -1 & 0 \\ 0 & 0 & 0 & -1 \end{matrix} \end{bmatrix};$$

$$\mathbf{F}_C^{(4)} := \begin{bmatrix} \mathbf{0} & \begin{matrix} -\sqrt{2} & 0 & 0 & 0 \\ 0 & -1 & 0 & 0 \\ -1 & 0 & -1 & 0 \\ 0 & -1 & 0 & -1 \\ 0 & 0 & -1 & 0 \\ 0 & 0 & 0 & -1 \end{matrix} \\ \begin{matrix} \sqrt{2} & 0 & 1 & 0 & 0 \\ 0 & 1 & 0 & 1 & 0 \\ 0 & 0 & 1 & 0 & 1 \\ 0 & 0 & 0 & 1 & 0 \\ 0 & 0 & 0 & 0 & 1 \end{matrix} & \mathbf{0} \end{bmatrix} \tag{4.25}$$

Denote the vectors and matrices appearing on the right sides of Eqs. (4.20) and 4.21 respectively by

$$\mathbf{y}_C^{(L)} := [\langle u_{pm}|_\Gamma H_z^{(\text{inc})} \cos\vartheta\rangle]; \quad \mathbf{y}_S^{(L)} := [\langle u_{pm}|_\Gamma H_z^{(\text{inc})} \sin\vartheta\rangle] \tag{4.26}$$

$$\mathbf{R}_C^{(L)} := [\langle u_{pm}|_\Gamma v_{ql} \cos\vartheta\rangle]; \quad \mathbf{R}_S^{(L)} := [\langle u_{pm}|_\Gamma v_{ql} \sin\vartheta\rangle] \tag{4.27}$$

and define

$$\mathbf{b}^{(L)} := \mathbf{F}_C^{(L)} \cdot \mathbf{y}_C^{(L)} + \mathbf{F}_S^{(L)} \cdot \mathbf{y}_S^{(L)}; \tag{4.28}$$

$$\mathbf{A}^{(L)} := \mathbf{F}_C^{(L)} \cdot \mathbf{R}_C^{(L)} + \mathbf{F}_S^{(L)} \cdot \mathbf{R}_S^{(L)} \tag{4.29}$$

then the AFP of Eq. (4.22) becomes

$$\mathbf{p}_z^{(L)} = -\frac{ik}{8}(\mathbf{b}^{(L)} + \mathbf{A}^{(L)} \cdot \mathbf{c}_z^{(L)}). \tag{4.30}$$

4.2. The Vector ABP and the Shape Reconstruction Algorithm

The introduction of the vector $X_1^{(L)}$-ABP is now straightforward.

Proposition 4.5. *Assume $\mathbf{p}_z^{(L)}$ is known, whereas $\mathbf{c}_z^{(L)}$ is not, and that*

$$\exists[[\mathbf{A}^{(L)}]^{\text{Trs}} \cdot \mathbf{A}^{(L)}]^{-1} \tag{4.31}$$

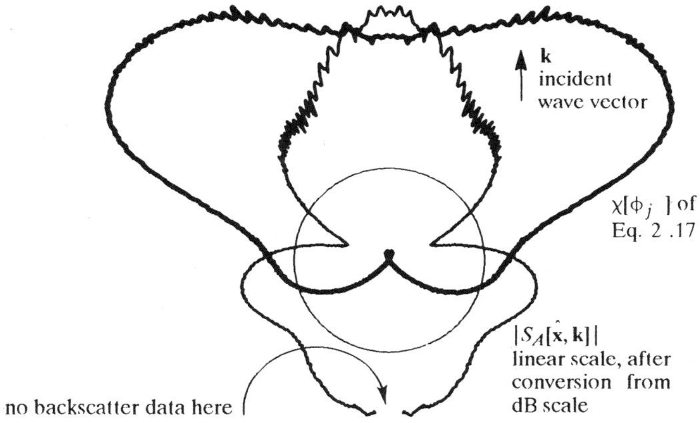

Figure 7. Polar diagrams of raw Ipswich H-polarization data from the **ips001/ips001hh.180** file.

then the algebraic system

$$[\mathbf{A}^{(L)}]^{\mathrm{Trs}} \cdot \left(\frac{\mathrm{i}8}{k} \mathbf{p}_z^{(L)} - \mathbf{b}^{(L)} \right) = [\mathbf{A}^{(L)}]^{\mathrm{Trs}} \cdot \mathbf{A}^{(L)} \cdot \mathbf{c}_z^{(L)} \tag{4.32}$$

of which $\mathbf{c}_z^{(L)}$ *is the solution, provides a representation of the* $\mathbf{p}_z^{(L)} \mapsto \mathbf{c}_z^{(L)}$ *ABP.*

As in Subsection 3.1, sufficiently wide classes of obstacles (other than disks) such that, Eq. (4.31) holds, are not known.

The reconstruction of the scatterer from single frequency experimental data is now stated as follows.

Problem 4.3. Given *the incident wave of Eq. (4.1), L,* Ψ_{ad} *and an Ipswich data set,* **find** $\psi^* \in \Psi_{\mathrm{ad}}$ *and* $\gamma_0{}^*$ *such that,* $B_{DH}^{(L)}$ *of Eq. (4.7) is minimized.*

The solution consists of implementing a version of Algorithm 2, where the estimated far field coefficients $\vec{\varphi}^{(L)}$ come from the counterpart of Eq. (3.4) and replace $\mathbf{p}_z^{(L)}$ in Eq. (4.32). Let the condition of Eq. (4.31) hold and $\vec{\xi}^{(L)}$ denote the backpropagated $\vec{\varphi}^{(L)}$, then $E_\tau^{(\mathrm{sc},L)}$, which shall appear in Eq. (4.7) is given by Eq. (4.24), where $\vec{\xi}^{(L)}$ replaces $\mathbf{c}^{(L)}$.

Preliminary numerical and graphical results are now presented and discussed.

Figure 7 above shows the polar diagrams of the raw Ipswich data **ips001/ips001hh.180** (horizontal polarization, $\phi_{\mathrm{inc}} = 180°$). The thickest curve is the raw phase angle. After the iterative optimization of γ_0, the polar diagrams of Fig. 8 above are obtained.

Figure 9 and Table 2 show results from the data set **ips001/ips001hh.200** ($\phi_{\mathrm{inc}} = 200°$), with $L = 7, I = 6, n_p = 255$ and $N_{\mathrm{main}} = 9$. The reference shape is the same as in Subsection 3.2.

Table 2. Some Numerical Values Related to Runs **1**, **2**, **8** and **9** of Fig. 9

r_0 denotes the radius of the initial shape at $\phi = \frac{\pi}{4}$. The best and worst results are labelled by **1** and **9** respectively.

1)	(thickest line)	$r_0 = .1728D+01$; $N_{\mathrm{main}} = 9$; $B = .2599D{+}01$; $\| \nabla B \| = .12D+2$; $\gamma_0 = .3-1$
2)	(thick line)	$r_0 = .1440D+01$; $N_{\mathrm{main}} = 9$; $B = .4100D{+}01$; $\| \nabla B \| = .38D+2$; $\gamma_0 = -.105$
8)	(medium line)	$r_0 = .5787D+00$; $N_{\mathrm{main}} = 9$; $B = .2939D{+}08$; $\| \nabla B \| = .77D+7$; $\gamma_0 = -.93$
9)	(thin line)	$r_0 = .4822D+00$; $N_{\mathrm{main}} = 9$; $B = .5793D{+}09$; $\| \nabla B \| = .16D+9$; $\gamma_0 = -.92$

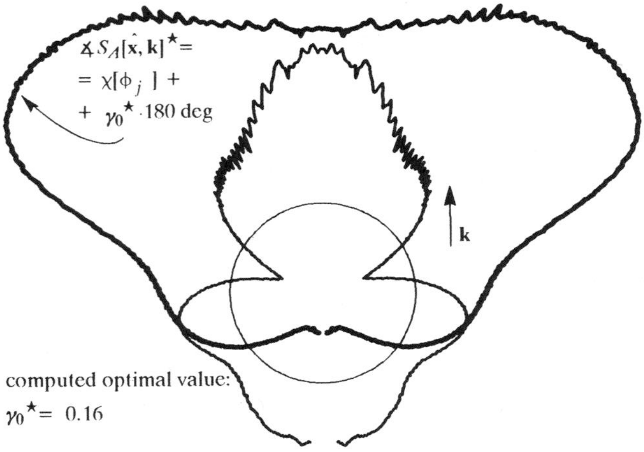

Figure 8. Polar diagrams after the optimization of γ_0.

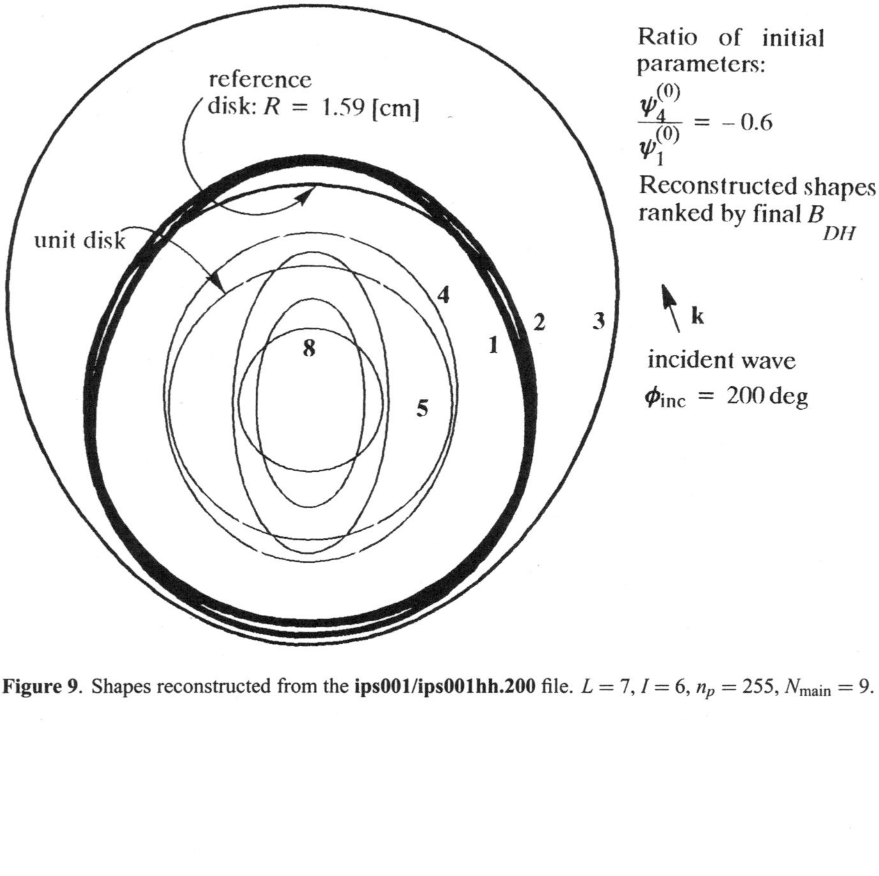

Figure 9. Shapes reconstructed from the **ips001/ips001hh.200** file. $L = 7$, $I = 6$, $n_p = 255$, $N_{main} = 9$.

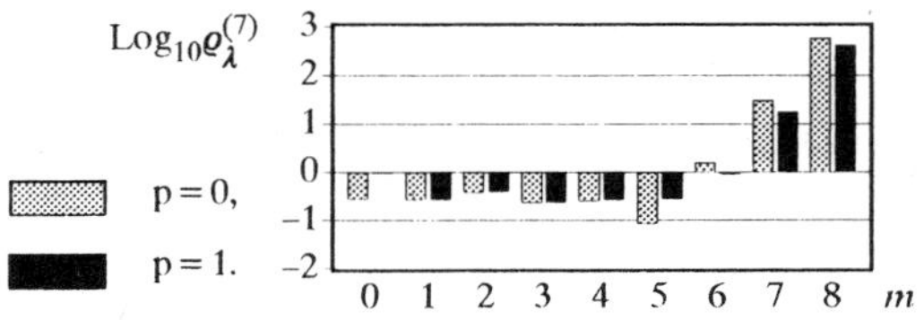

Figure 10. Bar chart of the relative estimation error affecting the far field coefficients of run **1** in Table 2.

Initial shapes have the ratio $\eta = -0.6$ in common (see Eq. (3.18)). The same representation criterion as in Fig. 3 applies. The best reconstructions are **1** and **2**.

As compared to the vertical polarization examples, only 3 out of 9 runs give rise to a low final value of $B_{DH}^{(7)}$. The other 6 are from 2 to 9 orders of magnitude above.

Estimation errors $\rho_\lambda^{(7)}$ (see Eq. (3.19)) are shown by the bar chart of Fig. 10.

The phase portrait obtained by letting η of Eq. (3.18) range between -0.8 and $+0.8$ and collecting the trajectories, is depicted by Fig. 11. The attraction domain of the reference shape is remarkably smaller than in the vertical polarization case. Many trajectories exhibit an apparently random behavior. This may be due to joint effects of approximation and numerical errors and still needs an explanation.

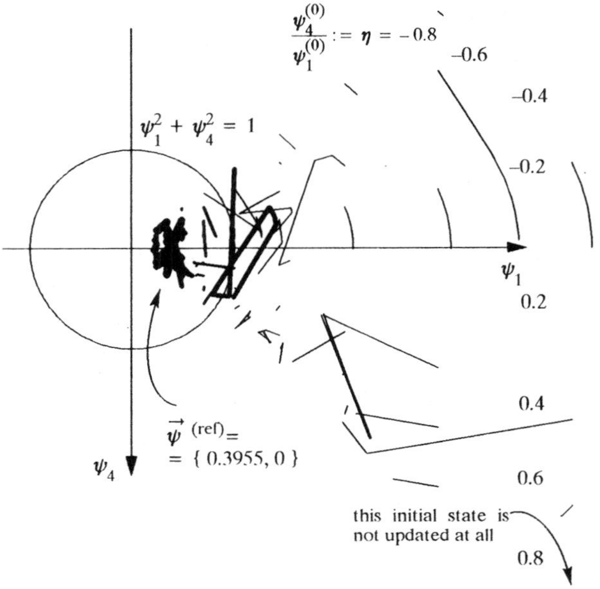

Figure 11. Collection of the trajectories of $\mathcal{S}$, where $\Psi_{\mathrm{ad}} \subset \mathbb{R}^6$ is projected onto $\{\psi_1, \psi_4\}$, the initial states lie on the rays of Eq. (3.18) with $-0.8 \leq \eta \leq 0.8$ and the raw data are the same as in Fig. 9.

DISCUSSION AND CONCLUSION

The following properties of both scalar and vector $X_1^{(L)}$-ABP algorithms are regarded as advantages ...

A.I. minimization affects a one term objective function based on the boundary defect i.e., there are neither a separate penalty term nor a far field error term, which are needed instead by other methods (see e.g., [3], for their classification);

A.II. the far field to boundary relation, which corresponds to an equality constraint, involves the coefficients and is represented by the ABP operator of Eqs. (3.6) or 4.32;

A.III. once $\psi^{(t)}$ has been determined, there is no need to compute the corresponding far scattered field;

A.IV. phase offset $\gamma_0$is the only unknown related to the far field;

... whereas these are the drawbacks:

D.I. the actual input used by the algorithm is the vector of estimated coefficients, $\varphi^{(L)}$, not the scattering amplitude, $S_A[\hat{\mathbf{x}}, \mathbf{k}]$, hence the procedure, which yields $\varphi^{(L)}$ from S_A must make small errors;

D.II. S_A must be known on the whole of S^{n-1} i.e., full aperture data are necessary.

The features, which have been presented for the first time herewith, are

F.I. the implementation of a scalar ABP algorithm in the 2-dimensional case;

F.II. the design and implementation of a vector ABP algorithm, which deals with electromagnetic inverse obstacle problems and horizontal polarization;

F.III. the application of both algorithms to the inversion of experimental data.

The availability of the Ipswich data has provided the opportunity to validate, at least at the computational level and on one reference shape, the above algorithms. These data, unlike the "noiseless" simulated ones, rule out every possibility of cross talk between the forward and the inverse solver.

All reconstruction examples have been deliberately carried out with one incident wave vector, with the purpose of determining the performance limits of the method.

Future developments include the application to other Ipswich data sets and the treatment of limited aperture data. This item will require the minimization of a two term objective function and therefore the implementation of the algorithm proposed by Ramm [11].

ACKNOWLEDGEMENTS

The author thanks Prof. A. G. Ramm for the invitation to the organized session *Inverse Problems* at *ISAAC '97* in Newark, DE and for many helpful suggestions about this research thread and this paper in particular.

This work and the related activities are being partially supported by DISAT (*Dipartimento di Scienze dell' Ambiente e del Territorio*), University of Milan. Most of the computations have been carried out by means of DISAT's *IBM RS/6000* (*53h* and *3ct*) machines.

REFERENCES

1. Barantsev, R. G., Kozachek, V. V., Issledovanie Matrizy Rasseyaniya na Ob'ektach Slozhnoi Formy (Investigation of the Scattering Matrix for Bodies of Complicated Form), *Vestnik Leningr Univers* # 7 71–77 (1968).
2. Bowman, J. J., Senior, T. B. A., Uslenghi, P. L. E., *Electromagnetic and Acoustic Scattering by Simple Shapes*, Hemisphere: New York (1987).
3. Colton, D., Kress, R., *Inverse Acoustic and Electromagnetic Scattering Theory*, Springer: Berlin (1992).
4. Crosta, G. F., The Backpropagation Method in Inverse Acoustics, in *Tomogra phy, Impedance Imaging and Integral Geometry*, **LAM 30**, M. Cheney, P. Kuchment, E .T. Quinto, eds., AMS: Providence, RI (1994a), pp 35–68.
5. Crosta, G. F., Inverse Obstacle Problem for the Scalar Helmholtz Equation, in *Proceedings of the SPIE***2241**, (*Inverse Optics III*) in M Fiddy, ed., SPIE: Bellingham, WA (1994b), pp 2–15.
6. Crosta, G. F, A Shape Optimization Problem in Inverse Acoustics, in *Control and Optimal Design of Distributed Parameter Systems*, J. Lagnese, D. L. Russel, L. White, eds., Springer-Verlag: New York (1995) pp 1–23.
7. Crosta, G. F., The Obstacle Reconstruction Problem in Acoustics: Error Analysis of an Inversion Algorithm Set in the Subspace of Outgoing Spherical Wave Functions in *Proceedings of the World Congress of Nonlinear Analysts — WCNA '96*,V. Lakshmikantham, ed., Elsevier: Exeter, UK (1997).
8. McGahan, R. V., Kleinman, R. E., Special Session on Image Reconstruction Using Real Data, *IEEE Antennas and Propagation Magazine***38** 39–40 (1996).
9. Ramm, A. G., *Scattering by Obstacles*, Reidel: Dordrecht (1986).
10. Ramm, A. G., *Multidimensional Inverse Scattering Problems*, Longman: Harlow (1992).
11. Ramm, A. G., A Numerical Approach to 3D Inverse Scattering Problems, *Appl. Math. Lett.* **7**# 2 57–61 (1994).
12. Sengupta, D. L., The Sphere, in *Electromagnetic and Acoustic Scattering by Simple Shapes*, Bowman, J. J., Senior, T. B. A., Uslenghi, P. L. E., eds., Hemisphere: New York (1987).
13. Waterman, P.C., New Formulation of Acoustic Scattering,*Journal of the Acoustical Soc of America* **45**1417–29 (1969).

3

SAMPLING IN PARALLEL-BEAM TOMOGRAPHY

Adel Faridani

Department of Mathematics
Oregon State University
Corvallis, OR
E-mail: faridani@math.orst.edu

ABSTRACT

We present Shannon sampling theory for functions defined on $\mathbb{T} \times \mathbb{R}$, where $\mathbb{T}$ denotes the circle group, prove a new estimate for the aliasing error, and apply the result to parallel-beam diffraction tomography. The class of admissible sampling lattices is characterized and general sampling conditions are derived which lead to the identification of new efficient sampling schemes. Corresponding results for x-ray tomography are obtained in the high-frequency limit.

1. INTRODUCTION

Sampling theorems provide interpolation formulas for functions whose Fourier transform is compactly supported. If the Fourier transform does not have compact support, a so-called aliasing error occurs. In this paper we present a new estimate for the aliasing error for functions defined on $\mathbb{T} \times \mathbb{R}$, where $\mathbb{T}$ denotes the circle group, and work out its application to computed tomography.

In computed tomography (CT) an object is exposed to radiation which is measured after passing through the object. From these measurements a function f characterizing the interaction of the object with the radiation is reconstructed, thus providing an image of the interior of the object. In practice only finitely many measurements can be taken, and the question arises of how to sample the data in order to obtain a desired resolution in the reconstructed image. This question can be addressed using Shannon sampling theory [2, 29]. We will characterize the class of practically relevant sampling lattices, derive sampling conditions which ensure that the data function Pf is essentially determined by the sampled values, and identify new efficient sampling schemes.

In diagnostic radiology, the classical application of CT, x-rays are used as radiation. The measurements are then line integrals of the x-ray absorption coefficient f. This leads

Inverse Problems, Tomography, and Image Processing, edited by Ramm,
Plenum Press, New York, 1998

to the mathematical problem of reconstructing a function from its line integrals, i.e., the inversion of the x-ray transform. When radiation of lower frequencies such as ultrasound or microwaves is used the mathematical model has to be generalized in order to include diffraction effects. A suitable generalization is the inverse scattering problem for the Helmholtz equation. The model we will investigate here results from linearizing this problem via the Born- or Rytov-approximations. This is called diffraction tomography [5, 12–14, 16, 19]. This model encompasses the x-ray transform which is obtained in the high-frequency limit.

The paper is organized as follows: In the next section we develop the Shannon sampling theory suitable for tomography. We characterize a class of admissible sampling lattices and obtain a new estimate for the aliasing error. The mathematical model underlying diffraction tomography is described briefly in the following section and the data function Pf is introduced. In Section 4 the essential support of the Fourier transform of Pf is determined. This allows to derive the sampling conditions in Section 5. It turns out that the required amount of data varies considerably for different sampling lattices. We identify a number of lattices which are more efficient than the usually employed standard scheme. In Section 6 the corresponding results for the x-ray transform are derived by taking a high-frequency limit.

2. SAMPLING ON $\mathbb{T} \times \mathbb{R}$

In this section we present Shannon sampling theory for functions of two variables which are 2π periodic in the first argument. Such functions can be viewed as being defined on the group $\mathbb{T} \times \mathbb{R}$, where $\mathbb{T}$ denotes the circle group. We will use the interval $[0, 2\pi)$ with addition modulo 2π as a model for $\mathbb{T}$. Sampling theorems provide exact reconstruction formulas for band-limited functions from function values on a discrete set. In the cases considered here the sampling sets are certain subgroups of $\mathbb{T} \times \mathbb{R}$. If the function to be reconstructed is not band-limited, an aliasing error occurs. The classical estimate for this error is given in Theorem 2.1. However, this estimate is not always convenient to evaluate. It turns out that a slight restriction on the admissible sampling sets allows for a sharper and more convenient estimate; see Proposition 2.3 and Theorem 2.4.

We begin with standard definitions and notation: Let $\mathbb{Z}, \mathbb{N}, \mathbb{R}, \mathbb{C}$ denote the integers, and the natural, real and complex numbers, respectively. $\mathbb{R}^n$ consists of n-tuples of real numbers, usually designated by single letters, $x = (x_1, \dots, x_n)^T, y = (y_1, \dots, y_n)^T$, etc. The inner product and absolute value are defined by $x \cdot y = \sum_{i=1}^n x_i y_i$ and $|x| = \sqrt{x \cdot x}$. The unit sphere S^{n-1} consists of the points of absolute value 1. For $a \in \mathbb{R}$ let $\lfloor a \rfloor$ and $\lceil a \rceil$ denote the largest integer $\leq a$ and the smallest integer $\geq a$, respectively.

The Fourier transform on $\mathbb{R}^n$ is defined by

$$\hat{f}(\xi) = (2\pi)^{-n/2} \int_{\mathbb{R}^n} f(x) e^{-ix\cdot\xi} dx$$

for integrable functions f, and is extended to larger classes of functions or distributions by continuity or duality. The Fourier transform of a function $g \in L_1(\mathbb{T} \times \mathbb{R})$ is given by

$$\begin{aligned}\hat{g}(\zeta) &= (2\pi)^{-1} \int_{\mathbb{T}\times\mathbb{R}} g(z) e^{-i\langle z,\zeta\rangle}\, dz \\ &= (2\pi)^{-1} \int_0^{2\pi} \int_{\mathbb{R}} g(\varphi, s) e^{-i(k\varphi+\sigma s)}\, ds\, d\varphi\end{aligned}$$

with $z = (\varphi, s) \in \mathbb{T} \times \mathbb{R}$, $\zeta = (k, \sigma) \in \mathbb{Z} \times \mathbb{R}$, and $\langle z, \zeta \rangle = k\varphi + \sigma s$. The corresponding inverse Fourier transform of a function G defined on $\mathbb{Z} \times \mathbb{R}$ is given by

$$\begin{aligned} \tilde{G}(z) &= (2\pi)^{-1} \int_{\mathbb{Z}\times\mathbb{R}} G(\zeta) e^{i\langle z,\zeta\rangle}\, d\zeta \\ &= (2\pi)^{-1} \sum_{k\in\mathbb{Z}} \int_{\mathbb{R}} G(k,\sigma) e^{i(k\varphi+\sigma s)}\, d\sigma. \end{aligned} \tag{2.1}$$

Definition 2.1. Let W be a non-singular (2,2)-matrix such that $(2\pi, 0)^T \in W\mathbb{Z}^2$, where $W\mathbb{Z}^2 = \left\{ W\binom{k}{l},\ k, l \in \mathbb{Z} \right\}$. The subgroup L of $T \times \mathbb{R}$ given by

$$L := (W\mathbb{Z}^2) \cap ([0, 2\pi) \times \mathbb{R})$$

is called the sampling lattice generated by W. The lattice $L^\perp = 2\pi W^{-T}\mathbb{Z}^2$ is called the dual lattice with respect to L. The lattice L does not uniquely determine the generator matrix W, but it does determine the determinant of W as well as the dual lattice. The lattice constant C_L is defined by

$$C_L = (2\pi)^{-1} |\det W|.$$

A sampling lattice L containing an element $(0, s)^T \in \mathbb{T} \times \mathbb{R}$ for some $s \neq 0$ is called an *admissible sampling lattice*.

The following theorem is the analogue of the well-known Petersen-Middleton theorem [23] for sampling on $\mathbb{T} \times \mathbb{R}$.

Theorem 2.1. *Let $g \in C_0^\infty(\mathbb{T} \times \mathbb{R})$, L a sampling lattice and K be a compact subset of $\mathbb{Z} \times \mathbb{R}$ such that its translates $K + \eta$, $\eta \in L^\perp$ are disjoint. Let χ_K denote the characteristic function of K. For $z \in \mathbb{T} \times \mathbb{R}$ define*

$$Sg(z) = C_L \sum_{y \in L} \tilde{\chi}_K(z - y) g(y). \tag{2.2}$$

Then

$$|g(z) - Sg(z)| \leq \pi^{-1} \int_{(\mathbb{Z}\times\mathbb{R})\setminus K} |\hat{g}(\zeta)|\, d\zeta. \tag{2.3}$$

Proof: See, e.g., [9] or [20, pp. 62–64].

The lattice $L^\perp$ has to be sufficiently sparse for the sets $K + \eta$, $\eta \in L^\perp$ to be disjoint. This translates into a condition for the lattice L to be sufficiently dense, since the densities of L and $L^\perp$ are inversely proportional to each other. The larger the set K, the more restrictive the requirement becomes. To allow for efficient sampling, K should be as small as possible, but on the other hand K must be sufficiently large for the right-hand side of the estimate (2.3) to be small. In this sense K can be viewed as essential support of $\hat{g}$.

Extensions of the theorem to sampling sets which are unions of cosets of a lattice have been proven in [8, 10]. In the remainder of this section we show that a sharper error estimate may be obtained for admissible sampling lattices. The next lemma gives a parameterization of the admissible lattices and provides two alternative normal forms for their generator matrices.

Lemma 2.2. *Let L be an admissible sampling lattice for $\mathbb{T}\times\mathbb{R}$. Then there exist $d>0$, $P,M,N\in\mathbb{N}\cup\{0\}$ with M a divisor of P, $0\le N<M$, $\gcd(M,N)=1$, such that $L=L(d,P,M,N)$ is generated by the matrices*

$$W_1=\begin{pmatrix} 2\pi/P & 0 \\ dN/M & d \end{pmatrix} \text{ and } W_2=\begin{pmatrix} 2\pi M/P & 2\pi N'/P \\ 0 & d/M \end{pmatrix} \tag{2.4}$$

where $0\le N'<M$, $NN'\equiv 1 \mod M$. Hence the lattice constant equals $C_L=d/P$, and the dual lattice is generated by

$$2\pi W_1^{-T}=\begin{pmatrix} P & -PN/M \\ 0 & 2\pi/d \end{pmatrix} \text{ and by } 2\pi W_2^{-T}=\begin{pmatrix} P/M & 0 \\ -2\pi N'/d & 2\pi M/d \end{pmatrix} \tag{2.5}$$

Proof: It was shown in [9], Lemma 2.4 that there exist $d>0$, $M,N',L'\in\mathbb{N}$, $0\le N'<M$, $\gcd(M,N')=1$, such that L is generated by the matrix

$$W=\begin{pmatrix} 2\pi/L' & 2\pi N'/(ML') \\ 0 & d/M \end{pmatrix}.$$

With $P=L'M$ this matrix equals W_2. Now let N be given by $0\le N<M$, $NN'\equiv 1 \mod M$. It remains to show that $W_1\mathbb{Z}^2=W_2\mathbb{Z}^2$, i.e., that $W_1^{-1}W_2\mathbb{Z}^2=\mathbb{Z}^2$. This is the case if and only if $W_1^{-1}W_2$ is an integer matrix and $|\det(W_1^{-1}W_2)|=1$. These conditions are readily verified. □

It follows from Lemma 2.2 that the admissible lattices have the general form

$$\begin{aligned} L &= L(d,P,M,N) \\ &= \{(\varphi_j,s_{jl})^T\in T\times\mathbb{R}:\varphi_j=2\pi j/P,\ j=0,\dots P-1, \\ &\qquad s_{jl}=d(l+jN/M),\ l\in\mathbb{Z}\}, \end{aligned} \tag{2.6}$$

i.e., for each of the P evenly distributed angles φ_j there are equidistant values s_{jl} with spacing d, which are shifted by the amount jdN/M. If $N\neq 0$ this shift varies with j and cycles effectively through M different values, since shifts by integer multiples of d have no effect.

Definition 2.2. For $g:\mathbb{T}\times\mathbb{R}\to\mathbb{C}$ and $\varphi\in\mathbb{T}$ let $g_\varphi:\mathbb{R}\to\mathbb{C}$ be given by $g_\varphi(s)=g(\varphi,s)$. Define

$$\epsilon^*(g,\tau)=(2\pi)^{-1/2}\sup_{\varphi\in\mathbb{T}}\int_{|\sigma|>\tau}|\widehat{g_\varphi}(\sigma)|d\sigma. \tag{2.7}$$

For $K\in\mathbb{Z}\times\mathbb{R}$ compact let $k_1=\max\{|k|:(k,\sigma)\in K\}$, $\sigma_1=\max\{|\sigma|:(k,\sigma)\in K\}$, and $M_1=\{(k,\sigma)\in\mathbb{Z}\times\mathbb{R}:|\sigma|\le\sigma_1\}\backslash K$; see Fig. 1.

We are now able to state the sampling theorem which will be used in later sections.

Proposition 2.3. *Let K be a compact subset of $\mathbb{Z}\times\mathbb{R}$ satisfying the condition that if $(k,\sigma)\in K$, then $(k',\sigma)\in K$ for all k' with $|k'|\le|k|$. Let $L=L(d,P,M,N)$ be an admissible sampling lattice such that the translated sets $K+\eta$, $\eta\in L^\perp$ are disjoint, $g\in C_0^\infty(\mathbb{T}\times\mathbb{R})$, Sg as in (2.2), $z\in\mathbb{T}\times\mathbb{R}$, $k_1,\sigma_1,M_1,\epsilon^*$ as in Definition 2.2, and $\sigma^*=\max\{\sigma_1,\frac{2\pi}{d}-\sigma_1\}$. Then*

$$\begin{aligned} |g(z)-Sg(z)| &\le \pi^{-1}\int_{M_1}|\hat{g}(\zeta)|d\zeta+\epsilon^*(g,\sigma_1) \\ &\quad +C(k_1,P)\left\lceil\frac{\sigma_1 d}{\pi}\right\rceil\epsilon^*(g,\sigma^*) \end{aligned}$$

with $C(k_1,P)=1+\frac{6k_1+3}{P}+\frac{2}{\pi}\ln(4k_1+2)$.

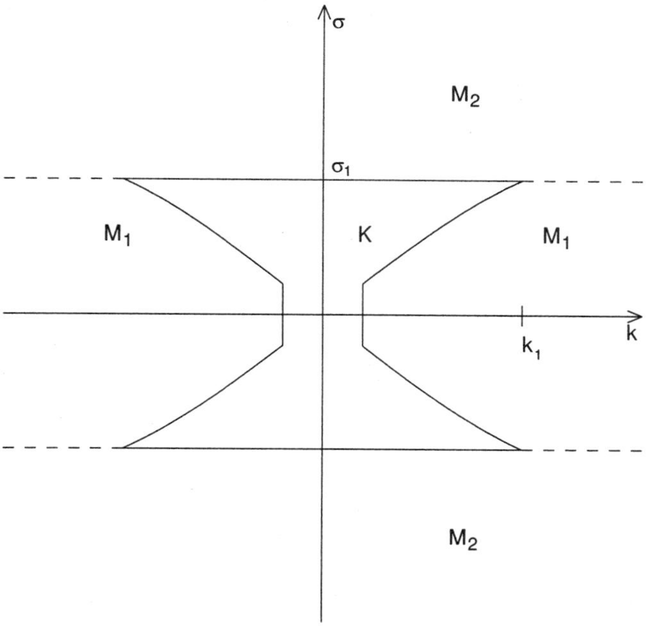

Figure 1. Example of a set K with the related quantities k_1, σ_1, M_1 as in Definition 2.2, and the set M_2 as used in the proof of Theorem 2.4.

Proposition 2.3 is a simplified version of Theorem 2.4 below, but is all that will be used later on. Readers not interested in the more general result or the proofs may safely move on to the next section.

Theorem 2.4. *Let* $g \in C_0^\infty(\mathbb{T}\times\mathbb{R})$*,* $K \subset \mathbb{Z}\times\mathbb{R}$ *compact and* $L = L(d,P,M,N)$ *an admissible sampling lattice such that the translated sets* $K+\eta$*,* $\eta \in L^\perp$ *are disjoint. Let* k_1, σ_1, M_1 *as in Definition 2.2,* $\sigma^* = \max\{\sigma_1, \frac{2\pi}{d} - \sigma_1\}$*, and* $\varphi_j = 2\pi j/P, j = 0, \ldots P-1$*. Then*

$$\begin{aligned}|g(\varphi,s) - Sg(\varphi,s)| \le \pi^{-1} &\int_{M_1} |\hat{g}(\zeta)|d\zeta \\ &+(2\pi)^{-1/2}\int_{\sigma>\sigma_1} |\widehat{g_\varphi}(\sigma)|\,d\sigma \\ &+\frac{C(K,P,\varphi)}{\sqrt{2\pi}}\left\lceil\frac{\sigma_1 d}{\pi}\right\rceil \max_{j=0,\ldots,P-1}\int_{|\sigma|>\sigma^*} |\widehat{g_{\varphi_j}}(\sigma)|\,d\sigma \end{aligned} \tag{2.8}$$

with

$$C(K,P,\varphi) = \frac{1}{P}\sum_{j=0}^{P-1}\max_{|\sigma|\le\sigma_1}\left|\sum_{k\in N(\sigma)} e^{ik(\varphi-\varphi_j)}\right|.$$

where $N(\sigma) = \{k : (k,\sigma) \in K\}$*.*

Proof: The Poisson summation formula for L reads

$$C_L \sum_{y\in L} g(y)e^{-i\langle y,\zeta\rangle} = \sum_{\eta\in L^\perp} \hat{g}(\zeta-\eta).$$

It implies that

$$\widehat{Sg}(\zeta) = \chi_K(\zeta) \sum_{\eta \in L^\perp} \hat{g}(\zeta - \eta). \tag{2.9}$$

Note that $\widehat{Sg}$ vanishes outside K. The Fourier inversion formula now gives

$$\begin{aligned} &|g(z) - Sg(z)| \\ &= \frac{1}{2\pi}\left|\int_{\mathbb{Z}\times\mathbb{R}} (\hat{g}(\zeta) - \widehat{Sg}(\zeta))e^{i\langle z,\zeta\rangle}\,d\zeta\right| \\ &\leq \frac{1}{2\pi}\left|\int_K (\hat{g}(\zeta) - \widehat{Sg}(\zeta))e^{i\langle z,\zeta\rangle}\,d\zeta\right| + \frac{1}{2\pi}\left|\int_{(\mathbb{Z}\times\mathbb{R})\setminus K} \hat{g}(\zeta)e^{i\langle z,\zeta\rangle}\,d\zeta\right| \end{aligned} \tag{2.10}$$

Let $M_2 = \{(k,\sigma) \in \mathbb{Z}\times\mathbb{R} : |\sigma| > \sigma_1\}$. Then $M_1 \cap M_2 = \emptyset$, and $(\mathbb{Z}\times\mathbb{R})\setminus K = M_1 \cup M_2$; see Fig. 1. Splitting the integral over $(\mathbb{Z}\times\mathbb{R})\setminus K$ into contributions coming from M_1 and M_2 and using the relation

$$(2\pi)^{-1/2}\sum_{k\in\mathbb{Z}} \hat{g}(k,\sigma)e^{ik\varphi} = \widehat{g_\varphi}(\sigma)$$

yields

$$\begin{aligned} &\frac{1}{2\pi}\left|\int_{(\mathbb{Z}\times\mathbb{R})\setminus K} \hat{g}(\zeta)e^{i\langle z,\zeta\rangle}\,d\zeta\right| \\ &\leq \frac{1}{2\pi}\int_{M_1} |\hat{g}(\zeta)|\,d\zeta + \frac{1}{2\pi}\left|\int_{|\sigma|>\sigma_1} \sum_{k\in\mathbb{Z}} \hat{g}(k,\sigma)e^{ik\varphi}e^{i\sigma s}\,d\sigma\right| \\ &\leq \frac{1}{2\pi}\int_{M_1} |\hat{g}(\zeta)|\,d\zeta + (2\pi)^{-1/2}\int_{\sigma>\sigma_1} |\widehat{g_\varphi}(\sigma)|\,d\sigma \end{aligned} \tag{2.11}$$

The theorem now follows from combining (2.10), (2.11), and the estimate

$$\begin{aligned} \frac{1}{2\pi}\left|\int_K (\hat{g}(\zeta) - \widehat{Sg}(\zeta))e^{i\langle z,\zeta\rangle}\,d\zeta\right| &= \frac{1}{2\pi}\left|\int_K \sum_{\eta\in L_0^\perp} \hat{g}(\zeta-\eta)e^{i\langle z,\zeta\rangle}\,d\zeta\right| \\ \leq \frac{1}{2\pi}\int_{M_1} |\hat{g}(\zeta)|\,d\zeta + \frac{C(K,P,\varphi)}{\sqrt{2\pi}} &\left\lceil \frac{\sigma_1 d}{\pi} \right\rceil \max_{j=0,\ldots,P-1} \int_{|\sigma|>\sigma^*} |\widehat{g_{\varphi_j}}(\sigma)|\,d\sigma \end{aligned} \tag{2.12}$$

where $L_0^\perp = L^\perp\setminus\{0\}$.

The first equation in (2.12) follows from (2.9). In order to prove the inequality note that $\zeta - \eta \in (\mathbb{Z}\times\mathbb{R})\setminus K = M_1 \cup M_2$ for $\zeta \in K$ and $\eta \in L_0^\perp$ since the sets $K+\eta$, $\eta \in L^\perp$ are disjoint. Hence

$$\frac{1}{2\pi}\left|\int_K \sum_{\eta\in L_0^\perp} \hat{g}(\zeta-\eta)e^{i\langle z,\zeta\rangle}\,d\zeta\right| \leq \frac{1}{2\pi}(I_1 + I_2) \tag{2.13}$$

with

$$I_j = \left|\int_K \sum_{\eta\in L_0^\perp} \hat{g}(\zeta-\eta)\chi_{M_j}(\zeta-\eta)e^{i\langle z,\zeta\rangle}\,d\zeta\right|, \quad j = 1,2.$$

Disjointness of the sets $K+\eta$, $\eta \in L^{\perp}$ implies

$$I_1 \leq \sum_{\eta \in L_0^{\perp}} \int_{K-\eta} |\hat{g}(\zeta)| \chi_{M_1}(\zeta) d\zeta \leq \int_{M_1} |\hat{g}(\zeta)| d\zeta \tag{2.14}$$

In order to estimate I_2 note that $K \subseteq [-k_1, k_1] \times [-\sigma_1, \sigma_1]$, and that by (2.5) any $\eta \in L^{\perp}$ has the form $\eta = (Pj - PNl/M,\ 2\pi l/d) = \eta_{jl}$ for some $j, l \in \mathbb{Z}$. Therefore, if $\zeta = (k, \sigma) \in K$ and $\eta_{jl} \in L_0^{\perp}$, then $\zeta - \eta_{jl} \in M_2$ if and only if $|\sigma - 2\pi l/d| > \sigma_1$. This is possible only if $l \neq 0$. It follows that

$$I_2 = \left| \int_{-\sigma_1}^{\sigma_1} \sum_{k \in N(\sigma)} \sum_{l \neq 0} \sum_{j \in \mathbb{Z}} \hat{g}\left(k - \frac{PNl}{M} - Pj,\ \sigma - \frac{2\pi l}{d}\right) e^{ik\varphi + i\sigma s} \chi_{\mathbb{R} \setminus [-\sigma_1, \sigma_1]}\left(\sigma - \frac{2\pi l}{d}\right) d\sigma \right| \tag{2.15}$$

The next step consists in transforming the sum over j using the Poisson summation formula for functions defined on $\mathbb{T}$, i.e.,

$$\frac{2\pi}{P} \sum_{j=0}^{P-1} G\left(\frac{2\pi j}{P}\right) e^{-2\pi i jk/P} = \sqrt{2\pi} \sum_{j \in \mathbb{Z}} \hat{G}(k + Pj).$$

Let

$$G_\tau(\varphi) = (2\pi)^{-1/2} \int_{\mathbb{R}} g(\varphi, s) e^{-is\tau} ds = \widehat{g_\varphi}(\tau).$$

With $\tau = \sigma - \frac{2\pi l}{d}$ and $\varphi_j = 2\pi j/P$ we have

$$\begin{aligned} \sum_{j \in \mathbb{Z}} \hat{g}\left(k - \frac{PNl}{M} - Pj,\ \sigma - \frac{2\pi l}{d}\right) &= \sum_{j \in \mathbb{Z}} \widehat{G_\tau}\left(k - \frac{PNl}{M} - Pj\right) \\ &= \frac{\sqrt{2\pi}}{P} \sum_{j=0}^{P-1} G_\tau\left(\frac{2\pi j}{P}\right) e^{-2\pi i j(k - PNl/M)/P} \\ &= \frac{\sqrt{2\pi}}{P} \sum_{j=0}^{P-1} \widehat{g_{\varphi_j}}\left(\sigma - \frac{2\pi l}{d}\right) e^{i(PNl/M - k)\varphi_j} \end{aligned} \tag{2.16}$$

Combining (2.15) and (2.16) yields

$$\begin{aligned} I_2 &\leq \frac{\sqrt{2\pi}}{P} \sum_{j=0}^{P-1} \left(\max_{|\sigma| \leq \sigma_1} \left| \sum_{k \in N(\sigma)} e^{ik(\varphi - \varphi_j)} \right| \right) \\ &\quad \sum_{l \neq 0} \int_{-\sigma_1}^{\sigma_1} \left| \widehat{g_{\varphi_j}}\left(\sigma - \frac{2\pi l}{d}\right) \right| \chi_{\mathbb{R} \setminus [-\sigma_1, \sigma_1]}\left(\sigma - \frac{2\pi l}{d}\right) d\sigma \\ &\leq \sqrt{2\pi} C(K, P, \varphi) \left\lceil \frac{\sigma_1 d}{\pi} \right\rceil \max_{j=0,\ldots,P-1} \int_{|\sigma| > \sigma^*} |\widehat{g_{\varphi_j}}(\sigma)| d\sigma \end{aligned} \tag{2.17}$$

The last inequality is obtained by observing that for almost all σ, σ' such that $|\sigma| \leq \sigma_1$, $|\sigma'| > \sigma^*$, there are at most $\lceil \frac{\sigma_1 d}{\pi} \rceil$ different values of l such that $(\sigma - 2\pi l/d) = \sigma'$. The estimate (2.12) now follows from (2.13), (2.14) and (2.17). □

An obvious but coarse estimate for the quantity $C(K,P,\varphi)$ is $C(K,P,\varphi) \le 2k_1+1$. The next lemma provides an estimate for $C(K,P,\varphi)$ in case the set K satisfies the condition of Proposition 2.3, i.e., if $(k,\sigma)\in K$, then $(k',\sigma)\in K$ for all k' with $|k'|\le|k|$. In this case $N(\sigma)=\{-n,\dots,n\}$ for some $0\le n\le k_1$, hence

$$\begin{aligned} C(K,P,\varphi) &\le \frac{1}{P}\sum_{j=0}^{P-1}\max_{0\le n\le k_1}\left|\sum_{k=-n}^{n} e^{ik(\varphi-\varphi_j)}\right| \\ &= \frac{1}{P}\sum_{j=0}^{P-1}\max_{0\le n\le k_1}\left|\frac{\sin((2n+1)(\varphi-\varphi_j)/2)}{\sin((\varphi-\varphi_j)/2)}\right|. \end{aligned} \tag{2.18}$$

Lemma 2.5. *Let*

$$g(\varphi)=\max_{0\le n\le k_1}\left|\frac{\sin((2n+1)\varphi/2)}{\sin(\varphi/2)}\right|.$$

Then

$$\frac{1}{P}\sum_{j=0}^{P-1} g(\varphi-2\pi j/P) \le \min\left(2k_1+1,\ 1+\frac{6k_1+3}{P}+\frac{2}{\pi}\ln(4k_1+2)\right). \tag{2.19}$$

Proof: Since $0\le g(\varphi)\le 2k_1+1$ it is clear that $P^{-1}\sum_{j=0}^{P-1} g(\varphi-2\pi j/P)\le 2k_1+1$. Let $\Delta\varphi=2\pi/P$, $\varphi^*=\min\left(\pi,\ 2\arcsin\left(\frac{1}{2k_1+1}\right)+\Delta\varphi\right)$, and $\varphi_j=j\Delta\varphi$. Consider first the case $\varphi^*=\pi$. Then

$$\pi=\varphi^*\le 2\arcsin\left(\frac{1}{2k_1+1}\right)+\frac{2\pi}{P}.$$

Multiplying by $(2k_1+1)/\pi$ and observing that $x\arcsin(1/x)\le\pi/2$ for $x\ge1$ gives $2k_1+1\le 1+(4k_1+2)/P$. Hence for $\varphi^*=\pi$ the right-hand side of (2.19) equals $2k_1+1$ and the assertion holds.

Now assume $\varphi^*<\pi$. Since g is 2π-periodic we may consider it a function on the interval $[-\pi,\pi)$. For $\varphi\in\mathbb{R}$ let $\varphi'\in[-\pi,\pi)$ such that $\varphi'\equiv\varphi \mod 2\pi$. Clearly,

$$g(\varphi)=g(\varphi')\le\begin{cases} 2k_1+1 & \text{for } |\varphi'|<\varphi^* \\ \frac{1}{\sin(\varphi'/2)} & \text{for } \varphi^*\le|\varphi'|\le\pi \end{cases}.$$

Since $|(\varphi-\varphi_j)'|<\varphi^*$ for at most $\left\lceil\frac{2\varphi^*}{\Delta\varphi}\right\rceil$ terms,

$$\begin{aligned} &\frac{1}{P}\sum_{j=0}^{P-1} g(\varphi-\varphi_j) \\ &\le \frac{2k_1+1}{P}\left\lceil\frac{2\varphi^*}{\Delta\varphi}\right\rceil+\frac{1}{P}\sum_{\varphi^*\le|(\varphi-\varphi_j)'|\le\pi}\frac{1}{\sin((\varphi-\varphi_j)'/2)} \\ &\le \frac{2k_1+1}{P}\left(\frac{2P\arcsin\left(\frac{1}{2k_1+1}\right)}{\pi}+3\right)+\frac{2}{P}\sum_{l=0}^{\lfloor\frac{\pi-\varphi^*}{\Delta\varphi}\rfloor}\frac{1}{\sin((\varphi^*+l\Delta\varphi)/2)} \\ &\le 1+\frac{6k_1+3}{P}+\frac{1}{\pi}\int_{\varphi^*-\Delta\varphi}^{\pi}\frac{1}{\sin(\varphi/2)}\,d\varphi. \end{aligned}$$

Evaluating the integral gives

$$\int_{\varphi^*-\Delta\varphi}^{\pi} \frac{1}{\sin(\varphi/2)}\,d\varphi = -2\ln(\tan((\varphi^*-\Delta\varphi)/4))$$
$$= 2\ln\left(2k_1+1+\sqrt{(2k_1+1)^2-1}\right)$$
$$\leq 2\ln(4k_1+2).$$

It is now clear that Proposition 2.3 follows from Theorem 2.4, Lemma 2.5 and (2.18).□

3. BRIEF INTRODUCTION TO DIFFRACTION TOMOGRAPHY

In order to obtain a mathematical model accounting for diffraction effects in a tomographic experiment, we assume that the Fourier amplitude $u(x,\omega)$ of the wavefield $U(x,t)$ satisfies the reduced wave equation

$$\Delta u + k_0^2(1+f(x))u = 0 \tag{3.1}$$

together with the Sommerfeld radiation condition. Here Δ denotes the Laplacian, and k_0 is the wavenumber of the incoming radiation. The compactly supported complex-valued function f describes the influence of the scatterer and is related to the index of refraction $n(x)$ by $f(x) = n^2(x) - 1$. Reconstructing f from measured values of u leads to the nonlinear inverse scattering problem for (3.1). In the framework of diffraction tomography the inverse scattering problem is usually linearized by means of the Born- or Rytov-approximations. Following [14, 18] these approximations can be motivated as follows:

Let w be a C^2-function to be specified later, u_0 an incoming plane wave,

$$u_0(x) = e^{ik_0\theta\cdot x},\quad \theta\in S^{n-1}$$

and

$$v := u_0\, w(u/u_0)$$

with u a solution of (3.1).

With $\alpha := \frac{u}{u_0}$ we have with (3.1):

$$(\Delta + k_0^2)v = -k_0^2 u_0\left[f + (\frac{dw}{d\alpha}\alpha - 1)f - k_0^{-2}\frac{d^2w}{d\alpha^2}(\nabla\alpha)^2\right] \tag{3.2}$$

If $w(\alpha) = \alpha - 1$, the third term in the bracket vanishes. Assuming $|u-u_0| \ll |u_0|$ and therefore neglecting the second term leads to the Born approximation with $v = u - u_0$ and

$$(\Delta + k_0^2)v = -k_0^2 u_0 f. \tag{3.3}$$

Setting $w(\alpha) = \ln\alpha$ leads to the Rytov approximation. Here the second term on the right-hand side of (3.2) vanishes. The third term is neglected, assuming that $|\nabla \ln \frac{u}{u_0}|^2 \ll k_0^2|f|$. We again get equation (3.3) with $v = u_0 \ln\frac{u}{u_0}$. The relative merits of these two approximations have been discussed extensively in the literature. Since both lead to the same equation (3.3) which is the starting point for our further considerations, we do not need to consider this point here.

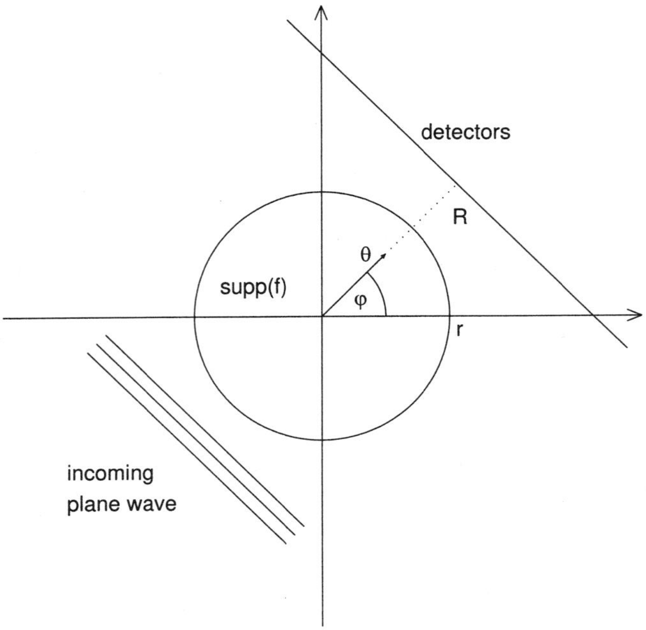

Figure 2. Parallel measurement geometry.

In the following we confine ourselves to two spatial dimensions and the so called 'parallel-beam' measurement geometry sketched in Fig. 2. The cross-section to be reconstructed is represented by the function f which is supported in the disk D_r of radius r with center in the origin. The object is irradiated with plane waves $u_0(x) = e^{ik_0\theta\cdot x}$ with wavenumber k_0 propagating in direction $\theta = (\cos\varphi, \sin\varphi)^T$. The scattered radiation is measured behind the object on a line orthogonal to θ with distance $R > r$ from the origin. So the detectors are located at points $R\theta + s\theta^\perp$ with $\theta^\perp = (-\sin\varphi, \cos\varphi)^T$ and $|s| \leq A$. Since for each direction θ one wishes to take more than one measurement, the admissible lattices defined in the previous section are precisely the lattices suitable for this case. We assume the aperture A to be sufficiently large, so that the effects of A being finite may be neglected. The data are assumed to consist of measured values of

$$Pf(\varphi,s) := k_0^{-1}\frac{v(R\theta+s\theta^\perp)}{u_0(R\theta+s\theta^\perp)} = k_0^{-1}e^{-ik_0R}v(R\theta+s\theta^\perp)$$

with v being the solution of (3.3) corresponding to the given boundary conditions. The appropriate Green's function is given by $-\frac{i}{4}H_0(k_0|x-x'|)$ where H_0 denotes the Hankel function of the first kind of order zero. This leads to the following definition of the 'propagation operator' P [6], which maps f into the data function Pf:

Definition 3.1. Throughout this paper, the letters θ and φ are related by θ being the unit vector in $\mathbb{R}^2$ with polar angle φ, i.e., $\theta = (\cos\varphi, \sin\varphi)^T$, and $\theta^\perp = (-\sin\varphi, \cos\varphi)^T$. The propagation operator $P : L_1(D_r) \to C^\infty(\mathbb{R}^2)$ is given by

$$Pf(\varphi,s) = \frac{i}{4}k_0e^{-ik_0R}\int_{D_r} H_0(k_0|R\theta+s\theta^\perp - y|)f(y)e^{ik_0\theta\cdot y}dy \tag{3.4}$$

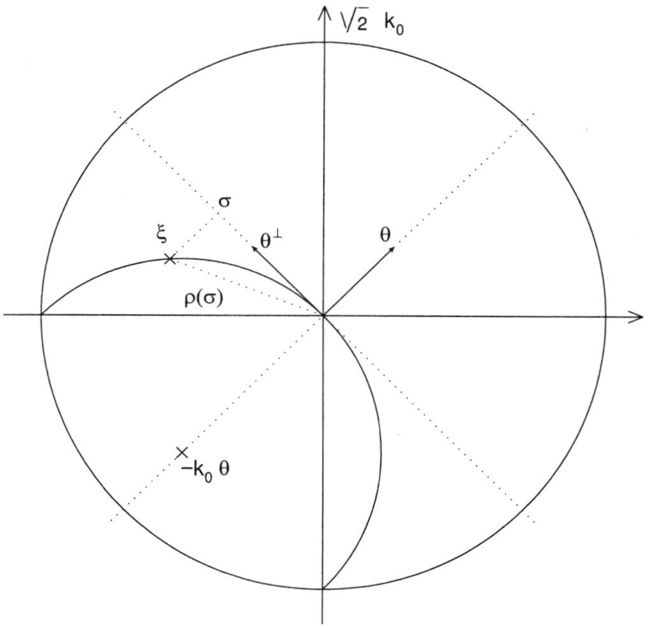

Figure 3. The Fourier transform $\widehat{P_\varphi f}(\sigma)$ is related to the Fourier transform of f at the point $\xi = (a(\sigma)-k_0)\theta + \sigma\theta^\perp$. For $-k_0 \le \sigma \le k_0$ the point ξ traverses a semicircle. As θ runs through S^1, this semicircle sweeps out a disk of radius $\sqrt{2}k_0$. The function ρ given in Definition 4.1 satisfies $\rho(\sigma) = |\xi|$.

Sometimes φ is kept fixed and Pf is considered a function of s alone. In this case we write $P_\varphi f(s)$ for $Pf(\varphi, s)$. Particularly useful is the Fourier transform

$$\widehat{P_\varphi f}(\sigma) = (2\pi)^{-1/2} \int_{\mathbb{R}} Pf(\varphi, s) e^{-i\sigma s} ds.$$

In diffraction tomography one tries to reconstruct an approximation to f from measured values of Pf. The following 'generalized projection theorem' [28] gives a relationship between the Fourier transforms of f and $P_\varphi f$:

Theorem 3.1. *For $\sigma \in \mathbb{R}$ let $a(\sigma) := \sqrt{k_0^2 - \sigma^2}$ so that $\Im a(\sigma) \ge 0$. If $f \in L_1(D_r)$,*

$$\widehat{P_\varphi f}(\sigma) = i\sqrt{\frac{\pi}{2}} k_0 \frac{e^{iR(a(\sigma)-k_0)}}{a(\sigma)} \hat{f}((a(\sigma)-k_0)\theta + \sigma\theta^\perp). \tag{3.5}$$

For a proof see e.g., [20, Chap. I].

For $-k_0 \le \sigma \le k_0$ the arguments $\xi = (a(\sigma)-k_0)\theta + \sigma\theta^\perp$ of $\hat{f}$ run over a semicircle with center at $-k_0\theta$, radius k_0, and top at the origin; see Fig. 3. By varying the direction θ the values of $\hat{f}(\xi)$ for $|\xi| \le \sqrt{2}k_0$ can thus be obtained from the data. By filtering and performing an inverse Fourier transform we can compute low-pass filtered versions of f with bandwidth $b \le \sqrt{2}k_0$. This is the basic idea underlying the standard reconstruction algorithms [5, 14, 22]. The achievement of resolution corresponding to a bandwidth greater than $\sqrt{2}k_0$ has been investigated in [26].

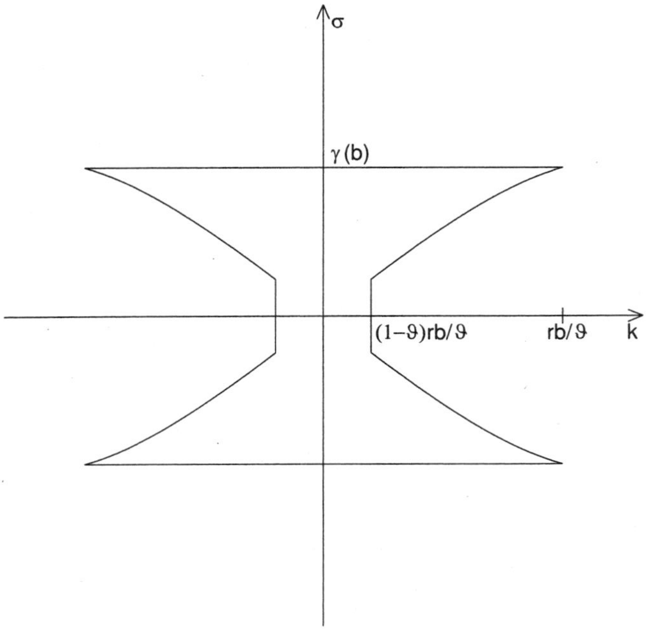

Figure 4. The set $K(\vartheta, b)$ of Definition 4.1 for $\vartheta = 0.8$ and $b = 1.2\,k_0$.

4. THE ESSENTIAL SUPPORT OF $\widehat{PF}$

We wish to apply the results of Section 2 to the data function Pf. This requires determination of a suitable set K and formulation of conditions on the lattice parameters d, P, M, N so that the translated sets $K + \eta$, $\eta \in L^\perp$ are disjoint.

Definition 4.1. For $k_0 > 0$ and $a(\sigma)$ as in Theorem 3.1 we define the functions $\rho : [-k_0, k_0] \to \mathbb{R}$ and $\gamma : \mathbb{R} \to \mathbb{R}$ as follows:

$$\rho(\sigma) := ((a(\sigma) - k_0)^2 + \sigma^2)^{\frac{1}{2}}, \quad |\sigma| \leq k_0$$

$$\gamma(\sigma) := \begin{cases} \sigma\sqrt{1 - (\frac{\sigma}{2k_0})^2} & |\sigma| \leq \sqrt{2}k_0 \\ k_0 \operatorname{sign}(\sigma) & |\sigma| > \sqrt{2}k_0 \end{cases}$$

Note that $\rho(\gamma(\sigma)) = |\sigma|$ for $|\sigma| \leq \sqrt{2}k_0$ and $\gamma(\rho(\sigma)) = |\sigma|$ for $|\sigma| \leq k_0$.

For $\vartheta, r, b, k_0 > 0$, $\vartheta < 1 \leq rb < \sqrt{2}rk_0$ define the set

$$K(\vartheta, b) := \left\{(k, \sigma) \in \mathbb{Z} \times \mathbb{R} : |\sigma| \leq \gamma(b),\ |k| < \frac{r}{\vartheta} \max(\rho(\sigma), (1 - \vartheta)b)\right\} \tag{4.1}$$

(see Fig. 4).

The next theorem will show that this is the set we are looking for.

Theorem 4.1. *For* $0 < b < \sqrt{2}k_0$, $0 < \vartheta < 1$ *let* $K = K(\vartheta, b)$ *as in (4.1). Let* $L = L(d, P, M, N)$ *be an admissible sampling lattice such that the sets* $K + \eta$, $\eta \in L^\perp$ *are disjoint. If* $f \in L_1(D_r)$,

$g = Pf$, Sg as in (2.2), and ϵ^* as in (2.7), then

$$|g(\varphi,s) - Sg(\varphi,s)| \leq 2^{-1/2} \, \|f\|_{L_1} \frac{be^{-\beta(\vartheta)rb}}{1-e^{-\alpha(\vartheta)}} + \epsilon^*(g,\gamma(b)) + c(\vartheta,b,P) \left\lceil \frac{\gamma(b)d}{\pi} \right\rceil \epsilon^*(g,\gamma^*). \tag{4.2}$$

where $\alpha(\vartheta) = (1-\vartheta^2)^{3/2}/3$, $\beta(\vartheta) = \alpha(\vartheta)(1-\vartheta)/\vartheta$, $c(\vartheta,b,P) = 1 + (3+6rb/\vartheta)/P + (2/\pi)\ln(2+4rb/\vartheta)$, *and* $\gamma^* = \max\{\gamma(b), \frac{2\pi}{d} - \gamma(b)\}$.

As discussed in conjunction with Theorem 2.1, a good choice for K should be small enough for the sampling to be efficient and large enough for the aliasing error to be small. The first term on the right-hand side of (4.2) decreases exponentially with b. It can be shown using (3.5) that $|\widehat{P_\varphi f}(\sigma)|$ decreases exponentially for $|\sigma| > k_0$ (evanescent waves), because f is supported in D_r and $R > r$. Hence $\epsilon^*(Pf,\gamma(b))$ will be small if $|\widehat{P_\varphi f}(\sigma)|$ is also small for $\gamma(b) \leq |\sigma| \leq k_0$. From (3.5) it follows that this will be the case if $|\hat{f}(\xi)|$ is small for $b \leq |\xi| \leq \sqrt{2}k_0$. This provides the criterion for choosing the parameter b, which may be interpreted as essential bandwidth of the function f.

It should be noted that the set K given here is minimal under the assumption that the only a priori information available on f is its essential bandwidth b. If more is known about f, smaller sets K may be possible. For example, in the extreme case that f is a radial function, $\widehat{Pf}(k,\sigma) = 0$ for $k \neq 0$ and the set K could be chosen as $\{(0,\sigma) : |\sigma| \leq \gamma(b)\}$.

The proof of Theorem 4.1 will occupy the rest of this section.

Lemma 4.2. *Under the hypotheses of Theorem 4.1 and with* $M_1 = \{(k,\sigma) \in \mathbb{Z} \times \mathbb{R} : |\sigma| \leq \gamma(b)\} \backslash K$,

$$\int_{M_1} |\hat{g}(\zeta)|\, d\zeta \leq \frac{\pi}{\sqrt{2}} \, \|f\|_{L_1} \frac{be^{-\beta(\vartheta)rb}}{1-e^{-\alpha(\vartheta)}}.$$

Proof: Let J_k denote the Bessel function of the first kind of integer order k. An integral representation is furnished by

$$J_k(w) = \frac{i^{-k}}{2\pi} \int_0^{2\pi} e^{iw\cos\varphi - ik\varphi}\, d\varphi, \quad w \in \mathbb{C}, \tag{4.3}$$

see [20, Formula VII.3.16] or [1, Formula 9.1.21]. Combining the upper bound [1, Formula 9.1.63] and a derivation given in [20, p. 198] yields the estimate

$$|J_k(tk)| \leq e^{-|k|(1-t^2)^{3/2}/3} = e^{-\alpha(t)|k|}, \quad 0 \leq t \leq 1. \tag{4.4}$$

For $|k| \geq b' = (1-\vartheta)rb/\vartheta$ let $I_k = \{\sigma \in \mathbb{R} : |\sigma| \leq \gamma(\min(\vartheta|k|/r, b))\}$. Then

$$\int_{M_1} |\hat{g}(\zeta)|\, d\zeta = \sum_{|k| \geq b'} \int_{I_k} |\hat{g}(k,\sigma)|\, d\sigma. \tag{4.5}$$

Using Theorem 3.1 and equation (4.3) one obtains for $|\sigma| \leq k_0$

$$|\hat{g}(k,\sigma)| = \frac{k_0}{2a(\sigma)} \left| \int_0^{2\pi} \hat{f}((a(\sigma)-k_0)\theta + \sigma\theta^\perp) e^{-ik\varphi} d\varphi \right|$$

$$= \frac{k_0}{2a(\sigma)} \left| \int_0^{2\pi} \hat{f}(\rho(\sigma)\theta) e^{-ik\varphi} d\varphi \right| \tag{4.6}$$

$$\leq \frac{k_0}{2\sqrt{k_0^2 - \sigma^2}} \int_{D_r} |f(y) J_k(|y|\rho(\sigma))| \, dy. \tag{4.7}$$

Using the substitution $u = r\rho(\sigma)$ and (4.4) we get

$$\int_{I_k} |\hat{g}(k,\sigma)| \, d\sigma$$

$$\leq \frac{k_0}{2} \|f\|_{L_1} \sup_{0 \leq t \leq 1} \int_{I_k} |J_k(tr\rho(\sigma))| \frac{d\sigma}{\sqrt{k_0^2 - \sigma^2}}$$

$$= \frac{k_0}{2} \|f\|_{L_1} \sup_{0 \leq t \leq 1} 2 \int_0^{\min(\vartheta|k|, rb)} (r^2 k_0^2 - u^2/4)^{-\frac{1}{2}} |J_k(tu)| \, du$$

$$\leq k_0 \|f\|_{L_1} \left(\sup_{0 \leq t \leq 1} |J_k(t\vartheta k)| \right) \int_0^{\min(\vartheta|k|, rb)} (r^2 k_0^2 - u^2/4)^{-\frac{1}{2}} \, du$$

$$\leq 2k_0 \arcsin\left(\frac{b}{2k_0}\right) \|f\|_{L_1} e^{-\alpha(\vartheta)|k|}$$

$$\leq \frac{\pi b}{2\sqrt{2}} \|f\|_{L_1} e^{-\alpha(\vartheta)|k|}. \tag{4.8}$$

The result now follows by inserting (4.8) into (4.5) and evaluating the sum over k. □

Lemma 4.3. $\widehat{Pf} \in L_1(\mathbb{Z} \times \mathbb{R})$.

Proof: Let $g = Pf$. We show that $\sum_{k \in \mathbb{Z}} \int_{\mathbb{R}} |\hat{g}(k,\sigma)| d\sigma < \infty$ by establishing that $\int_{\mathbb{R}} |\hat{g}(k,\sigma)| d\sigma = O(|k|^{-n})$ for all $n \in \mathbb{N}$. Let

$$q(\varphi, \sigma, x) := -ix \cdot \left((a(\sigma) - k_0)\theta + \sigma\theta^\perp \right).$$

Then

$$|k^n \hat{g}(k,\sigma)| = \left| (2\pi)^{-1/2} \int_0^{2\pi} \left(\frac{d^n}{d\varphi^n} \hat{g}_\varphi(\sigma) \right) e^{-ik\varphi} d\varphi \right|$$

$$= \frac{k_0}{2} |a(\sigma)|^{-1} \left| e^{iRa(\sigma)} \right|$$

$$\times \left| \int_0^{2\pi} \left(\frac{d^n}{d\varphi^n} \hat{f}\left((a(\sigma) - k_0)\theta + \sigma\theta^\perp \right) \right) e^{-ik\varphi} d\varphi \right|$$

$$\leq \frac{k_0}{2} \| f \|_{L_1} |a(\sigma)|^{-1} \left| e^{iRa(\sigma)} \right| \sup_{x \in D_r, \varphi \in T} \left| \frac{d^n}{d\varphi^n} e^q \right|.$$

We have $\sup_{x,\varphi} \left| \frac{d^l}{d\varphi^l} q \right| \leq \sqrt{2} r |\sigma|$. The real part of q satisfies

$$|\mathrm{Re} q| \begin{cases} = 0 & |\sigma| \leq k_0 \\ \leq r\sqrt{\sigma^2 - k_0^2} & |\sigma| > k_0 \end{cases}.$$

Therefore

$$\sup_{x\in D_r,\varphi\in\mathbb{T}}\left|\frac{d^n}{d\varphi^n}e^q\right|\le\begin{cases}P_n(\sqrt{2}r|\sigma|) & \sigma\le k_0\\ P_n(\sqrt{2}r|\sigma|)e^{r\sqrt{\sigma^2-k_0^2}} & \sigma>k_0\end{cases}$$

with P_n a polynomial of degree at most n. Now let $h(\sigma)=1$ for $\sigma\le k_0$ and $h(\sigma)=e^{-(R-r)\sqrt{\sigma^2-k_0^2}}$ for $\sigma>k_0$. Then

$$\begin{aligned}\int_{\mathbb{R}}|\hat{g}(k,\sigma)d\sigma&\le|k|^{-n}\frac{k_0}{2}\|f\|_{L_1}\int_{\mathbb{R}}|a(\sigma)|^{-1}P_n(\sqrt{2}r|\sigma|)h(\sigma)d\sigma\\&=C(n)|k|^{-n}.\end{aligned}$$

□

Proof of Theorem 4.1: For $\epsilon>0$ define $g^\epsilon(\varphi,s)=g(\varphi,s)\psi(\epsilon s)$ with $\psi\in C_0^\infty(\mathbb{R})$, $0\le\psi(s)\le1$, $\psi(s)=1$ for $|s|\le1$, and $\psi(s)=0$ for $|s|>2$. The theorem follows by applying Proposition 2.3 to g^ϵ with $\sigma_1=\gamma(b)$, $k_1=rb/\vartheta$, letting $\epsilon\to0$, and using Lemma 4.2. Note that in the limit $\epsilon\to0$ the estimates for g^ϵ turn into their counterparts for g because of Lemma 4.3 and the fact that $\widehat{g^\epsilon_\varphi}$ and $\widehat{g^\epsilon}(k,\cdot)$ converge in the L_1 -sense to $\widehat{g_\varphi}$ and $\hat{g}(k,\cdot)$, respectively. □

An earlier version of Theorem 4.1 was given in [7] with a proof based on Theorem 2.1. Proposition 2.3 allows both the sharper estimate and the considerably less complicated proof presented here.

5. SAMPLING CONDITIONS

In this section we translate the condition that the sets $K+\eta$, $\eta\in L^\perp$ be disjoint into conditions on the lattice parameters d,P,M,N. (Recall the general form (2.6) of an admissible lattice $L(d,P,M,N)$.) In order to avoid technicalities coming from working with subsets of $\mathbb{Z}\times\mathbb{R}$ we introduce the following subset of $\mathbb{R}^2$:

$$K'(\vartheta,b):=\left\{(k,\sigma)\in\mathbb{R}^2:|\sigma|\le\gamma(b),\ |k|\le\frac{r}{\vartheta}\max(\rho(\sigma),(1-\vartheta)b)\right\},\tag{5.1}$$

with $0<\vartheta<1\le rb<\sqrt{2}rk_0$. Clearly, $K'\cap\mathbb{Z}\times\mathbb{R}$ contains the set K of (4.1), and disjointness of $K'+\eta$, $\eta\in L^\perp$ implies disjointness of $K+\eta$, $\eta\in L^\perp$. We obtain the following sampling conditions.

Proposition 5.1. *Let $L=L(d,P,M,N)$ be an admissible sampling lattice and $K'=K'(\vartheta,b)$ as in (5.1). The sets $K'+\eta$, $\eta\in L^\perp$ are disjoint if and only if*

$$d<\frac{\pi M}{\gamma(b)}\quad\textit{and}\tag{5.2}$$

$$P>\max_{0\le l\le l_0}c_l^{-1}\left(F(\gamma(b))+F\left(\frac{2\pi l}{d}-\gamma(b)\right)\right),\tag{5.3}$$

where

$$\begin{aligned}l_0&=\lfloor d\gamma(b)/\pi\rfloor,\\F(\sigma)&=\frac{r}{\vartheta}\max\{\rho(\sigma),\ (1-\vartheta)b\},\quad|\sigma|\le\gamma(b),\end{aligned}$$

and

$$c_l = \begin{cases} 1, & l = 0 \\ \min_{k\in\mathbb{Z}} \left|k - \frac{Nl}{M}\right|, & l \neq 0 \end{cases}.$$

Before proving the Proposition we discuss some of its consequences. First it is worthwhile to note that F is an even function and

$$F(\gamma(b)) = \frac{rb}{\vartheta}.$$

Since always $l_0 \geq 0$, a necessary condition on the number of views is $P > c_0^{-1}(F(\gamma(b)) + F(-\gamma(b))$, i.e.,

$$P > 2rb/\vartheta. \tag{5.4}$$

On the other hand, sufficient conditions are

$$d < \frac{\pi}{\gamma(b)}, \quad P > \frac{2rb}{\vartheta}, \tag{5.5}$$

independently of M and N. This follows from (5.2) and (5.3) since $d < \pi/\gamma(b)$ implies $l_0 = 0$. We may use the lattice constant

$$C_L = (2\pi)^{-1}|\det W| = d/P$$

as a measure of the overall sampling efficiency, since it is inversely proportional to the density of sampling points. The larger C_L, the fewer points are needed, and hence the more efficient the lattice.

The most often used lattice which we call the standard lattice is obtained for $M = 1$, $N = 0$. The condition (5.2) for d reads $d < \pi/\gamma(b)$. As shown above this means that the condition for P simplifies to $P > 2rb/\vartheta$. Hence the sampling conditions for the standard lattice are exactly the conditions (5.5) which are always sufficient. Hence the standard lattice, although it needs a minimal number of views, is not the most efficient lattice. The sampling conditions imply that for the standard lattice

$$C_L < \frac{\pi\vartheta}{2rb\gamma(b)}. \tag{5.6}$$

Choosing $M = 2$ and $N = 1$ gives a lattice which we call the efficient lattice. The condition (5.2) becomes $d < 2\pi/\gamma(b)$, hence d may be chosen up to twice as large as in case of the standard lattice. If $\pi/\gamma(b) \leq d < 2\pi/\gamma(b)$ then $l_0 = 1$, $c_0 = 1$, $c_1 = 1/2$ and (5.3) reads

$$P > \frac{2rb}{\vartheta} + 2F\left(\frac{2\pi}{d} - \gamma(b)\right). \tag{5.7}$$

If d is sufficiently close to its maximum value of $2\pi/\gamma(b)$, then $F\left(\frac{2\pi}{d} - \gamma(b)\right) = (1-\vartheta)rb/\vartheta$, and the condition on P reads $P > (2-\vartheta)2rb/\vartheta$. For the efficiency it follows that for these values of d and P

$$C_L < \frac{2}{2-\vartheta}\frac{\pi\vartheta}{2rb\gamma(b)}. \tag{5.8}$$

Hence, for ϑ close to 1 this lattice is nearly twice as efficient as the standard lattice.

The truly two-dimensional nature of the sampling conditions is manifested by the dependence of the condition (5.3) for P on the parameter d. As a consequence, increasing the amount of sampled data may make things worse instead of better in some cases. E.g., consider the efficient lattice with d close to $2\pi/\gamma(b)$, and P close to $(2-\vartheta)2rb/\vartheta$. If P is kept fixed and d is sufficiently decreased but still larger than $\pi/\gamma(b)$, the condition (5.7) will be violated. This effect is caused by the non-rectangular shape of the set K'.

In order to find new lattices of high efficiency, let $M > 1$ and observe that if d satisfies (5.2) then $l_0 \leq M-1$, and $c_l \in \{j/M, j = 1, \dots, M\}$ for $0 \leq l \leq l_0$. Hence the smallest possible value for c_l is $1/M$. Furthermore,

$$c_l^{-1}\left(F(\gamma(b))+F\left(\frac{2\pi l}{d}-\gamma(b)\right)\right)\begin{cases} > MF(\gamma(b)) & \text{if } c_l = 1/M \\ \leq MF(\gamma(b)) & \text{if } c_l \geq 2/M \end{cases}.$$

Assume that d is chosen close to its maximum value of $M\pi/\gamma(b)$. Then $l_0 = M-1$ and the maximum in (5.3) is assumed for $l \in \{l_1, l_2\}$ where l_1, l_2 are the two values of l for which $c_l = 1/M$. Since $F(\sigma)$ increases with $|\sigma|$, it follows that the parameter N should be chosen such that $\max_{j=1,2} |2\pi l_j/d - \gamma(b)|$ is small. This means that l_1, l_2 should both be close to $M/2$. A class of lattices which satisfies this condition is obtained by choosing

$$M > 1, \quad M \text{ odd}, \quad N = 2. \tag{5.9}$$

In this case, if d is close $M\pi/\gamma(b)$, $c_l = 1/M$ for $l \in \{(M-1)/2,\ (M+1)/2\}$ and (5.3) reads

$$P > M(F(\gamma(b)) + F(\pi(M+1)/d - \gamma(b)))$$

In the limiting case $d = M\pi/\gamma(b)$ this becomes

$$P > M(F(\gamma(b)) + F(\gamma(b)/M))$$

If M is large enough such that $\rho(\gamma(b)/M) < (1-\vartheta)b$, then the lattice is as efficient as the efficient lattice.

Sampling conditions for the standard lattice have also been derived in [22, 27]. The qualitative argument used in [22] for the condition on P has been made precise in Lemma 4.2. The approach taken in [27] assumes that $\hat{f}$ has already been computed via the generalized projection theorem. Hence only the condition for the number of views can be compared to the results derived here. Translated into our terminology, the condition is $P \geq 2r\gamma(b)$ for the minimum number of views. For b close to $\sqrt{2}k_0$ this is significantly lower than our condition $p > 2rb$, while the two conditions differ not very much for $b < k_0$. From the theory developed above it follows that there could be aliasing in the data when the sampling is such that the sets $K+\eta$, $\eta \in L^\perp$ overlap and if $\widehat{Pf}(\zeta)$ is not negligibly small in the part of K being overlapped. In such a case, our theoretical as well as numerical results indicate that the condition $p > 2rb$ cannot be weakened. We attribute the discrepancy to the result of [27] to the fact that the approach taken there is based on the approximative Carson's rule rather than on an exact theorem. However, for many objects the essential support of $\widehat{Pf}$ does not occupy all of K, so that some overlap of the sets $K+\eta$, $\eta \in L^\perp$ can be accepted without consequences. Then the required number of views for the standard lattice may be much lower than $2rb$.

The remainder of this section will be devoted to the proof of Proposition 5.1.

Lemma 5.2. *Let K' and F be as in Proposition 5.1 and $\eta = (\eta_1, \eta_2) \in \mathbb{Z} \times \mathbb{R}$. Then $K' \cap (K' + \eta) = \emptyset$ if and only if one of the following two conditions is satisfied.*

$$i)\ |\eta_2| > 2\gamma(b) \tag{5.10}$$

$$ii)\ |\eta_2| \leq 2\gamma(b), \quad |\eta_1| > F(\gamma(b)) + F(|\eta_2| - \gamma(b)) \tag{5.11}$$

Proof: Since $(k, \sigma) \in K'$ implies $|\sigma| \leq \gamma(b)$ it is clear that condition $i)$ is sufficient. Consider the case that $i)$ does not hold, i.e., that $0 \leq |\eta_2| \leq 2\gamma(b)$. Assume first that $\eta_1 \geq 0$ and $0 < \eta_2 \leq 2\gamma(b)$. Let S be the strip

$$S = \mathbb{R} \times [\eta_2 - \gamma(b), \gamma(b)].$$

Clearly, $K' \cap (K' + \eta) \subset S$. The left and right boundaries of the set K' are partly flat and partly curved towards the interior of K', cf. Fig. 4. Therefore the part of K' intersecting S lies to the left of the line segment joining the two boundary points $(F(\eta_2 - \gamma(b)),\ \eta_2 - \gamma(b))$ and $(F(\gamma(b)),\ \gamma(b))$ of K'. Similarly, the part of $K' + \eta$ intersecting S lies to the right of the line segment joining the two boundary points $(\eta_1 - F(\gamma(b)),\ \eta_2 - \gamma(b)), (\eta_1 - F(\eta_2 - \gamma(b)),\ \gamma(b))$ of $K' + \eta$. Since these two line segments are parallel, a sufficient condition for disjointness of K' and $K' + \eta$ is $\eta_1 - F(\gamma(b)) > F(\eta_2 - \gamma(b))$, i.e., $\eta_1 > F(\gamma(b)) + F(\eta_2 - \gamma(b))$. If this condition is violated, then the line segment joining $(-F(\gamma(b)),\ \gamma(b))$ and $(F(\gamma(b)),\ \gamma(b))$ which is contained in K' intersects the segment joining $(\eta_1 - F(\eta_2 - \gamma(b)),\ \gamma(b))$ and $(\eta_1 + F(\eta_2 - \gamma(b)),\ \gamma(b))$ which is contained in $K' + \eta$, hence $K' \cap (K' + \eta) \neq \emptyset$.

Because of the symmetry of the set K', analogous arguments can be used to prove the assertion for the cases $\eta_1 \geq 0$, $-2\gamma(b) \leq \eta_2 \leq 0$, and $\eta_1 < 0$, $|\eta_2| \leq 2\gamma(b)$. □

Proof of Proposition 5.1: Since $(K' + \eta) \cap (K' + \eta') \neq \emptyset$ implies $K' \cap (K' + (\eta' - \eta)) \neq \emptyset$, it suffices to find conditions such that $K' \cap (K' + \eta) = \emptyset$ for $0 \neq \eta \in L^\perp$. By Lemma 5.2 $K' \cap (K' + (\eta_1, \eta_2)) = \emptyset$ if and only if (5.10) or (5.11) are satisfied.

Note that $L^\perp = 2\pi W_1^{-T}\mathbb{Z}^2 = 2\pi W_2^{-T}\mathbb{Z}^2$ with W_1, W_2 as in Lemma 2.2. Using W_2, any $\eta \in L^\perp$ can be written as $\eta = (Pk/M,\ 2\pi(lM - kN')/d)$ for some $k, l \in \mathbb{Z}$. For $k = 0$, $l = 1$ this gives $\eta = (\eta_1, \eta_2) = (0, 2\pi M/d)$. Hence (5.11) is not satisfied and therefore (5.10) yields the necessary condition $d < \pi M/\gamma(b)$. Now assume that this condition is satisfied and represent $\eta \in L^\perp$ using W_1, i.e., $\eta = (P(k - Nl/M),\ 2\pi l/d)$ for some $k, l \in \mathbb{Z}$. We have $|\eta_2| = |2\pi l/d| > 2\gamma(b)$ if and only if $|l| > \lfloor d\gamma(b)/\pi \rfloor = l_0$. For $|l| \leq l_0$ condition (5.11) has to be satisfied. Since $d < \pi M/\gamma(b)$, $l_0 \leq M - 1$. For $|l| \leq l_0$ and $0 \neq \eta \in L^\perp$ we have

$$\min_{\substack{k \in \mathbb{Z} \\ (k,l) \neq (0,0)}} |\eta_1| = P \min_{\substack{k \in \mathbb{Z} \\ (k,l) \neq (0,0)}} \left| k - \frac{Nl}{M} \right| = Pc_l.$$

Hence the required condition is

$$P > c_l^{-1} \left(F(\gamma(b)) + F\left(\frac{2\pi|l|}{d} - \gamma(b) \right) \right), \quad |l| \leq l_0.$$

Observing that $c_{-l} = c_l$ gives the condition (5.3). □

6. SAMPLING CONDITIONS FOR THE X-RAY TRANSFORM

In the high-frequency limit $k_0 \to \infty$ diffraction effects are negligible and the radiation can be assumed to propagate along lines. Accordingly, the propagation operator turns into a line integral of f. This is the model underlying x-ray tomography. For an overview over the mathematical aspects of x-ray tomography see, e.g., [11,20,24] and the references given there. Because of its practical importance it is worthwhile to state our results for this case explicitly. For simplicity assume that $f \in C_0^\infty$.

Definition 6.1. Let $f \in C_0^\infty(\mathbb{R}^2)$. Then

$$\tilde{P}f(\varphi,s) = \int_{\mathbb{R}} f(s\theta^\perp + t\theta)dt \tag{6.1}$$

is called the x-ray transform of f.

Clearly $\tilde{P}f$ is the integral of f over the line with direction θ and signed distance s from the origin. Note that

$$\lim_{k_0\to\infty} (-2i)Pf(\varphi,s) = \tilde{P}f(\varphi,s), \tag{6.2}$$

$$\lim_{k_0\to\infty} \rho(\sigma) = |\sigma|, \tag{6.3}$$

$$\lim_{k_0\to\infty} \gamma(\sigma) = \sigma. \tag{6.4}$$

A proof of (6.2) can be found in [20, p. 7]. Equations (6.3) and (6.4) imply that the set $K'(\vartheta,b)$ given in (5.1) turns into the set

$$\tilde{K}(\vartheta,b) = \left\{(k,\sigma) \in \mathbb{R}^2 : |\sigma| \le b,\ |k| \le \frac{r}{\vartheta}\max\left(|\sigma|,\ (1-\vartheta)b\right)\right\}, \tag{6.5}$$

which corresponds to the set defined in [20, p. 71, Theorem III.3.1]. Taking the high-frequency limit in Theorem 4.1 yields

Corollary 6.1. *For $0 < \vartheta < 1 \le rb$ let $\tilde{K}(\vartheta,b)$ as in (6.5). Let $L = L(d,P,M,N)$ be an admissible sampling lattice such that the sets $\tilde{K}+\eta$, $\eta \in L^\perp$ are disjoint. If $f \in C_0^\infty(D_r)$, $g = \tilde{P}f$, and Sg as in (2.2), then*

$$|g(\varphi,s) - Sg(\varphi,s)| \le 2^{1/2}\,\|f\|_{L_1}\frac{be^{-\beta(\vartheta)rb}}{1-e^{-\alpha(\vartheta)}} + \epsilon^*(g,b) + c(\vartheta,b,P)\left\lceil\frac{bd}{\pi}\right\rceil\epsilon^*(g,b^*), \tag{6.6}$$

where $\alpha(\vartheta) = (1-\vartheta^2)^{3/2}/3$, $\beta(\vartheta) = \alpha(\vartheta)(1-\vartheta)/\vartheta$, $c(\vartheta,b,P) = 1 + (3+6rb/\vartheta)/P + (2/\pi)\ln(2+4rb/\vartheta)$, and $b^* = \max\{b, \frac{2\pi}{d} - b\}$.

The estimate (6.6), which is based on Proposition 2.3 sharpens the corresponding estimate in [20, Theorem III.3.1] which was derived using Theorem 2.1. This can most easily be seen by observing that the quantity $\epsilon_0(f,b)$ in [20, Theorem III.3.1] becomes infinite if f has discontinuities, while the right-hand side of (6.6) remains finite for some discontinuous functions, e.g. for f being the characteristic function of a disk. The general sampling conditions for the x-ray transform read as follows:

Corollary 6.2. *Let $L = L(d,P,N,M)$ be an admissible sampling lattice and $\tilde{K}(\vartheta,b)$ as in (6.5). The sets $\tilde{K}+\eta$, $\eta \in L^{\perp}$ are disjoint if and only if*

$$d < \frac{\pi M}{b} \quad \textit{and} \tag{6.7}$$

$$P > \max_{0\le l\le l_0} c_l^{-1}\left(F(b)+F\left(\frac{2\pi l}{d}-b\right)\right), \tag{6.8}$$

where

$$l_0 = \lfloor db/\pi \rfloor,$$
$$F(\sigma) = \frac{r}{\vartheta}\max\{|\sigma|,\ (1-\vartheta)b\}, \qquad |\sigma| \le b,$$

and c_l as in Proposition 5.1.

The discussion of the various lattices and their relative efficiency given in the previous section applies here as well. In particular, the choice of parameters (5.9) again leads to new efficient lattices.

While sampling the x-ray transform has received considerable attention, investigations in the literature concentrated on the standard and the efficient lattice. The general sampling conditions and the discussion of other lattices given here seem to be new. The efficient lattice was first suggested in [3] based on a geometrical argument. It was rediscovered in [17,25] by using Shannon sampling theory, and a rigorous mathematical treatment was given in [20]. Error estimates for reconstructions from x-ray data sampled on the efficient lattice have been derived in [9, 15] and additional numerical experiments can be found in [11]. Use of the efficient lattice for diffraction tomography was suggested and supported by numerical experiments in [7]. Parallel-beam sampling schemes were the sampling set is a union of cosets of a lattice where investigated in [8] and applied in [4]. Sampling conditions for the so-called fan-beam geometry were derived in [21].

ACKNOWLEDGMENT

This research has been supported by NSF grant DMS-9404436.

REFERENCES

1. M. Abramowitz and I. A. Stegun. “Handbook of Mathematical Functions,” U.S. Dept. of Commerce (1972).
2. P. L. Butzer, W. Splettstößer and R. L. Stens, The sampling theorem and linear prediction in signal analysis, Jahresber. Deutsch. Math.-Verein. 90:1 (1988).
3. A. M. Cormack, Sampling the Radon transform with beams of finite width, *Phys. Med. Biol.* 23:1141 (1978).
4. L. Desbat, Efficient sampling on coarse grids in tomography, *Inverse Problems* 9:251 (1993).
5. A. J. Devaney, A filtered backpropagation algorithm for diffraction tomography, *Ultrasonic Imaging* 4:336 (1982).
6. A. J. Devaney, Reconstructive tomography with diffracting wavefields, *Inverse Problems* 2:161 (1986)
7. A. Faridani. “Abtastbedingungen und Auflösung in der Beugungstomographie.” Ph.D. Dissertation, University of Münster, Germany (1988).
8. A. Faridani, An application of a multidimensional sampling theorem to computed tomography, *in*: “Integral Geometry and Tomography,” E. Grinberg and E.T Quinto, eds., Contemp. Math., vol. 113, Amer. Math. Soc., Providence, R.I., (1990), pp.65-80.

9. A. Faridani, Reconstructing from efficiently sampled data in parallel-beam tomography, *in*: "Inverse Problems and Imaging," G.F. Roach, ed., Pitmans Research Notes in Mathematics Series, vol. 245, (1991), pp. 68-102.
10. A. Faridani, A generalized sampling theorem for locally compact abelian groups, *Math. Comp.* 63:307 (1994).
11. A. Faridani, Results, old and new, in computed tomography, *in*: "Inverse Problems in Wave Propagation," G. Chavent et al., ed., Springer, New York (1997), pp. 167-193.
12. J. F. Greenleaf, Computerized tomography with ultrasound, *Proc. IEEE* 71:330 (1983).
13. A. C. Kak and M. Slaney. " Principles of Computerized Tomographic Imaging," IEEE Press, New York (1988).
14. M. Kaveh , M. Soumekh and J. F. Greenleaf, Signal processing for diffraction tomography, *IEEE Trans. Sonics and Ultrasonics* 31:230 (1984).
15. H. Kruse, Resolution of reconstruction methods in computerized tomography, *SIAM J. Sci. Stat. Comput.* 10:447 (1989).
16. K. J. Langenberg, Applied inverse problems for acoustic, electromagnetic and elastic wave scattering, *in*: "Basic Methods of Tomography and Inverse Problems," P. C. Sabatier, ed., Adam Hilger, Bristol (1987), pp. 125-467.
17. A. G. Lindgren and P. A. Rattey, The inverse discrete Radon transform with applications to tomographic imaging using projection data, *Advances in Electronics and Electron Physics* 56:359 (1981).
18. Z. Q. Lu, Multidimensional structure diffraction tomography for varying object orientation through generalized scattered waves, *Inverse Problems* 1:339 (1985).
19. R. K. Mueller, M. Kaveh and G. Wade, Reconstructive tomography and applications to ultrasonics, *Proc. IEEE* 67:567 (1979).
20. F. Natterer. "The Mathematics of Computerized Tomography," Wiley, New York (1986).
21. F. Natterer, Sampling in fan-beam tomography, *SIAM J. Appl. Math.* 53:358 (1993).
22. S. X. Pan and A. C. Kak, A computational study of reconstruction algorithms for diffraction tomography: interpolation versus filtered backpropagation, *IEEE Trans. Acoust. Speech Signal Processing* 31:1262 (1983).
23. D. P. Petersen and D. Middleton, Sampling and reconstruction of wave-number-limited functions in N-dimensional euclidean space, *Inf. Control* 5:279 (1962).
24. A. G. Ramm and A. I. Katsevich. "The Radon Transform and Local Tomography," CRC Press, Boca Raton (1996).
25. P. A. Rattey and A. G. Lindgren, Sampling the 2-D Radon transform, *IEEE Trans. Acoust. Speech Signal Processing* 29:994 (1981).
26. A. Schatzberg and A. J. Devaney, Super-resolution in diffraction tomography, *Inverse Problems* 8:149 (1992).
27. M. Soumekh and J.-H. Choi, Reconstruction in diffraction imaging, *IEEE Trans. Ultrason. Ferroelec. Freq. Contr.* 36:93 (1989).
28. E. Wolf, Three-dimensional structure determination of semi-transparent objects from holographic data, *Opt. Commun.* 1:153 (1969).
29. A. I. Zayed. "Advances in Shannon's Sampling Theory," CRC Press, Boca Raton (1993).

MULTIDIMENSIONAL INVERSE SCATTERING PROBLEM WITH NON-REFLECTING BOUNDARY CONDITIONS

Semion Gutman

Department of Mathematics
University of Oklahoma
Norman, OK

ABSTRACT

We discuss an algorithm for the refraction coefficient recovery in 2-D and 3-D inverse scattering problems. Suppose that a small object is illuminated by plane acoustic waves. Given data on a circular boundary of the region of interest, we employ a Regularized Quasi-Newton method (RQN) to construct an iterative recovery algorithm. The main new feature of the method is the utilization of non-reflective boundary conditions. The convergence of the algorithm is established for exact and for noisy data. Explicit estimation of the recovered coefficient is obtained, with a detailed analysis for a cylindrically configured geometry. We also present results of several numerical experiments illustrating the method's performance.

1. INTRODUCTION

Let $B_a = \left\{x \in \mathbf{R}^2 \middle| |x| \le a\right\}$ be the ball of a radius $a > 0$ in $\mathbf{R}^2$, and let Γ be its boundary. Here $|\cdot|$ denotes the Euclidean distance in $\mathbf{R}^2$. Let S^1 be the unit circle in $\mathbf{R}^2$. Then $u_0(x, \nu) = e^{ik\langle x, \nu\rangle}$ is the scalar incident planar wave of frequency $k > 0$ propagating in the direction of the vector $\nu \in S^1$. Here $\langle\cdot,\cdot\rangle$ denotes the inner product in $\mathbf{R}^2$. Let $\varepsilon(x)$ be a real valued function with $\varepsilon(x) = 0$ for $x \in \mathbf{R}^2 \setminus B_a$, and let $u(x, \nu) = e^{ik\langle x,\nu\rangle} + \tilde{u}(x, \nu)$, where $x \in \mathbf{R}^2$ and $\nu \in S^1$. Then the system

$$\Delta u(x, \nu) + k^2(1 + \varepsilon(x))u(x, \nu) = 0, \qquad x \in \mathbf{R}^2 \tag{1.1}$$

$$\lim_{r\to\infty} \sqrt{r}\left(\frac{\partial \tilde{u}(x, \nu)}{\partial r} - ik\tilde{u}(x, \nu)\right) = 0, \qquad r = |x| \tag{1.2}$$

Inverse Problems, Tomography, and Image Processing, edited by Ramm,
Plenum Press, New York, 1998

describes the scattering of the incident wave $u_0(x,\nu)$ by an object in B_a, for which the perturbation of the refraction coefficient is given by $\varepsilon(x)$. Equation (1.1) is the Helmholtz equation for the total field u, and condition (1.2) is the Sommerfeld radiation condition for the scattered field $\tilde{u}(x,\nu)$. While the above scattering problem as well as the consequent results are stated for the 2-dimensional case, similar results can be obtained for problems in a 3-D setting.

Suppose that the measurement functions

$$g_0(\phi,\nu) = u(x,\nu)\Big|_{\Gamma},$$

where ϕ is the angular polar coordinate on Γ, are known for some or all direction vectors $\nu \in S^1$. In an Inverse Scattering Problem one seeks to recover the unknown potential function $\varepsilon(x)$ from the given measurements $g_0(\phi,\nu)$. More precisely, we have

The ISP Statement

Let the wave number $k =$ constant > 0 be given. Determine the potential function $\varepsilon(x)$ in (1.1) such that the solution $u(x,\nu)$ satisfies (1.1)–(1.2) and

$$u(x,\nu)\Big|_{\Gamma} = g_0(\phi,\nu) \tag{1.3}$$

Concerning the uniqueness of this ISP, see [1, 2, 8] We are concerned with the weak scattering case, that is, the unknown spatial variations of the medium, represented by the coefficient $\varepsilon(x)$, are assumed to be small. See [3, 4] for physical examples of the weak scattering. See surveys [5, 6] on the numerical solutions.

2. NON-REFLECTING BOUNDARY CONDITIONS AND THE QUASI-NEWTON METHOD

The Inverse Scattering Problem (1.1)–(1.3) is stated in the entire plane $\mathbf{R}^2$, while the inhomogeneity $\varepsilon(x)$ is concentrated in the ball B_a. A numerical solution of such a problem would necessarily be inefficient, unless a reduction of (1.1)–(1.3) to a finite region is attained. Such a reduction and an algorithm for the ISP is presented in this paper, however, first, we have to describe the appropriate boundary conditions.

Let $\nu \in S^1$, $g(\phi,\nu)$ be a continuous function on Γ, and let $\tilde{u}(x,\nu)$ be the solution of the exterior problem

$$\Delta\tilde{u}(x,\nu) + k^2\tilde{u}(x,\nu) = 0, \qquad x \in \mathbf{R}^2 \setminus B_a \tag{2.1}$$

$$\tilde{u}(x,\nu)\Big|_{\Gamma} = g(\phi,\nu), \tag{2.2}$$

satisfying the Sommerfeld radiation condition.

Definition 2.1. Given $\nu \in S^1$, the Dirichlet to Neumann Map $M(g)$ is defined as

$$M(g) = \frac{\partial \tilde{u}}{\partial r},$$

where $\tilde{u}$ is defined as above.

Definition 2.2. A function $u(x,\nu)$, $x \in B_a$, $\nu \in S^1$ is said to satisfy the Non-reflecting Boundary Conditions on Γ, if

$$M(u\Big|_{\Gamma}) = \frac{\partial u}{\partial r}.$$

For a similar construction based on the Dirichlet-to-Neumann map see [9].

To obtain an explicit representation of the operator M we can argue as follows. Let $g(\phi,\nu)$ be a continuous function on Γ. Then it can be expanded into its Fourier series

$$g(\phi,\nu) = \sum_{-\infty}^{\infty} b_m(\nu) e^{im\phi}.$$

Let (r,ϕ) be the polar coordinates of the variable x and $\tilde{u}(x,\nu) = \tilde{u}(r,\phi,\nu)$. Then the solution of the exterior problem (2.1)-(2.2) is

$$\tilde{u}(r,\phi,\nu) = \sum_{-\infty}^{\infty} a_m(\nu) H_m^{(1)}(kr) e^{im\phi}, \qquad r > a,$$

where $H_m^{(1)}(z)$ is the Hankel function of the first kind. Thus,

$$\tilde{u}(r,\phi,\nu)\Big|_{\Gamma} = \sum_{-\infty}^{\infty} a_m(\nu) H_m^{(1)}(ka) e^{im\phi}.$$

Therefore

$$a_m(\nu) = \frac{b_m(\nu)}{H_m^{(1)}(ka)}$$

for all integer m. Note that here $H_m^{(1)}(ka) \neq 0$ since the Wronskian

$$J_m(ka)Y_m'(ka) - J_m'(ka)Y_m(ka) = \frac{2}{\pi ka} \neq 0.$$

On the other hand,

$$\frac{\partial \tilde{u}(r,\phi,\nu)}{\partial r} = \sum_{-\infty}^{\infty} a_m(\nu) k H_m^{(1)\prime}(kr) e^{im\phi}$$

and

$$\frac{\partial \tilde{u}(r,\phi,\nu)}{\partial r}\Big|_{\Gamma} = \sum_{-\infty}^{\infty} a_m(\nu) k H_m^{(1)\prime}(ka) e^{im\phi}.$$

Therefore,

$$M(g)(\phi,\nu) = \frac{\partial \tilde{u}(r,\phi,\nu)}{\partial r}\Big|_{\Gamma} = \sum_{-\infty}^{\infty} a_m(\nu) k H_m^{(1)\prime}(ka) e^{im\phi}.$$

Letting

$$M(g)(\phi,\nu) = \frac{\partial \tilde{u}(r,\phi,\nu)}{\partial r}\Big|_{\Gamma} = \sum_{-\infty}^{\infty} c_m(\nu) e^{im\phi} \tag{2.3}$$

we obtain

$$c_m(\nu) = \frac{k H_m^{(1)\prime}(ka)}{H_m^{(1)}(ka)} b_m(\nu) \tag{2.4}$$

for $m = 0, \pm 1, \pm 2, \ldots$, which is the desired explicit expression of $M(g)$.

Using the non-reflecting boundary conditions we can restate our original system (1.1)–(1.3) as the following system on the bounded domain B_a

$$\Delta \tilde{u}(x,\nu) + k^2(1+\varepsilon(x))\tilde{u}(x,\nu) + k^2\varepsilon(x)u_0(x,\nu) = 0, \qquad x \in B_a \tag{2.5}$$

$$\tilde{u}(x,\nu)\Big|_{\Gamma} = g(\phi,\nu) \tag{2.6}$$

$$\frac{\partial \tilde{u}(x,\nu)}{\partial r}\Big|_{\Gamma} = M(g)(\phi,\nu) \tag{2.7}$$

where $g(\phi,\nu) = g_0(\phi,\nu) - \left(u_0(x,\nu)\Big|_{\Gamma}\right)$, and $u(x,\nu) = u_0(x,\nu) + \tilde{u}(x,\nu)$.

Equation (2.5) can be viewed as a nonlinear equation in a Banach space $\mathbf{X}$. One can attempt to solve this equation by the Quasi-Newton method (also known as Newton–Kantorovich method), see [7]. The solution is sought as the limit of the sequence $\{z_n\}_{n=0}^{\infty}$ defined iteratively by

$$z_{n+1} = z_n - \left[A'(z_0)\right]^{-1} A z_n \qquad n \geq 0 \tag{2.8}$$

provided an initial guess $z_0 \in \mathbf{X}$.

First, we need to introduce the Banach space $\mathbf{X}$. Denote by Q^0 the subspace of $L^2(B_a \times S^1)$ of functions having the finite norm $||f||_{Q^0}$, defined by

$$||f||_{Q^0} = \text{ess} - \sup\left\{ ||f(\cdot,\nu)||_{L^2(B_a)} : \nu \in S^1 \right\}.$$

Let

$$\mathbf{X} = L^2(B_a) \times Q^0$$

with the norm

$$||z||_{\mathbf{X}} = ||(\varepsilon,u)||_{\mathbf{X}} = ||\varepsilon||_{L^2(B_a)} + ||u||_{Q^0}$$

for $\forall z = (\varepsilon, u) \in \mathbf{X}$. Then $\mathbf{X}$ is a Banach space.

For $(\varepsilon,\tilde{u}) \in \mathbf{X}$ and $\Delta\tilde{u} \in Q^0$, let

$$A(\varepsilon,\tilde{u}) = \Delta\tilde{u} + k^2(1+\varepsilon)\tilde{u} + k^2\varepsilon u_0$$

Then (2.5) is just $A(\varepsilon,\tilde{u}) = 0$ under the restrictions (2.6) and (2.7). We introduce the operator $\mathbf{T} = I - [A'(z_0)]^{-1} A$. Writing (2.8) as

$$z_{n+1} = \mathbf{T}(z_n)$$

implies that the convergence of the sequence $\{z_n\}_{n=0}^{\infty}$ can be analyzed in the general framework of the fixed point type arguments for the equation

$$z = \mathbf{T}(z)$$

where $z_0 = (0,0) \in \mathbf{X}$ is our initial guess. Here $A'(z_0)$ is the Frechet derivative of $A(\varepsilon, \tilde{u})$ at z_0 and it is computed, for any $z = (h, H) \in \mathbf{X}$ and $\Delta H \in Q^0$, as follows

$$A'(z_0)z = A'(z_0)(h,H) = \Delta H + k^2 H + k^2 h u_0 .$$

This follows from

$$\frac{||A(h,H) - A(0,0) - A'(z_0)(h,H)||_{L^2(B_a)}}{||(h,H)||_{\mathbf{X}}} = k^2 \frac{||hH||_{L^2(B_a)}}{||(h,H)||_{\mathbf{X}}},$$

and one can easily prove that $||(h,H)||_{\mathbf{X}} \to 0$ implies

$$\frac{||hH||_{L^2(B_a)}}{||(h,H)||_{\mathbf{X}}} \to 0$$

under the above conditions (note, that $hH \in L^2(B_a)$).

Now $\mathbf{T} = I - [A'(z_0)]^{-1} A = [A'(z_0)]^{-1} (A'(z_0) - I)$. Writing $z_n = (\varepsilon_n, \tilde{u}_n)$, equation $z_n = \mathbf{T}(z_{n-1})$ becomes

$$A'(z_0)(\varepsilon_n, \tilde{u}_n) = (A'(z_0) - A)(\varepsilon_{n-1}, \tilde{u}_{n-1}).$$

That is

$$\begin{aligned}
&\Delta\tilde{u}_n + k^2\tilde{u}_n + k^2\varepsilon_n u_0 \\
&= \Delta\tilde{u}_{n-1} + k^2\tilde{u}_{n-1} + k^2\varepsilon_{n-1}u_0 - \left[\Delta\tilde{u}_{n-1} + k^2(1+\varepsilon_{n-1})\tilde{u}_{n-1} + k^2\varepsilon_{n-1}u_0\right] \\
&= -k^2\varepsilon_{n-1}\tilde{u}_{n-1}.
\end{aligned}$$

Thus, starting at an initial guess $z_0 = (\varepsilon_0, \tilde{u}_0)$, at each step, we need to solve

$$\Delta\tilde{u}_n + k^2\tilde{u}_n + k^2\varepsilon_n u_0 = -k^2\varepsilon_{n-1}\tilde{u}_{n-1} \tag{2.9}$$

$$\tilde{u}(x,\nu)\Big|_{\Gamma} = g(\phi,\nu) \tag{2.10}$$

$$\frac{\partial\tilde{u}(x,\nu)}{\partial r}\Big|_{\Gamma} = M(g)(\phi,\nu).$$

Our algorithm for the solution of (2.9)–(2.11) is described in the next section.

3. THE RQN (REGULARIZED QUASI-NEWTON) ALGORITHM

Rewrite (2.9)- (2.11) in the form

$$\Delta\tilde{u}_n + k^2\tilde{u}_n = -k^2\varepsilon_n u_0 - k^2\varepsilon_{n-1}\tilde{u}_{n-1}$$

$$\tilde{u}(x,\nu)\Big|_{\Gamma} = g(\phi,\nu)$$

$$\frac{\partial\tilde{u}(x,\nu)}{\partial r}\Big|_{\Gamma} = M(g)(\phi,\nu)$$

where ε_{n-1} and $\tilde{u}_{n-1}$ are known at the nth iteration. For the convenience of our description, let's get rid of the subscript n and consider the system

$$\Delta v + k^2 v = -k^2 \varepsilon u_0 + f(r, \phi, \nu) \tag{3.1}$$

$$v(x, \nu)\Big|_{\Gamma} = g(\phi, \nu) \tag{3.2}$$

$$\frac{\partial v(x, \nu)}{\partial r}\Big|_{\Gamma} = M(g)(\phi, \nu). \tag{3.3}$$

where $f(r, \phi, \nu) \in L^2(B_a \times S^1)$ is assumed to be given.

Let $\mu \in \mathbf{R}^2$. Multiply (3.1) by $e^{ik\langle x, \mu\rangle}$ and integrate the result over B_a to get

$$\begin{aligned} &\iint_{B_a} e^{ik\langle x,\mu\rangle} \Delta v\, dx + k^2 \iint_{B_a} v e^{ik\langle x,\mu\rangle}\, dx \\ &= -k^2 \iint_{B_a} \varepsilon e^{ik\langle x,\mu+\nu\rangle}\, dx + \iint_{B_a} f \cdot e^{ik\langle x,\mu\rangle}\, dx. \end{aligned} \tag{3.4}$$

Using the second Green's formula

$$\int_D u \Delta v\, dx = \int_D v \Delta u\, dx - \int_{\partial D} (v \frac{\partial u}{\partial n} - u \frac{\partial v}{\partial n})\, ds,$$

we obtain

$$\begin{aligned} &\iint_{B_a} e^{ik\langle x,\mu\rangle} \Delta v\, dx \\ &= \iint_{B_a} v \Delta e^{ik\langle x,\mu\rangle}\, dx - \int_\Gamma \left(v \frac{\partial e^{ik\langle x,\mu\rangle}}{\partial n} - e^{ik\langle x,\mu\rangle} \frac{\partial v}{\partial n} \right) ds \\ &= -k^2 |\mu|^2 \iint_{B_a} v e^{ik\langle x,\mu\rangle}\, dx - \int_\Gamma \left(\frac{ik\langle x,\mu\rangle}{|x|} v - \frac{\partial v}{\partial n} \right) e^{ik\langle x,\mu\rangle}\, ds. \end{aligned}$$

Substitute it into (3.4).

$$\begin{aligned} k^2 \iint_{B_a} \varepsilon e^{ik\langle x,\mu+\nu\rangle}\, dx &= -k^2(1 - |\mu|^2) \iint_{B_a} v e^{ik\langle x,\mu\rangle}\, dx \\ &+ \int_\Gamma \left(\frac{ik\langle x,\mu\rangle}{|x|} v - \frac{\partial v}{\partial n} \right) e^{ik\langle x,\mu\rangle}\, ds + \iint_{B_a} f e^{ik\langle x,\mu\rangle}\, dx. \end{aligned}$$

Let $|\mu| = 1$. We obtain

$$\begin{aligned} \iint_{B_a} \varepsilon e^{ik\langle x,\mu+\nu\rangle}\, dx = \frac{1}{k^2} \Big\{ &\int_\Gamma \left(\frac{ik\langle x,\mu\rangle}{|x|} v - \frac{\partial v}{\partial n} \right) e^{ik\langle x,\mu\rangle}\, ds \\ &+ \iint_{B_a} f e^{ik\langle x,\mu\rangle}\, dx \Big\}. \end{aligned}$$

Since $\varepsilon(x) = 0$ outside B_a, we have

$$\begin{aligned} \iint_{\mathbf{R}^2} \varepsilon e^{ik\langle x,\mu+\nu\rangle}\, dx = \frac{1}{k^2} \Big\{ &\int_\Gamma \left(\frac{ik\langle x,\mu\rangle}{|x|} v - \frac{\partial v}{\partial n} \right) e^{ik\langle x,\mu\rangle}\, ds \\ &+ \iint_{B_a} f e^{ik\langle x,\mu\rangle}\, dx \Big\}. \end{aligned}$$

On the boundary Γ, $v = g$ is assumed to known for any ν with $|\nu| = 1$. Since $\varepsilon(x)$ does not depend on ν, we can compute the Fourier transform of $\varepsilon(x)$

$$\widehat{\varepsilon}(\xi) = \frac{1}{2\pi k^2}\left\{\int_\Gamma \left(\frac{ik\langle x,\mu\rangle}{|x|}v - \frac{\partial v}{\partial n}\right) e^{ik\langle x,\mu\rangle}\,ds + \int\int_{B_a} f e^{ik\langle x,\mu\rangle}\,dx\right\}$$

at any point $\xi = k(\mu+\nu)$ within $|\xi| \leq 2k$.

We use the inversion of $\widehat{\varepsilon}(\xi)$ on B_{2k} to approximate $\varepsilon(x)$

$$\varepsilon(x) = \frac{1}{2\pi}\int\int_{B_{2k}} e^{-i\langle x,\xi\rangle}\widehat{\varepsilon}(\xi)\,d\xi.$$

Let $\Phi(x,y) = \frac{i}{4}H_0^{(1)}(k|x-y|)$ be the fundamental solution of (1.1)–(1.3) (with $\varepsilon(x) = 0$). For the approximation of $v(x,\nu)$, we use

$$\begin{aligned} v(x,\nu) = &\int_\Gamma \left\{\frac{\partial v}{\partial n(y)}\Phi(x,y) - v\frac{\partial \Phi(x,y)}{\partial n(y)}\right\} ds(y) \\ &- \int\int_{B_a} \left\{\Delta v(y,\nu) + k^2 v(y,\nu)\right\}\Phi(x,y)\,dy \end{aligned}$$

for any $x \in B_a$, where $v(x,\nu)\Big|_\Gamma = g(\phi,\nu)$ and $\frac{\partial v(x,\nu)}{\partial n(y)} = \frac{\partial v(x,\nu)}{\partial r} = M(g)$. See [1, formula (2.4)]. Summarizing the above results, we present the RQN algorithm here.

The RQN algorithm:

Given an initial guess $z_0 = (\varepsilon_0(y), \tilde{u}_0(y,\nu))$, the RQN algorithm for the system (2.5)–(2.7) is the following procedure:

For $n = 1,2,3,\ldots$, compute the sequence $\{z_n\} = \{(\varepsilon_n(x), \tilde{u}_n(x,\nu)\}$ iteratively by

$$\varepsilon_n(x) = \frac{1}{2\pi}\int\int_{B_{2k}} e^{-i\langle x,\xi\rangle}\widehat{\varepsilon}_n(\xi)\,d\xi \tag{3.5}$$

where

$$\begin{aligned} \widehat{\varepsilon}_n(\xi) = &-\frac{1}{2\pi}\int\int_{B_a} \varepsilon_{n-1}(y)\tilde{u}_{n-1}(y,\nu)e^{ik\langle y,\mu\rangle}\,dy + \\ &+\frac{1}{2\pi k^2}\int_\Gamma \left[\frac{ik\langle y,\mu\rangle}{a}g(y,\nu) - (Mg)(y,\nu)\right] e^{ik\langle y,\mu\rangle}\,ds(y) \end{aligned} \tag{3.6}$$

where $\xi = k(\mu+\nu)$, and

$$\begin{aligned} \tilde{u}_n(x,\nu) = k^2 &\int\int_{B_a} \left[\varepsilon_n(y)u_0(y,\nu) + \varepsilon_{n-1}(y)\tilde{u}_{n-1}(y,\nu)\right]\Phi(x,y)\,dy + \\ &+ \int_\Gamma \left\{(Mg)(y,\nu)\Phi(x,y) - g(y,\nu)\frac{\partial \Phi(x,y)}{\partial n(y)}\right\} ds(y) \end{aligned} \tag{3.7}$$

where $n(y)$ denotes an outward normal vector on the circle Γ.

4. PROPERTIES OF THE RQN ALGORITHM

Denote by Q^0 the subspace of $L^2(B_a \times S^1)$ of functions having the finite norm $||f||_{Q^0}$, defined by

$$||f||_{Q^0} = ess - sup\left\{||f(\cdot,\nu)||_{L^2(B_a)} : \nu \in S^1\right\}.$$

Let

$$\mathbf{X} = L^2(B_a) \times Q^0$$

with the norm

$$||x||_{\mathbf{X}} = ||(\varepsilon,u)||_{\mathbf{X}} = ||\varepsilon||_{L^2(B_a)} + ||u||_{Q^0}$$

for all $x = (\varepsilon,u) \in \mathbf{X}$. Let $\Phi(x,y) = \frac{i}{4}H_0^{(1)}(k|x-y|)$ be the fundamental solution of (1.1)–(1.3). The operator $\mathbf{T}$ is introduced by

Definition 4.1. The operator $\mathbf{T} : \mathbf{X} \to \mathbf{X}$ is defined as

$$\mathbf{T}(\varepsilon,u) = (K_1(\varepsilon,u), K_2(\varepsilon,u)) \tag{4.1}$$

for all $(\varepsilon,u) \in \mathbf{X}$ where the operators $K_1 : \mathbf{X} \to L^2(B_a)$ and $K_2 : \mathbf{X} \to Q^0$ are defined respectively by

$$K_1(\varepsilon,u) = \frac{1}{2\pi}\int\int_{B_{2k}} e^{-i\langle x,\xi\rangle}\widehat{\varepsilon}(\xi)\,d\xi \tag{4.2}$$

where

$$\begin{aligned}\widehat{\varepsilon}(\xi) = &-\frac{1}{2\pi}\int\int_{B_a} \varepsilon(y)u(y,\nu)e^{ik\langle y,\mu\rangle}\,dy + \\ &+\frac{1}{2\pi k^2}\int_{\Gamma}\left[\frac{ik\langle y,\mu\rangle}{a}g(y,\nu) - (Mg)(y,\nu)\right]e^{ik\langle y,\mu\rangle}\,ds(y)\end{aligned} \tag{4.3}$$

where $\xi = k(\mu+\nu)$, and

$$\begin{aligned}K_2(\varepsilon,u) = k^2 &\int\int_{B_a} [K_1(\varepsilon,u)u_0(y,\nu) + \varepsilon(y)u(y,\nu)]\,\Phi(x,y)\,dy + \\ &+\int_{\Gamma}\left\{(Mg)(y,\nu)\Phi(x,y) - g(y,\nu)\frac{\partial\Phi(x,y)}{\partial n(y)}\right\}ds(y)\end{aligned} \tag{4.4}$$

where $n(y)$ denotes an outward normal vector on the circle Γ.

Note that both $K_1(\varepsilon,u)$ and $K_2(\varepsilon,u)$ are well defined for all $x \in \mathbf{R}^2$.

Suppose that the measurements $\tilde{u}(x,\nu)\Big|_{\Gamma} = g(\phi,\nu) \in C(\Gamma \times S^1)$. Given any initial guess z_0, The RQN algorithm produces a sequence $z_n = \mathbf{T}(z_{n-1})$. Using the framework of the fixed point type arguments we can obtain the following results.

Lemma 4.1. *For any $(\varepsilon_i, u_i) \in \mathbf{X}, i = 1$ and 2, we have*

$$\begin{aligned}&\| \mathbf{T}(\varepsilon_2,u_2) - \mathbf{T}(\varepsilon_1,u_1) \|_{\mathbf{X}} \\ &= ||K_1(\varepsilon_2,u_2) - K_1(\varepsilon_1,u_1)||_{L^2(B_a)} + ||K_2(\varepsilon_2,u_2) - K_2(\varepsilon_1,u_1)||_{Q^0} \\ &\leq E(k,a)\left\{||u_2||_{Q^0}\,||\varepsilon_2 - \varepsilon_1||_{L^2(B_a)} + ||\varepsilon_1||_{L^2(B_a)}\,||u_2 - u_1||_{Q^0}\right\}.\end{aligned}$$

where $E(k,a) = k^2\left[\frac{a}{\sqrt{\pi}} + (a^2k^2+1)C(k,a)\right]$ *and*

$$C(k,a) = \left\{\frac{1}{8\pi}\left[2(e^{-1}+\sqrt{2})^2a^2 + (2e^{-1}+2\sqrt{2}+1)\frac{1}{k^2}\right]\right\}^{\frac{1}{2}}.$$

Now we are ready for the convergence theorem.

Theorem 4.2. *Let the operator $\mathbf{T} : \mathbf{X} \to \mathbf{X}$ be defined as in (4.1)–(4.4) and $u_0 = e^{ik\langle x,\nu\rangle}$ where $\nu \in S^1$. Let $\delta = (2E(k,a))^{-1}$ where $E(k,a)$ is as in Lemma 4.1. Denote $x_0 = (0,0) \in \mathbf{X}$. Let $U = \left\{x \in \mathbf{X} \,\middle|\, ||x||_{\mathbf{X}} \leq \delta\right\}$. Furthermore, we suppose that the solution (ε, u) of (1.1)–(1.3) is in the space $\mathbf{X}$. If*

$$||\varepsilon||_{L^2(B_a)} \leq \left\{\frac{k^2}{4\pi}C(k,a) + \frac{4\sqrt{\pi}aE(k,a)}{\delta}\right\}^{-1},$$

then, under the exact data $\tilde{u}\Big|_{\Gamma} = g$ and $\frac{\partial \tilde{u}}{\partial r}\Big|_{\Gamma} = Mg$, the following statements are valid

(1). $\mathbf{T}$ is a contraction in U and

$$||\mathbf{T}(x_2) - \mathbf{T}(x_1)||_{\mathbf{X}} \leq \frac{1}{2}\,||x_2 - x_1||_{\mathbf{X}}$$

for any $x_1, x_2 \in U$.

(2). $\mathbf{T}(x_0) \in U$ and $||\mathbf{T}(x_0)||_{\mathbf{X}} \leq \frac{\delta}{4}$.

(3). $\mathbf{T}(U) \subset U$.

(4). The sequence $\{z_n\}_{n=0}^{\infty}$ defined by $z_{n+1} = \mathbf{T}(z_n), n = 0,1,2,3\ldots$ converges for any initial guess $z_0 = (\varepsilon_0, \tilde{u}_0) \in U$.

(5). The limit point q of $\{z_n\}_{n=0}^{\infty}$ is the unique fixed point of the operator $\mathbf{T}$ in U and

$$||z_n - q||_{\mathbf{X}} \leq \frac{1}{2^{n-1}}\,||z_1 - z_0||_{\mathbf{X}}.$$

While the previous Theorem addresses the issue of the convergence of the RQN algorithm, the quality of this process is discussed below. To recall, the RQN algorithm produces a sequence $\{z_n\}_{n=0}^{\infty}$ which is identified by $z_{n+1} = \mathbf{T}(z_n), n = 0,1,2,\ldots$, and under the hypothesis of Theorem 4.2, it converges to a fixed point in the space $\mathbf{X}$ with the topology defined by $||\cdot||_{\mathbf{X}}$. We denote this fixed point by $q \in \mathbf{X}$. Let $q = (\varepsilon_q, \tilde{u}_q)$. The function ε_q is called the recovered potential. Since $q \in \mathbf{X}$, the recovered potential $\varepsilon_q \in L^2(B_a)$. Throughout the rest of the paper, we will denote the solution of (2.5)–(2.7) by $s = (\varepsilon, \tilde{u})$. Let U be the closed subset of $\mathbf{X}$ defined in Theorem 4.2. Also let δ be as in Theorem 4.2, and let $\bar{\delta} = \bar{\delta}(\delta, k, a)$ be appropriately chosen. The following theorem describes the approximation of the true potential ε by the recovered potential ε_q.

Theorem 4.3. *Let $s = (\varepsilon, \tilde{u})$ be the solution of (2.5)-(2.7) with*

$$||\varepsilon||_{L^2(B_a)} \leq \bar{\delta},$$

where $\bar{\delta} = \bar{\delta}(\delta, k, a)$, and let q be the unique fixed point of $\mathbf{T}$ in U. Then

$$||\varepsilon - \varepsilon_q||_{L^2(B_a)} \leq \frac{1}{13}\left[18 + 5\sqrt{\pi} a k^2 C(k,a)\right] ||\varepsilon - K_1(\varepsilon, \tilde{u})||_{L^2(B_a)}.$$

We can provide a further analysis of the difference $||\varepsilon - K_1(\varepsilon, \tilde{u})||_{L^2(B_a)}$.
By the definition

$$K_1(\varepsilon, u) = \frac{1}{2\pi} \int\int_{B_{2k}} e^{-i\langle x, \xi\rangle} \widehat{\varepsilon}(\xi)\, d\xi$$

where $\widehat{\varepsilon}(\xi) = \frac{1}{2\pi} \int\int_{B_a} \varepsilon(y) e^{i\langle y, \xi\rangle}\, dy$. Therefore, $K_1(\varepsilon, u)$ can be viewed as an approximation of $\varepsilon(x)$ through its Fourier transformation on a finite domain. Theorem 4.3 states that the absolute error of RQN algorithm is bounded, in the L^2 sense, by the difference between the potential $\varepsilon(x)$ and its Fourier transformation on the finite domain B_{2k} where k is the wave number.

Suppose that the exact potential $\varepsilon(x) \in L^2(B_a)$. Let us examine how the exact potential $\varepsilon(x)$ can be approximated by its Fourier transform on B_{2k}.

Lemma 4.4. *For any $\varepsilon(x) \in L^2(B_a)$, let*

$$\bar{\varepsilon}(x) = \begin{cases} \varepsilon(x) & \text{if } x \in B_a \\ 0 & \text{if } x \notin B_a. \end{cases}$$

and B be any open ball which contains the closure of B_a. If $\bar{\varepsilon}(x) \in H^2(B)$, then

$$||\varepsilon - K_1(\varepsilon, \tilde{u})||_{L^2(B_a)} \leq \frac{a}{4k} ||\Delta\bar{\varepsilon}(x)||_{L^2(B)}$$

where $\Delta\bar{\varepsilon}(x)$ is the Laplacian of $\bar{\varepsilon}(x)$ in the distributional sense.

Moreover, if $\varepsilon(x) \in C_0^2(B_a)$, then

$$||\varepsilon - K_1(\varepsilon, \tilde{u})||_{L^2(B_a)} \leq \frac{a}{4k} ||\Delta\varepsilon(x)||_{L^2(B_a)}$$

where $\Delta\varepsilon(x)$ is the regular Laplacian of $\varepsilon(x)$.
For the special case, when

$$\varepsilon(x) = h(r),$$

where $r = |x|$, we can establish

Lemma 4.5. *For any $\varepsilon(x) = h(r) \in L^2(B_a)$, we have*

$$K_1(\varepsilon, \tilde{u})(x) = \int_0^a r h(r) \left\{ \int_0^{2k} s J_0(rt) J_0(|x|t)\, dt \right\} dr \tag{4.5}$$
$$= \int_0^a r h(r) F\, dr$$

where

$$F(\alpha,\beta)=\begin{cases}\frac{2k}{\alpha^2-\beta^2}\{\beta J_{-1}(2k\beta)J_0(2k\alpha)-\alpha J_{-1}(2k\alpha)J_0(2k\beta)\} & \text{if } \alpha\neq\beta\\ \frac{(2k)^2}{2}\{J_0^2(2k\alpha)+J_1^2(2k\alpha)\} & \text{if } \alpha=\beta\end{cases}$$

In particular, if

$$\varepsilon(x)=\begin{cases}\rho=\text{constant} & |x|\leq b\\ 0 & \text{otherwise}\end{cases}$$

where $0<b\leq a$, *we have*

$$K_1(\varepsilon,\tilde{u})(x)=\rho b\int_0^{2k}J_0(|x|t)J_1(bt)\,dt$$

and

$$\varepsilon(x)-K_1(\varepsilon,\tilde{u})(x)=\begin{cases}\rho b\int_{2k}^{\infty}J_0(|x|t)J_1(bt)\,dt & \text{if } |x|\neq b\\ \frac{\rho}{2}\left[1+J_0^2(2bk)\right] & \text{if } |x|=b.\end{cases}$$

5. ANALYSIS OF THE RQN ALGORITHM FOR NOISY DATA

Practically speaking, the measurement data $\tilde{u}\Big|_\Gamma=g(\phi,\nu)$ of the scattered field is not exact. Like in the last two sections, we will denote the exact data on the boundary Γ by $\tilde{u}\Big|_\Gamma=g(\phi,\nu)$, while use $\tilde{u}\Big|_\Gamma=g_s(\phi,\nu)$ for the noisy data. Our question can be stated as:

If $g(\phi,\nu)$ and $g_s(\phi,\nu)$ are close, does our RQN algorithm still converge? If it does, how far is the limit point from the original refraction coefficient ε?

Let $\mathbf{T}$ be the operator defined under the exact data as before. Denote $(Mg)_s=M(g_s)$ and the operator $\mathbf{T}$ under the noisy data by $\mathbf{T}_s$.

Definition 5.1. The operator $\mathbf{T}_s:\mathbf{X}\to\mathbf{X}$ is defined as

$$\mathbf{T}_s(\varepsilon,u)=(K_{1s}(\varepsilon,u),K_{2s}(\varepsilon,u))$$

for any $(\varepsilon,u)\in\mathbf{X}$, where the operators $K_{1s}:\mathbf{X}\to L^2(B_a)$ and $K_{2s}:\mathbf{X}\to Q^0$ are defined respectively by

$$K_{1s}(\varepsilon,u)=\frac{1}{2\pi}\int\int_{B_{2k}}e^{-i\langle x,\xi\rangle}\widehat{\varepsilon}_s(\xi)\,d\xi,$$

where

$$\widehat{\varepsilon}_s(\xi)=-\frac{1}{2\pi}\int\int_{B_a}\varepsilon(y)u(y,\nu)e^{ik\langle y,\mu\rangle}\,dy$$
$$+\frac{1}{2\pi k^2}\int_\Gamma\left[\frac{ik\langle y,\mu\rangle}{a}g_s(y,\nu)-(Mg)_s(y,\nu)\right]e^{ik\langle y,\mu\rangle}\,ds(y),$$

where $\xi=k(\mu+\nu)$. And

$$K_{2s}(\varepsilon,u)=k^2\int\int_{B_a}\left[K_{1s}(\varepsilon,u)u_0(y,\nu)+\varepsilon(y)u(y,\nu)\right]\Phi(x,y)\,dy$$
$$+\int_\Gamma\left\{(Mg)_s(y,\nu)\Phi(x,y)-g_s(y,\nu)\frac{\partial\Phi(x,y)}{\partial n(y)}\right\}ds(y),$$

where $n(y)$ denotes an outward normal vector on the circle Γ.

Hölder spaces $C^{i,\alpha}(\Gamma), i=0,1$ (see e.g. [1]) are used to formulate the regularity properties of these boundary potentials $g(y,\nu)$ and $g_s(y,\nu)$. It is shown in [3, Theorem 3.11] that *the Dirichlet-to-Neumann map M is a bounded operator from* $C^{1,\alpha}(\Gamma)$ *to* $C^{0,\alpha}(\Gamma)$.

Let

$$C^{1,\alpha,\infty}(\Gamma) = \left\{ g(x,\nu) \in C^{1,\alpha}(\Gamma) \middle| \sup_{\nu \in S^1} \| g \|_{1,\alpha} < \infty \right\}$$

and

$$\| g \|_{1,\alpha,\infty} = \sup_{\nu \in S^1} \| g \|_{1,\alpha} .$$

Now we can briefly summarize our results for the noisy data.

Lemma 5.1. *Let* $x_0 = (0,0) \in \mathbf{X}$ *and* $g(x,\nu), g_s(x,\nu) \in C^{1,\alpha,\infty}$. *Then*

$$||K_{1s}(x_0) - K_1(x_0)||_{L^2(B_a)} \le c \| g_s - g \|_{1,\alpha,\infty}$$

where c is a constant which only depends on the radius a and the wave number k.

Lemma 5.2. *For any* $x \in \mathbf{R}^2$, *let*

$$f(x) = \int_\Gamma \phi(y)\Phi(x,y)\, ds(y)$$

be the acoustic single-layer potential with density $\phi(y) \in L^2(\Gamma)$. *Then*

$$f(x) \in L^\infty(\mathbf{R}^2)$$

and, for any $x \in \mathbf{R}^2$,

$$|f(x)| \le \alpha(k,a)\, ||\phi||_{L^2(\Gamma)}$$

where $\alpha(k,a)$ *only depends on the radius a and the wave number k.*

The above Lemmas are used to obtain

Theorem 5.3. *Let the operator* $\mathbf{T}_s : \mathbf{X} \to \mathbf{X}$ *be defined as in Definition 5.1. Let* δ, U *and* ε *satisfy the conditions of Theorem 4.2. Moreover, we assume that* $g(x,\nu), g_s(x,\nu) \in C^{1,\alpha,\infty}(\Gamma)$. *Then there exists a number* $\tilde{\delta} > 0$, *which depends only on the radius a and the wave number k, such that, if*

$$\| g_s - g \|_{1,\alpha,\infty} \le \tilde{\delta},$$

then the following statements hold.

1. $\mathbf{T}_s$ *is a contraction in U and*

$$||\mathbf{T}_s(x_2) - \mathbf{T}_s(x_1)||_{\mathbf{X}} \le \frac{1}{2} ||x_2 - x_1||_{\mathbf{X}}$$

for any $x_1, x_2 \in U$.

Table 1.

Iteration no.	1	2	3	4	5
Ft. rel. error	0.2665×10^{-2}	0.1820×10^{-3}	0.1689×10^{-3}	0.1678×10^{-3}	0.1677×10^{-3}
Iter. rel. error	0.1000×10^{1}	0.2225×10^{-2}	0.8257×10^{-5}	0.2613×10^{-7}	0.8696×10^{-10}

2. $\mathbf{T}_s(x_0) \in U$ *and* $||\mathbf{T}_s(x_0)||_{\mathbf{X}} \leq \frac{\delta}{2}$ *where* $x_0 = (0,0) \in U$.
3. $\mathbf{T}_s(U) \subset U$.
4. *The sequence* $\{z_n\}_{n=0}^{\infty}$ *defined by* $z_{n+1} = \mathbf{T}_s(z_n), n = 0,1,2,3\ldots$ *converges for any initial guess* $z_0 = (\varepsilon_0, \tilde{u}_0) \in U$.
5. *The limit point* $q_s = (\varepsilon_{q_s}, \tilde{u}_{q_s}$ *of* $\{z_n\}_{n=0}^{\infty}$ *is the unique fixed point of the operator* $\mathbf{T}_s$ *in* U *and*
$$||z_n - q_s||_{\mathbf{X}} \leq \frac{1}{2^{n-1}} ||z_1 - z_0||_{\mathbf{X}}.$$
6. *If* $||\varepsilon||_{L^2(B_a)} \leq \bar{\delta}$ *where* $\bar{\delta}$ *is defined in Theorem 4.2, then*
$$||\varepsilon - \varepsilon_{q_s}||_{L^2(B_a)} \leq \frac{1}{13}\left[18 + 5\sqrt{\pi}ak^2C(k,a)\right] ||\varepsilon - K_1(\varepsilon,\tilde{u})||_{L^2(B_a)}.$$

6. NUMERICAL EXPERIMENTS

To evaluate the numerical performance, we conducted several numerical experiments. Three of them are presented here. Assume that the function $\varepsilon(x)$ in (1.1) is known. We obtain the measurements $g(\phi, \nu)$ by solving the forward scattering problem. While it is difficult to solve the forward problem for an arbitrary distribution of the refraction coefficient represented by $1 + \varepsilon(x)$, it is quite easy to do so when $\varepsilon(x)$ depends only on the radius variable r. We emphasize that this restriction is caused by the difficulty of solving the forward problem while our RQN Algorithm works for any $\varepsilon(x) \in L^2(B_a)$ in the weak scattering case. The following is a brief description of how we solve the forward problem for radially dependent function $\varepsilon(x) = \varepsilon(r)$.

Let

$$\varepsilon(r) = \begin{cases} c & \text{if } r \leq b \leq a \\ 0 & \text{otherwise} \end{cases}$$

where c is a constant. Then the scattering field is given by

$$u(x,\nu) = \begin{cases} e^{ik\langle x,\nu\rangle} + \sum_{m=-\infty}^{\infty} a_m H_m^{(1)}(kr)e^{im(\phi-\alpha)} & \text{if } r > b \\ \sum_{m=-\infty}^{\infty} b_m J_m(k_1 r)e^{im(\phi-\alpha)} & \text{if } r \leq b \end{cases}$$

where $k_1 = k \cdot \sqrt{1+c}$ and J_m and $H_m^{(1)}$ are the Bessel and Hankel functions. The coefficients a_m and b_m are computed by

$$a_m = \frac{i^m k_1 J_m(ka)J_m'(k_1 a) - k i^m J_m'(ka)J_m(k_1 a)}{-k_1 H_m^{(1)}(ka)J_m'(k_1 a) + kH_m^{(1)\prime}(ka)J_m(k_1 a)}$$

$$b_m = i^m \frac{J_m(ka)}{J_m(k_1 a)} + a_m \frac{H_m^{(1)}(ka)}{J_m(k_1 a)}$$

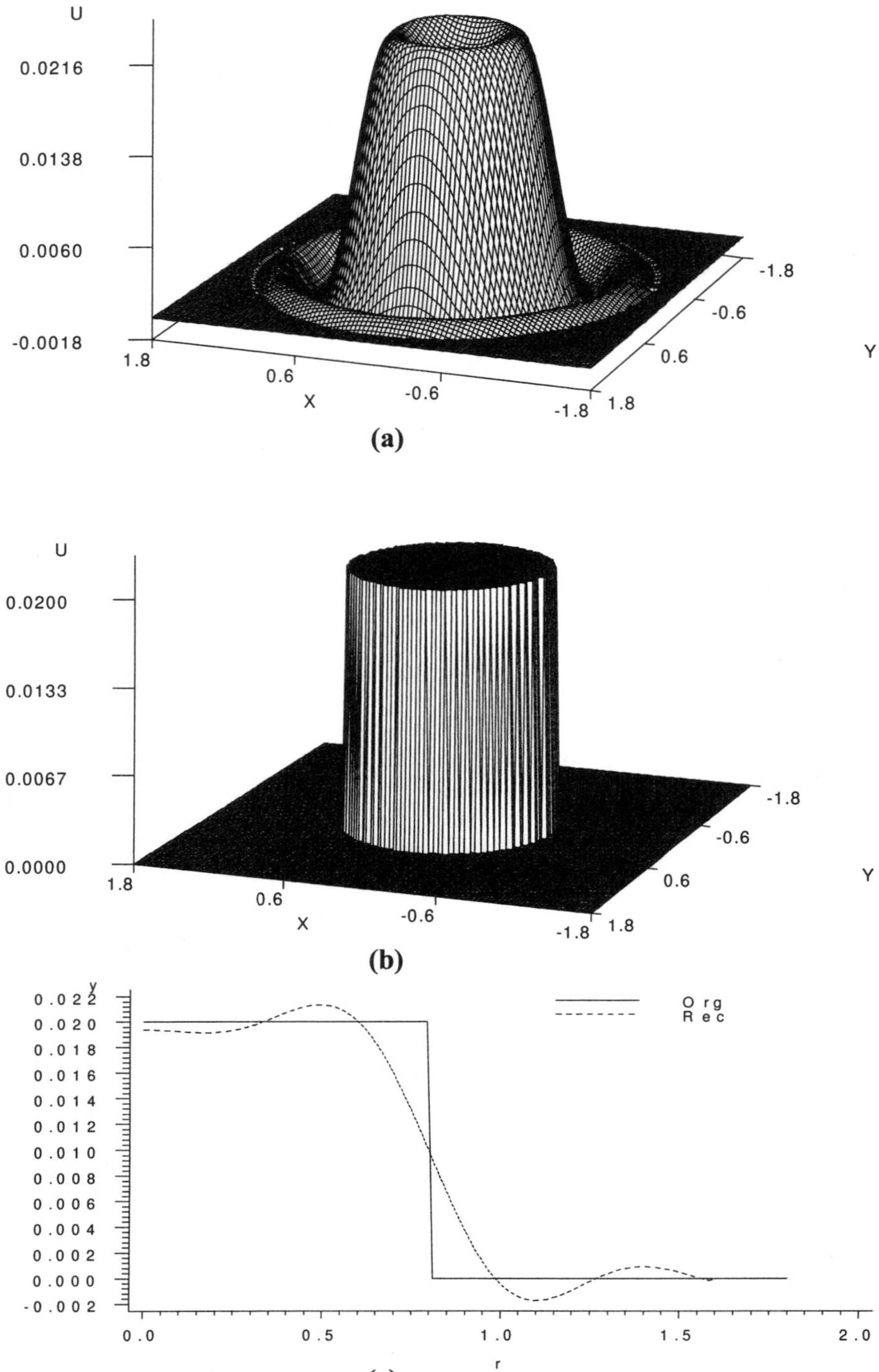

Figure 1. **(a)** Recovered; **(b)** original; **(c)** cross section. $k = 5.300000$, $a = 1.600000$, Fourier transform relative error $= 0.1677 \times 10^{03}$, $p = 357$, $p' = 1373$, no. of iteration $= 5$.

Table 2.

Iteration no.	1	2	3	4	5
Ft. rel. error	0.1292×10^{-1}	0.3074×10^{-2}	0.4134×10^{-2}	0.3455×10^{-2}	0.3614×10^{-2}
Iter. rel. error	0.1000×10^{1}	0.2947×10^{-1}	0.3075×10^{-2}	0.4258×10^{-3}	0.7331×10^{-4}

for any integer m. This formula is obtained by solving the Helmholtz equation both inside and outside of B_b. The coefficients are found from the compatibility (continuity) conditions for the solution u and its normal derivative at $r = b$. A similar method can be applied to the case when $\varepsilon(r)$ is a step function. Finally, an arbitrary function $\varepsilon(r) \in L^2$ can be approximated by a step function. Then we solve the forward problem for that step function. In this way we simulated data $g(\phi, \nu)$, and conducted the following numerical experiments:

Experiment 1. The original function $\varepsilon(x)$ is

$$\varepsilon(x) = \begin{cases} 0.02 & \text{if } |x| \le \frac{a}{2} \\ 0 & \text{otherwise} \end{cases}$$

where $a = \frac{\pi}{2}$. The wave number $k = 5.3$. Please refer to the **Figure 1**. In the figure, the graph **(a)** shows the recovered function. The graph **(b)** is the original function $\varepsilon(x)$. Graph **(c)** is a vertical cross-section version of those two functions. In **(c)**, the solid graph is the original function $\varepsilon(x)$ while the dotted graph is the recovered function. Here p and p' are numbers of points used in the quadrature formula for integrals on the domain B_a and B_{2k} respectively. **Table 1** shows the errors obtained during the iterations.

Explanations for Table 1: Ft. rel. error is computed as

$$\text{Ft. rel. error} = \sqrt{\frac{\sum_{i=1}^{p'} |\widehat{\varepsilon}(\xi_i) - \widehat{\varepsilon}^n(\xi_i)|^2}{\sum_{i=1}^{p'} |\widehat{\varepsilon}(\xi_i)|^2}}$$

and Iter. rel. error is computed as

$$\text{Iter. rel. error} = \sqrt{\frac{\sum_{i=1}^{p} |\varepsilon^n(\xi_i) - \varepsilon^{n-1}(\xi_i)|^2}{\sum_{i=1}^{p} |\varepsilon^n(\xi_i)|^2}}.$$

The function $\widehat{\varepsilon}(\xi)$ is the Partial Fourier Transform of the original function $\varepsilon(x)$ on the domain B_{2k}. The function $\widehat{\varepsilon}^n(\xi)$ is defined by (3.6), which can be viewed as the Partial Fourier Transform of the function $\varepsilon^n(x)$ on the domain B_{2k} and the function $\varepsilon^n(x)$ is the recovered function at the nth iteration. One can see that the algorithm converges very fast in the weak scattering case.

Experiment 2. The original function $\varepsilon(x)$ is

$$\varepsilon(x) = \begin{cases} 0 & \text{if } |x| \le \frac{a}{4} \\ 0.04 & \text{if } \frac{a}{4} < |x| \le \frac{3a}{4} \\ 0 & \text{otherwise} \end{cases}$$

where $a = \frac{\pi}{2}$. The wave number $k = 5.3$. Please refer to **Figure 2** for the results. **Table 2** shows the errors obtained during the iterations.

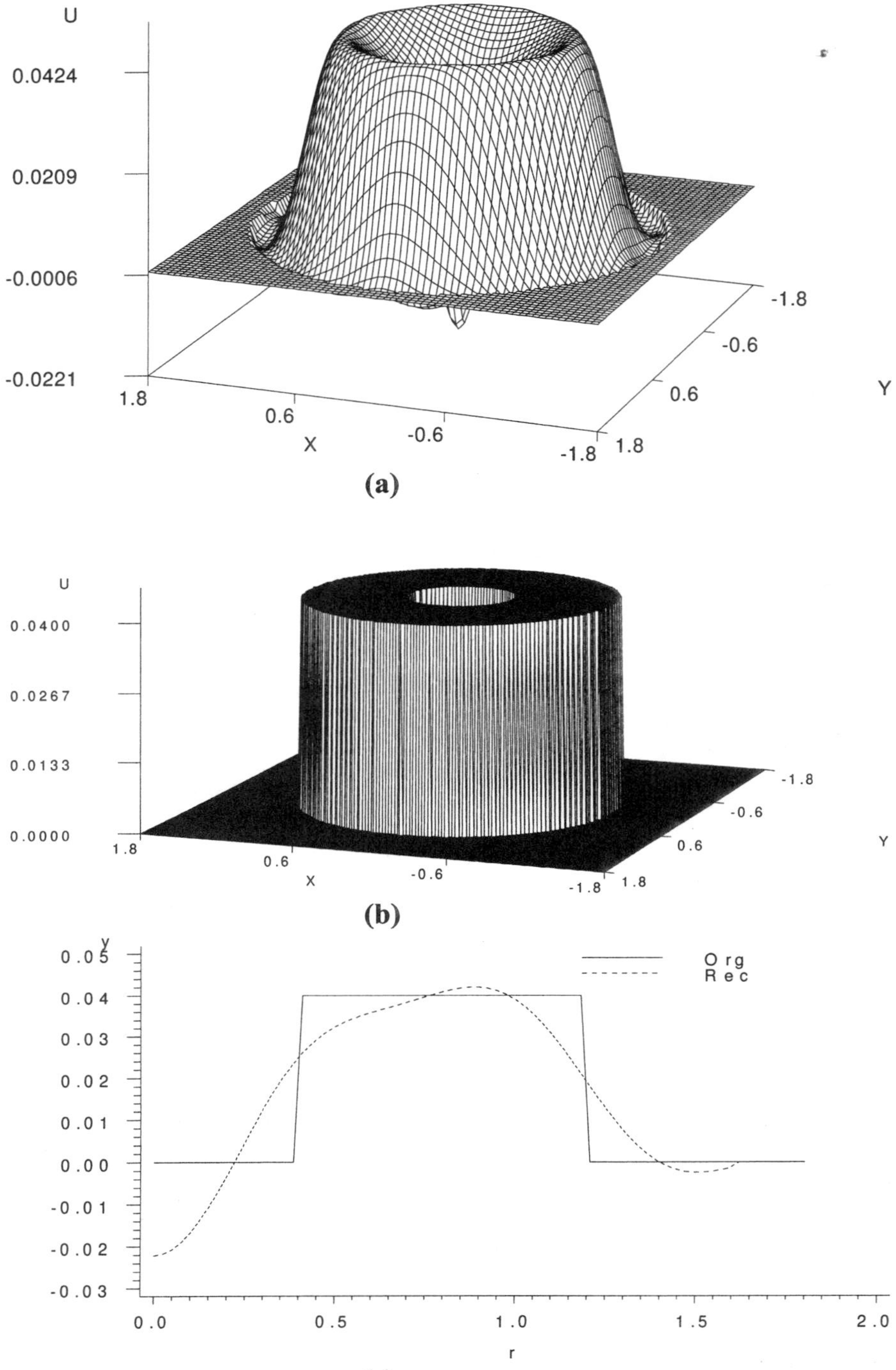

Figure 2. **(a)** Recovered; **(b)** original; **(c)** cross section. $k = 5.300000$, $a = 1.600000$, Fourier transform relative error $= 0.1484 \times 10^{02}$, $p = 553$, $p' = 1373$, no. of iteration $= 5$.

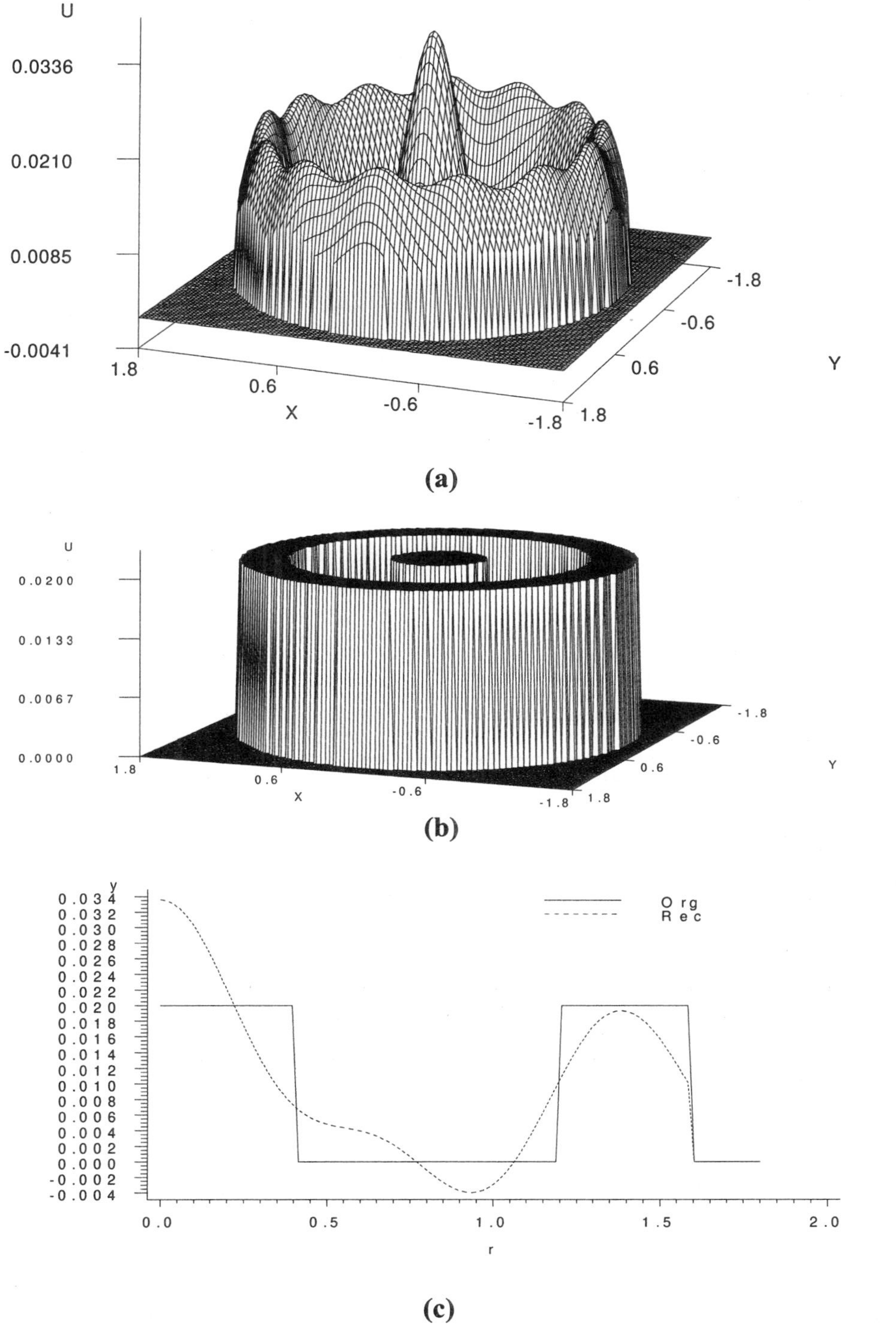

Figure 3. **(a)** Recovered; **(b)** original function; **(c)** cross section. $k = 5.300000$, $a = 1.600000$, relative error $= 0.958510^{02}$, $p = 357$, $p' = 1373$, no. of iteration $= 4$.

Table 3.

Iteration no.	1	2	3	4
Ft. rel. error	0.8609×10^{-1}	0.1041×10^{-1}	0.9992×10^{-2}	0.9585×10^{-2}
Iter. rel. error	0.1000×10^{1}	0.2300×10^{-1}	0.1773×10^{-2}	0.1340×10^{-3}

Experiment 3. The original function $\varepsilon(x)$ is

$$\varepsilon(x) = \begin{cases} 0.02 & \text{if } |x| \le \frac{a}{4} \\ 0 & \text{if } \frac{a}{4} < |x| \le \frac{3a}{4} \\ 0.02 & \text{if } \frac{3a}{4} < |x| \le a \\ 0 & \text{otherwise} \end{cases}$$

where $a = \frac{\pi}{2}$. The wave number $k = 5.3$. Please refer to **Figure 3** for the results. **Table 3** shows the errors obtained during the iterations.

ACKNOWLEDGMENT

The author would like to thank Dr. B. Zhou for his help during the work on this project.

REFERENCES

1. David Colton, Rainer Kress, *Inverse Acoustic and Electromagnetic Scattering Theory*, Springer-Verlag, New York, (1992).
2. A Ramm, "Recovery of the potential from fixed-energy scattering data," *Inverse Problems*, **4**, 877–886 (1988).
3. B. Crosignani and P di Porto, "Coupled-mode theory approach to depolarization associated with propagation in turbulent medium," *Scattering and Propagation in Random Media. AGARD-CP-419, meeting held in Rome, Italy, May 1987,*, (1988).
4. A. Ishimaru, *Wave Propagation and Scattering in Random Media, Vol. 1*, Academic Press, New York, (1978).
5. M. Cheney, "A review of multi-dimensional inverse potential scattering," *Inverse Problems in Partial Differential Equations, SIAM. (Edited by D. Colton, R. Ewing and W. Rundell*, (1990).
6. D. Colton and P. Monk, "The inverse scattering problem for acoustic waves in an inhomogeneous medium," *Inverse Problems in Partial Differential Equations, SIAM. (Edited by D. Colton, R. Ewing and W. Rundell*, (1990).
7. S. Gutman and M. Klibanov, "Regularized Quasi-Newton Method for Inverse Scattering Problems," *Mathl. Comput. Modelling*, **18, No. 1**, 5–31 (1993).
8. A. G. Ramm, *Multidimensional Inverse Scattering Problems*, Longman Scientific and Wiley, New York, (1992).
9. A. G. Ramm, "Finding potential from fixed-energy scattering data via D–N map," *J. Inv and Ill-Posed Prob*, **4, No. 2**, 145–152 (1996).

5

LOCAL TOMOGRAPHY WITH NONSMOOTH ATTENUATION II

Alexander Katsevich*

Department of Mathematics
University of Central Florida
Orlando, FL
E-mail: katsev@pegasus.cc.ucf.edu

ABSTRACT

We continue investigation of local tomography with nonsmooth attenuation, which was proposed earlier by the author. Our main result is a new and simple characterization of the wave front of the local tomography function $\tilde{f}_\Lambda^{(\Phi)}$, which holds under fairly general conditions on the density function f and the attenuation coefficient μ.

1. INTRODUCTION

The theory of Single Photon Emission Computed Tomography (SPECT), which is widely used in nuclear medicine, is based on the attenuated Radon transform:

$$\hat{f}^{(\Phi)}(\theta,p) = \int_{-\infty}^{\infty} f(p\Theta + t\Theta^\perp)\exp\left(-\int_t^\infty \mu(p\Theta + s\Theta^\perp)ds\right)dt,$$
$$\Theta = (\cos\theta, \sin\theta),\ \Theta^\perp = (-\sin\theta, \cos\theta). \tag{1.1}$$

Here $f(x)$ is the density of some radioactive isotope inside a patient, and the coefficient $\mu(x)$ characterizes attenuating properties of tissues. The coefficient $\mu(x)$ is assumed to be known, and f is to be determined from the data $\hat{f}^{(\Phi)}(\theta,p), \theta \in [0,2\pi), p \in \mathbb{R}$. If $\mu = 0$, the problem of inverting transform (1.1) is equivalent to inverting the classical Radon transform and can be easily solved. In most cases, however, the attenuating properties of the medium cannot be neglected [2, p. 17]. Moreover, no inversion formula for transform (1.1) is known in the case when μ is a function of x. The difficulty can be avoided if one confines himself to reconstructing singularities of f. This can be done by reconstructing not f, but $\mathcal{B}f$, where $\mathcal{B}$ is an elliptic

*This research was supported by NSF grant DMS-9704285

Inverse Problems, Tomography, and Image Processing, edited by Ramm,
Plenum Press, New York, 1998

pseudodifferential operator (PDO). Since PDO's are pseudolocal, all information about the singularities of f is contained in $\mathcal{B}f$. Moreover, if $\mathcal{B}$ is appropriately chosen, calculation of $\mathcal{B}f$ is local: to compute $\mathcal{B}f$ at a point x one uses the tomographic data $\hat{f}^{(\Phi)}(\theta,p)$ for $\theta \in [0,2\pi)$ and $|p-\Theta\cdot x| < \epsilon$, where $\epsilon > 0$ can be taken arbitrarily small. If the order of $\mathcal{B}$ is positive (in practice, the order of $\mathcal{B}$ equals one), the singularities of f are better visible in $\mathcal{B}f$. As an example, consider the following function:

$$\tilde{f}_\Lambda^{(\Phi)}(x) := -\frac{1}{4\pi}\int_0^{2\pi} \frac{\partial^2}{\partial p^2}\hat{f}^{(\Phi)}(\theta,p)\bigg|_{p=\Theta\cdot x} d\theta. \tag{1.2}$$

One can show that $\tilde{f}_\Lambda^{(\Phi)} = \mathcal{B}f$, where $\mathcal{B}$ is a classical elliptic PDO of order one [8], [7]. More precisely, one has

$$\tilde{f}_\Lambda^{(\Phi)}(x) = \frac{1}{(2\pi)^2}\int_0^\infty \int_0^{2\pi} \int_{\mathbb{R}^2} b(y,\theta)f(y)e^{-i\sigma\Theta\cdot(x-y)}dyd\theta\sigma^2 d\sigma, \tag{1.3}$$

where

$$b(y,\theta) = \frac{1}{2}\left[\exp\left\{-\int_0^\infty \mu(y+t\Theta^\perp)dt\right\} + \exp\left\{-\int_0^\infty \mu(y-t\Theta^\perp)dt\right\}\right]. \tag{1.4}$$

Here and throughout the paper the variables $\theta \in [0,2\pi)$ and $\Theta, \Theta^\perp \in S^1$ are related as follows: $\Theta = (\cos\theta, \sin\theta), \Theta^\perp = (-\sin\theta, \cos\theta)$. S^1 denotes the unit sphere in $\mathbb{R}^2$. As is seen from equation (1.2), calculation of $\tilde{f}_\Lambda^{(\Phi)}$ is purely local. The function $\tilde{f}_\Lambda^{(\Phi)}$ was introduced for the generalized Radon transform with C^∞ weight in [8].

A group of methods based on computing $\mathcal{B}f$ is known as Local Tomography (see [9], [3], and references therein). Usually one assumes that the coefficient μ is C^∞ (see, e.g., [8]), because in this case $\mathcal{B}$ is a bona fide elliptic PDO. However, if $\mu \notin C^\infty$, the resulting PDO's have nonsmooth amplitudes. The nonsmoothness of the amplitude has undesirable consequences. In particular, such operators no longer enjoy the pseudolocal property. The first investigation of local tomography with nonsmooth attenuation was undertaken in [6]. It was shown that the singular support of the local tomography function $\tilde{f}_\Lambda^{(\Phi)}$ consists of two parts: 'genuine' singularities – $\text{singsupp} f \cup \text{singsupp}\,\mu$, and 'extra' singularities, that cause artifacts in the tomographic reconstruction. Behavior of $\tilde{f}_\Lambda^{(\Phi)}$ near 'genuine' singularities was obtained and it was shown how to extract values of jumps of f knowing $\tilde{f}_\Lambda^{(\Phi)}$. In [5] the behavior of $\tilde{f}_\Lambda^{(\Phi)}$ near the 'extra' singularities was obtained. It was shown that in most cases the latter are smoother then the genuine singularities. Therefore, they do not cause considerable artifacts in the reconstructions based on $\tilde{f}_\Lambda^{(\Phi)}$. These theoretical results together with numerical experiments presented in [6] demonstrate that the ideas of local tomography can be successfully used even in the case of nonsmooth attenuation.

In the present paper we continue investigation of local tomography with nonsmooth attenuation. Our main result is a new and simple characterization of the wave front of $\tilde{f}_\Lambda^{(\Phi)}$, which holds under fairly general conditions on f and μ (only $\text{singsupp}\tilde{f}_\Lambda^{(\Phi)}$ was found in [6]). These conditions are more general than those considered in [6]. Also, the proof given here is simpler than the one in [6].

In Section 2 the main theorem is stated and proved. Some auxiliary lemmas are proved in Section 3.

2. THE MAIN RESULT

Suppose that f and μ can be represented in the form

$$f(x) = \sum_k f_k(x)\chi_{f,k}(x), \ \mu(x) = \sum_k \mu_k(x)\chi_{\mu,k}(x), \tag{2.1}$$

where the sums are finite, $f_k, \mu_k \in C^\infty(\mathbb{R}^2)$, and $\chi_{f,k}, \chi_{\mu,k}$ are the characteristic functions of the bounded open sets $D_{f,k}, D_{\mu,k}$, respectively. Denote

$$S := \bigcup_k \partial D_{f,k}, \ \Gamma := \bigcup_k \partial D_{\mu,k}. \tag{2.2}$$

Let us introduce the following conventions which will be used throughout the paper. Let $\mathcal{C}$ be a curve. We say that $\mathcal{C}$ is smooth at $x^{(0)} \in \mathcal{C}$ if there is an open set $U, x^{(0)} \in U \subset \mathbb{R}^2$, such that $\mathcal{C} \cap U$ is diffeomorphic to an open interval. A curve segment is smooth if it is diffeomorphic to an interval. The line $\Theta \cdot x = p$ is tangent to $\mathcal{C}$ at $x^{(0)} \in \mathcal{C}$ if it contains $x^{(0)}$ and either $\mathcal{C}$ is not smooth at $x^{(0)}$ or the vector Θ is conormal to $\mathcal{C}$ at $x^{(0)}$. The dual curve $\hat{\mathcal{C}} \in S^1 \times \mathbb{R}$ is defined as the set of all $(\Theta,p), \Theta \in S^1, p \in \mathbb{R}$, such that the line $\Theta \cdot x = p$ is tangent to $\mathcal{C}$. Here S^1 is the unit sphere in $\mathbb{R}^2$. Thus, if $\mathcal{C}$ is not smooth at $x^{(0)}$, then $(\Theta, \Theta \cdot x^{(0)}) \in \hat{\mathcal{C}}, \forall \Theta \in S^1$. Clearly, $\hat{\Gamma}, \hat{S} \subset \widehat{S \cup \Gamma}$. Our definition of the dual curve is very close to the generalized Legendre transform introduced in [11], [10]. We say that the line L is transversal to $\mathcal{C}$ if either $L \cap \mathcal{C} = \varnothing$ or $\mathcal{C}$ is smooth at $L \cap \mathcal{C}$ and $N_x^* L \cap N_x^* \mathcal{C} = \{0\}, \forall x \in L \cap \mathcal{C}$. Here $N_x^* L$ and $N_x^* \mathcal{C}$ denote the spaces conormal to L at x and to $\mathcal{C}$ at x, respectively. For convenience of notation, we consider wave fronts of distributions as subsets of $\mathbb{R}^2 \times S^1$.

Theorem 2.1. *Let f and μ be as above. Suppose that for any $x^{(0)} \in \Gamma$ there exists a neighborhood $U \ni x^{(0)}$ such that*

A1. *$S \cap U = \Gamma \cap U$ if $x^{(0)} \in S$, and*

A2. *Either Γ is smooth at $x^{(0)}$ or $\Gamma \cap U$ is a union of two C^∞ curve segments which share common endpoint $x^{(0)}$ and otherwise do not intersect. In the latter case the limiting tangents to Γ at $x^{(0)}$ are supposed to be different, that is the case of cusp on Γ is excluded.*

Define the set

$$\Upsilon := \{(\Theta,p) \in \hat{\Gamma} : \widehat{S \cup \Gamma} \text{ is not smooth at } (\Theta,p)\}. \tag{2.3}$$

Then one has:

$$WF(\tilde{f}_\Lambda^{(\Phi)}) \subset WF(f) \cup WF(\mu) \cup E(f,\mu), \tag{2.4}$$

where

$$E(f,\mu) := \{(x,\Theta) \in \mathbb{R}^2 \times S^1 : (\Theta, \Theta \cdot x) \in \Upsilon\}. \tag{2.5}$$

Proof: Fix a point $(\Theta_0, p_0) \notin \Upsilon$. According to the definition of the set Υ, either $(\Theta_0, p_0) \notin \hat{\Gamma}$ or $(\Theta_0, p_0) \in \hat{\Gamma}$ and $\widehat{S \cup \Gamma}$ is a smooth curve at (Θ_0, p_0).

Case I: $(\Theta_0, p_0) \notin \hat{\Gamma}$. Let $V := \Omega \times P$ be a sufficiently small rectangular neighborhood of (Θ_0, p_0) so that $V \cap \hat{\Gamma} = \varnothing$ (this is possible, because our assumptions imply that $\hat{\Gamma}$ is compact and, therefore, $\text{dist}((\Theta_0, p_0), \hat{\Gamma}) > 0$). Thus, all the lines $\Theta \cdot x = p, (\Theta, p) \in V$, intersect Γ transversally. Here Ω is open, $\Theta_0 \in \Omega \subset S^1$, and $P, p_0 \in P \subset \mathbb{R}$, is an open interval. Using (1.3), define the function

$$g_\chi(x) = \int_0^\infty \int_\Omega \int_{\mathbb{R}^2} \chi(\Theta, \Theta \cdot y) b(y, \theta) f(y) e^{-i\sigma\Theta\cdot(x-y)} dy d\theta \sigma^2 d\sigma, \quad \chi(\Theta, p) \in C_0^\infty(V). \tag{2.6}$$

Consider now the subset of S the dual of which is $\hat{S} \cap V$ (provided that $\hat{S} \cap V \neq \varnothing$), that is:

$$S_V := \{x \in S: \text{the line } \Theta \cdot y = p \text{ is tangent to } S \text{ for some } (\Theta, p) \in V\}. \tag{2.7}$$

By assumption A1 in Theorem 2.1, if $S_V \cap \Gamma \neq \varnothing$, then there exists a neighborhood U of $S_V \cap \Gamma$ such that Γ and S coincide inside U. This implies that $V \cap \hat{\Gamma} \neq \varnothing$. Since this contradicts the assumption $V \cap \hat{\Gamma} = \varnothing$, we have $S_V \cap \Gamma = \varnothing$. If $\overline{S_V} \cap \Gamma \neq \varnothing$, where the overbar denotes closure, take $x \in \overline{S_V} \setminus S_V$ such that $x \in \Gamma$. $S_V \subset S$, hence $x \in S \cap \Gamma$. By assumption A1, there exists an open $U \ni x$ such that S and Γ coincide in U. By construction, $S_V \cap U \neq \varnothing$, therefore $S_V \cap \Gamma \neq \varnothing$. This contradiction implies that $\overline{S_V} \cap \Gamma = \varnothing$. Since $\overline{S_V}$ and Γ are compact, there exists a function $w_1 \in C_0^\infty$ which equals 1 in a neighborhood of Γ and equals 0 in a neighborhood of S_V. Since $\text{supp}\,\chi \subset V$ and $\hat{\Gamma} \cap V = \varnothing$, any line $\Theta \cdot x = p$ for which $\chi(\Theta, p) \neq 0$ is transversal to Γ. Lemma 3.2 in Section 3 asserts that in this case

$$\int_0^\infty \int_\Omega \int_{\mathbb{R}^2} \chi(\Theta, \Theta \cdot y) b(y, \theta)(w_1(y) f(y)) e^{-i\sigma\Theta\cdot(x-y)} dy d\theta \sigma^2 d\sigma \in C^\infty(\mathbb{R}^2). \tag{2.8}$$

The function $\chi(\Theta, \Theta \cdot y) b(y, \theta)(1 - w_1(y))$ defines a conventional amplitude. Since PDO's are pseudolocal, we have

$$WF\left(\int_0^\infty \int_\Omega \int_{\mathbb{R}^2} \chi(\Theta, \Theta \cdot y) b(y, \theta)(1 - w_1(y)) f(y) e^{-i\sigma\Theta\cdot(x-y)} dy d\theta \sigma^2 d\sigma\right) \subset WF(f). \tag{2.9}$$

Combining (2.8) and (2.9) gives

$$WF(g_\chi) \subset WF(f). \tag{2.10}$$

If $\hat{S} \cap V = \varnothing$, we can take $w_1 \equiv 1$ in (2.8). By Lemma 3.2, $g_\chi \in C^\infty$; therefore, $WF(g_\chi) = \varnothing$, and (2.10) is trivially satisfied.

Case II: $(\Theta_0, p_0) \in \hat{\Gamma}$, *$\widehat{S \cup \Gamma}$ is smooth near (Θ_0, p_0), and $(\Theta_0, p_0) \notin \hat{S}$.* Using the notation of Case I and the results of Lemma 3.1 ($\hat{\Gamma} \subset \Pi := \widehat{S \cup \Gamma}$, so Lemma 3.1 applies), we conclude that there exists a sufficiently small rectangle V such that $(\Theta_0, p_0) \in V = \Omega \times P$, and $\hat{\Gamma} \cap V$ is a smooth curve segment. Take now any $(\Theta', p') \in \hat{\Gamma} \cap V$. If $(\Theta', p') \in \hat{S} \cap V$, then Lemma 3.1 applies because $\hat{S} \subset \Pi := \widehat{S \cup \Gamma}$. Lemma 3.1 yields that $\hat{S}$ is smooth and $\hat{S} = \hat{\Gamma}$ near (Θ', p'). Using that $\hat{S}$ is compact, moving from (Θ', p') towards (Θ_0, p_0) along $\hat{\Gamma}$, and applying Lemma 3.1 repeatedly, we conclude that $\hat{S} = \hat{\Gamma}$ near (Θ_0, p_0). This contradiction proves that

$V \cap \hat{S} = \varnothing$, that is all the lines $\Theta \cdot x = p, (\Theta,p) \in V$, are transversal to S. Let $x^{(0)} \in \Gamma$ be a point where the line $\Theta_0 \cdot x = p_0$ is tangent to Γ. Obviously, $x^{(0)} \notin S$, because otherwise S and Γ would coincide near $x^{(0)}$, which would lead to a false statement $(\Theta_0, p_0) \in \hat{S}$.

Combining Lemma 3.1 of Section 3 and assumption A2, we see that the point $x^{(0)}$ is determined uniquely and it suffices to consider only two cases:

IIa. Γ_V is smooth and has nonvanishing curvature, and

IIb. Γ_V has a corner at $x^{(0)}$ and the limiting normals to Γ_V at $x^{(0)}$ are outside of Ω.

Here $\Gamma_V \subset \Gamma$ is the set the dual of which coincides with $\hat{\Gamma} \cap V$ (cf. (2.7)). Let χ and g_χ be the same as before.

Case IIa: *Γ_V is smooth and has nonvanishing curvature.* Using the assumptions about μ, denote

$$\mu_{ns}(x) := \sum_{k: x^{(0)} \in \partial D_{\mu,k}} \mu_k(x) \chi_{\mu,k}(x), \quad \mu_{sm} := \mu - \mu_{ns}. \tag{2.11}$$

Clearly, $\mu = \mu_{sm} + \mu_{ns}$, and the function μ_{sm} has the property

$$\text{the lines } \Theta \cdot x = p, (\Theta,p) \in V, \text{ intersect discontinuities of } \mu_{sm} \text{ transversally.} \tag{2.12}$$

By Lemma 3.1, the equation of Γ_V is given by $p = p_0(\theta)$ for some $p_0(\theta) \in C^\infty(\Omega)$. Let $x^{(0)}(\theta)$ denote the point where the line $\Theta \cdot x = p_0(\theta), \Theta \in \Omega$, is tangent to Γ_V. Fix any $(\Theta,p) \in V$ such that the line $\Theta \cdot x = p$ intersects Γ_V. Let $t = a(\theta,p)$ and $t = b(\theta,p)$ be the points of intersection of the line $\{p\Theta + t\Theta^\perp, t \in \mathbb{R}\}$ and Γ_V in a neighborhood of $x^{(0)}(\theta)$ (that is, $a(\theta,p), b(\theta,p) \to x^{(0)}(\theta) \cdot \Theta^\perp$ as $p \to p_0(\theta)$). Since Γ_V has nonvanishing curvature, there are precisely two such points provided that p is sufficiently close to $p_0(\theta)$. Put $y = p\Theta + t\Theta^\perp$ in (2.6) and rewrite the integral with respect to y in (2.6) as follows:

$$I(\sigma, \Theta) = \int_{-\infty}^{\infty} \chi(\Theta,p) G(\theta,p) e^{i\sigma p} dp, \tag{2.13}$$

where

$$G(\theta,p) = \int_{-\infty}^{\infty} b(p\Theta + t\Theta^\perp, \theta) f(p\Theta + t\Theta^\perp) dt. \tag{2.14}$$

By construction, any line $\Theta \cdot x = p, (\Theta,p) \in V = \Omega \times P, p \neq p_0(\theta)$, is transversal to Γ. This implies that $G(\theta, \cdot) \in C^\infty(P \setminus p_0(\theta))$. Let us investigate the singularity of $G(\theta,p)$ as $p \to p_0(\theta)$. By modifying, if necessary, the functions μ_{sm} and μ_{ns} in such a way that $\mu = \mu_{sm} + \mu_{ns}$ and property (2.12) holds, we can assume without loss of generality that μ_{ns} vanishes on the exterior side of Γ_V:

1. $\mu_{ns} \equiv 0$ on any line $\Theta \cdot x = p, (\Theta,p) \in V$, that does not intersect Γ_V, and

2. $\mu_{ns}(p\Theta + t\Theta^\perp) \equiv 0, t \notin [a(\theta,p), b(\theta,p)]$, if $(\Theta,p) \in V$ and the line $p\Theta + t\Theta^\perp, t \in \mathbb{R}$, intersects Γ_V.

Indeed, if $\mu_{ns} \neq 0$ on the exterior side of Γ_V in a neighborhood of $x^{(0)}$, take any $\mu'(x) \in C_0^\infty(\mathbb{R}^2)$ which coincides with μ_{ns} on the exterior side of Γ_V, and represent μ as follows: $\mu = (\mu_{sm} + \mu') + (\mu_{ns} - \mu')$. Using an appropriate partition of unity one deals with the case when μ_{ns} does not vanish away from Γ_V. Since $x^{(0)} \notin S$, there exists an open $U \ni x^{(0)}$ such that $S \cap U = \varnothing$. Therefore, we may assume without loss of generality that the rectangle V is sufficiently small, i.e.

3. Any line segment $p\Theta + t\Theta^\perp, t \in [a(\theta,p), b(\theta,p)]$, does not intersect S provided that $(\Theta,p) \in V$.

Substituting (1.4) into (2.14) and using properties 1, 2, and 3 above, we find for p sufficiently close to $p_0(\theta)$:

$$\begin{aligned}
2G(\theta,p) = &\int_{-\infty}^{a} \exp\left\{-\int_a^b \mu_{ns} ds\right\} f_+(y)dt + \int_{-\infty}^{a} f_-(y)dt \\
&+ \int_a^b \exp\left\{-\int_t^b \mu_{ns} ds\right\} f_+(y)dt + \int_a^b \exp\left\{-\int_a^t \mu_{ns} ds\right\} f_-(y)dt \\
&+ \int_b^\infty f_+(y)dt + \int_b^\infty \exp\left\{-\int_a^b \mu_{ns} ds\right\} f_-(y)dt, \\
y = y(t) = &\, p\Theta + t\Theta^\perp,
\end{aligned} \tag{2.15}$$

where we have dropped the arguments of a and b, used the convention $\int \mu ds = \int \mu(p\Theta + s\Theta^\perp)ds$, and denoted

$$f_+(y) := \exp\left(-\int_t^\infty \mu_{sm} ds\right) f(y);\ f_-(y) := \exp\left(-\int_{-\infty}^t \mu_{sm} ds\right) f(y). \tag{2.16}$$

In (2.15) it is assumed that if Θ and p are such that the line $\Theta \cdot x = p$ does not intersect the support of μ_{ns}, then the integral of μ_{ns} along the line equals zero and the right side of (2.15) becomes just $\int_{-\infty}^{\infty} f_+(y)dt + \int_{-\infty}^{\infty} f_-(y)dt$. This allows us not to worry about the fact that $a(\theta,p)$ and $b(\theta,p)$ are not defined for such θ and p. Proposition 2 in Section 8 of [7] and Theorem 4.5.1 in [9, p. 106] (see also [9, pp. 112–114]) imply that on the domain of the functions a and b the following equalities hold

$$\begin{aligned}
(a(\theta,p) + b(\theta,p))/2 &= \psi_1(\theta,p),\ \psi_1 \in C^\infty(V), \\
b(\theta,p) - a(\theta,p) &= \psi_2(\theta,p)(p - p_0(\theta))_\pm^{0.5},\ \psi_2 \in C^\infty(V),
\end{aligned} \tag{2.17}$$

where $(p - p_0(\theta))_\pm = \max(\pm(p - p_0(\theta)), 0)$. Let $x^{(0)}(\theta)$ be the point where the line $\Theta \cdot x = p$ is tangent to Γ. Then $+$ in the above formulas is chosen if Θ's, $\Theta \in \Omega$, are inward normals to Γ at $x^{(0)}(\theta)$, and $-$ is chosen otherwise. Using the same idea as in the proof of Lemma 3.2, one can show that the first equation in (2.17) implies that on the domain of the functions a and b the integrals

$$\int_{-\infty}^{(a+b)/2} f_+(y)dt,\ \int_{-\infty}^{(a+b)/2} f_-(y)dt,\ \int_{(a+b)/2}^{\infty} f_+(y)dt,\ \int_{(a+b)/2}^{\infty} f_-(y)dt \tag{2.18}$$

coincide with some $C^\infty(V)$ functions. Changing variables $v = t - (a+b)/2$ in (2.15), expanding $\mu_{ns}(x)$ in the Taylor series in a neighborhood of $x = x^{(0)}(\theta)$, using the series representation for the exponentials containing μ_{ns}, and taking into account (2.17), (2.18), we prove that $G(\theta,p)$ admits an expansion in smoothness of the type $G(\theta,p) \sim \sum_{k\ge 1} g_k(\theta)[(p-p_0(\theta))_\pm^{0.5}]^k, p \to p_0(\theta)$, where $g_k(\theta) \in C^\infty(\Omega)$. This is equivalent to the existence of two functions $\varphi_{1,2}$ such that

$$G(\theta,p) = \varphi_1(\theta,p)(p-p_0(\theta))_\pm^{0.5} + \varphi_2(\theta,p),\ \varphi_{1,2} \in C^\infty(V). \tag{2.19}$$

Substituting (2.19) into (2.13), changing variables $t = p - p_0(\theta)$, using that $p_0(\theta) \in C^\infty(\Omega)$ and $\chi(\Theta,p) \in C_0^\infty(V)$, and appealing to the Erdelyi lemma, we find

$$I(\sigma,\Theta) = \Psi_1(\sigma,\theta)e^{i\sigma p_0(\theta)},\ \Psi_1 \in C^\infty([0,\infty)\times\Omega),\ \Psi_1(\sigma,\cdot) \in C_0^\infty(\Omega), \tag{2.20}$$

$$\Psi_1(\sigma,\theta) \sim \sum_{k\ge 0} \frac{c_k(\theta)}{\sigma^{k+1.5}},\ \sigma \to \infty,\ c_k \in C_0^\infty(\Omega). \tag{2.21}$$

Clearly, the expansion in (2.21) can be differentiated with respect to θ. Substituting into (2.6), we get

$$g_\chi(x) = \int_0^\infty \int_\Omega \Psi_1(\sigma,\theta)e^{i\sigma(p_0(\theta)-\Theta\cdot x)}d\theta\sigma^2 d\sigma. \tag{2.22}$$

Using (2.20)–(2.22) and appealing to Lemma 3.3, we prove the desired assertion: $WF(g_\chi) \subset WF(\mu)$.

Case IIb: *Γ_V has a corner at $x^{(0)}$ and the limiting normals to Γ_V at $x^{(0)}$ are outside of Ω.* By assumption A2, Γ_V can be represented in the form $\Gamma_{2,-}\cup\Gamma_{2,+} = \Gamma_V$, where $\Gamma_{2,-}$ and $\Gamma_{2,+}$ are C^∞ curve segments which share common endpoint $x^{(0)}$ and otherwise do not intersect. Using (2.11), represent μ in the form $\mu = \mu_{sm} + \mu_{ns}$, where the function μ_{sm} has property (2.12). As in the preceding case, we can assume without loss of generality that μ_{ns} vanishes on the exterior side of Γ_V. Moreover, since the limiting normals to Γ_V at $x^{(0)}$ are outside Ω, we can assume also that either supp μ_{ns} lies on one side of any line in the family $\Theta\cdot(x-x^{(0)}) = 0, \Theta \in \Omega$, or $\Gamma_{2,-}$ and $\Gamma_{2,+}$ lie on opposite sides of any line in the family.

Suppose first that supp μ_{ns} lies on one side of any line in the family. The proof in this case follows the lines of Case IIa. Equations (2.13)–(2.16) remain unchanged (as before, we assume that the line segments $p\Theta + t\Theta^\perp, t \in [a(\theta,p), b(\theta,p)], (\Theta,p) \in V$, do not intersect S), and the analog of (2.17) becomes

$$\begin{aligned}(a(\theta,p)+b(\theta,p))/2 &= \psi_1(\theta,p),\ \psi_1 \in C^\infty(V),\\ b(\theta,p)-a(\theta,p) &= \psi_2(\theta,p)(p-p_0(\theta))_\pm,\ \psi_2 \in C^\infty(V).\end{aligned} \tag{2.23}$$

In the last equation, $+$ is chosen if the vectors $\Theta \in \Omega$ point inward at the vertex of the wedge formed by the limiting tangents to Γ at $x^{(0)}$, and $-$ is chosen otherwise. As usual, the latter equalities are assumed to hold only on the domain of the functions $a(\theta,p)$ and $b(\theta,p)$. Inclusions (2.18) still hold, and equation (2.19) is transformed as follows:

$$G(\theta,p) = \varphi_1(\theta,p)(p-p_0(\theta))_\pm + \varphi_2(\theta,p),\ \varphi_{1,2} \in C^\infty(V). \tag{2.24}$$

The Erdelyi lemma yields

$$I(\sigma,\Theta) = \Psi_1(\sigma,\theta)e^{i\sigma p_0(\theta)},\ \Psi_1 \in C^\infty([0,\infty)\times\Omega),\ \Psi_1(\sigma,\cdot) \in C_0^\infty(\Omega), \tag{2.25}$$

$$\Psi_1(\sigma,\theta) \sim \sum_{k\ge 0} \frac{c_k(\theta)}{\sigma^{k+2}},\ \sigma \to \infty,\ c_k \in C_0^\infty(\Omega), \tag{2.26}$$

and the desired assertion follows from Lemma 3.3: $WF(g_\chi) \subset WF(\mu)$.

Suppose now that $\Gamma_{2,-}$ and $\Gamma_{2,+}$ lie on opposite sides of any line in the family $\Theta \cdot (x - x^{(0)}) = 0, \Theta \in \Omega$. To fix the notation, let $\Gamma_{2,-}$ and $\Gamma_{2,+}$ be the segments that belong to the half-planes $\Theta \cdot x \leq p_0(\theta), \forall \Theta \in \Omega$, and $\Theta \cdot x \geq p_0(\theta), \forall \Theta \in \Omega$, respectively. Further, let $t = a(\theta,p)$ and $t = b(\theta,p)$ be the points of intersection of the line $x(t) = p\Theta + t\Theta^\perp, (\Theta,p) \in V$, with $\Gamma_{2,-}$ (when $p \leq p_0(\theta)$) and $\Gamma_{2,+}$ (when $p \geq p_0(\theta)$), respectively. Clearly,

$$\begin{aligned}
&2G(\theta,p) \\
&= \int_{-\infty}^{a} \exp\left\{-\int_{t}^{a} \mu_{ns} ds\right\} f_+(y)dt + \int_{-\infty}^{a} \exp\left\{-\int_{-\infty}^{t} \mu_{ns} ds\right\} f_-(y)dt \\
&+ \int_{a}^{\infty} f_+(y)dt + \int_{a}^{\infty} \exp\left\{-\int_{-\infty}^{a} \mu_{ns} ds\right\} f_-(y)dt, \; p \leq p_0(\theta), \\
&2G(\theta,p) \\
&= \int_{-\infty}^{b} \exp\left\{-\int_{t}^{b} \mu_{ns} ds\right\} f_+(y)dt + \int_{-\infty}^{b} \exp\left\{-\int_{-\infty}^{t} \mu_{ns} ds\right\} f_-(y)dt \\
&+ \int_{b}^{\infty} f_+(y)dt + \int_{b}^{\infty} \exp\left\{-\int_{-\infty}^{b} \mu_{ns} ds\right\} f_-(y)dt, \; p \geq p_0(\theta),
\end{aligned} \tag{2.27}$$

where we have assumed without loss of generality that $\mu_{ns}(p\Theta + t\Theta^\perp) \equiv 0$ if $t \geq a(\theta,p), p \leq p_0(\theta)$, or $t \geq b(\theta,p), p \geq p_0(\theta)$. Using (2.23), we conclude that $G(\theta,p)$ is C^∞ in V provided that $p \neq p_0(\theta)$, $G(\theta,p)$ is continuous at $p = p_0(\theta)$, and derivatives of $G(\theta,p)$ with respect to p have finite jumps across $p = p_0(\theta)$. Therefore, equations (2.25) and (2.26) still hold and the assertion $WF(g_\chi) \subset WF(\mu)$ follows from Lemma 3.3.

Case III: $(\Theta_0,p_0) \in \hat{\Gamma}$, $\widehat{S \cup \Gamma}$ *is smooth near* (Θ_0,p_0), *and* $(\Theta_0,p_0) \in \hat{S}$. Let $x^{(0)} \in \Gamma$ be the point where the line $\Theta_0 \cdot x = p_0$ is tangent to Γ. By Lemma 3.1, $\hat{S} = \hat{\Gamma}$ near (Θ_0,p_0) and $x^{(0)} \in S$. By assumption A1, $S = \Gamma$ near $x^{(0)}$. As usual, let V be a sufficiently small rectangle, $(\Theta_0,p_0) \in V = \Omega \times P$, such that $\hat{S} \cap V = \hat{\Gamma} \cap V$ is a smooth curve segment. Let $S_V \subset S$ and $\Gamma_V \subset \Gamma$ be such that their duals are $\hat{S} \cap V$ and $\hat{\Gamma} \cap V$, respectively (cf. (2.7)). Then, $S_V = \Gamma_V$ and, as in Case II, Lemma 3.1 implies that the point $x^{(0)}$ is unique and it suffices to consider only two cases:

IIIa. Γ_V is smooth and has nonvanishing curvature, and

IIIb. Γ_V has a corner at $x^{(0)}$ and the limiting normals to Γ_V at $x^{(0)}$ are outside of Ω.

Let χ and g_χ be the same as before.

Case IIIa: Γ_V *is smooth and has nonvanishing curvature.* Similarly to (2.11), we can represent μ and f in the form $\mu = \mu_{sm} + \mu_{ns}$ and $f = f_{sm} + f_{ns}$, where the functions μ_{sm}, μ_{ns} and f_{sm}, f_{ns} have the following properties.

1. The lines $\Theta \cdot x = p, (\Theta,p) \in V$, intersect the discontinuities of μ_{sm} and f_{sm} transversally; and
2. μ_{ns} and f_{ns} are identically zero on the exterior side of Γ_V (cf. properties 1 and 2 formulated below (2.14)).

As before, we may assume without loss of generality that the rectangle V is sufficiently small, i.e.

3. Any line segment $p\Theta + t\Theta^{\perp}, t \in [a(\theta,p), b(\theta,p)]$, does not intersect discontinuities of f_{sm} provided that $(\Theta,p) \in V$.

Using (2.6), define two functions:

$$g_{ns}(x) = \int_0^{\infty}\int_{\Omega}\int_{\mathbb{R}^2} \chi(\Theta,\Theta\cdot y)b(y,\theta)f_{ns}(y)w(y)e^{-i\sigma\Theta\cdot(x-y)}dyd\theta\sigma^2 d\sigma,$$
$$g_{sm}(x) = \int_0^{\infty}\int_{\Omega}\int_{\mathbb{R}^2} \chi(\Theta,\Theta\cdot y)b(y,\theta)f_{sm}(y)w(y)e^{-i\sigma\Theta\cdot(x-y)}dyd\theta\sigma^2 d\sigma. \qquad (2.28)$$

Clearly, $g_{\chi} = g_{sm} + g_{ns}$. Using the results of Case IIa, $WF(g_{sm}) \subset WF(\mu)$. To find the wave front of g_{ns}, we replace f by f_{ns} in equations (2.14) and (2.16). Since f_{ns} vanishes identically on the exterior side of S_V, the analog of (2.15) becomes

$$2G(\theta,p) = \int_a^b \exp\left\{-\int_t^b \mu_{ns}ds\right\}f_+(y)dt + \int_a^b \exp\left\{-\int_a^t \mu_{ns}ds\right\}f_-(y)dt. \qquad (2.29)$$

Using the argument that follows (2.18), we prove that G admits representation (2.19) with $\varphi_2 \equiv 0$, and the rest of the argument goes without changes. This yields the inclusion $WF(g_{ns}) \subset WF(\mu)$. Combining the functions g_{sm} and g_{ns}, we prove the assertion $WF(g_{\chi}) \subset WF(\mu)$.

Case IIIb: *Γ_V has a corner at $x^{(0)}$ and the limiting normals to Γ_V at $x^{(0)}$ are outside of Ω.* As in the preceding case, represent μ and f in the form $\mu = \mu_{sm} + \mu_{ns}$ and $f = f_{sm} + f_{ns}$, where the functions μ_{sm} and f_{sm} have properties 1 and 2 formulated above (2.28). Using the result of Case IIa, we have: $WF(g_{sm}) \subset WF(\mu)$. Let us now find $WF(g_{ns})$. Suppose first that $\operatorname{supp}\mu_{ns}$ lies on one side of any line in the family $\Theta\cdot(x - x^{(0)}) = 0, \Theta \in \Omega$ (in this case we also make assumption 3 stated above (2.28)). It is easy to see that equation (2.29) holds and G admits representation (2.24) with $\varphi_2 \equiv 0$. Therefore, $WF(g_{ns}) \subset WF(\mu)$. If $\Gamma_{2,-}$ and $\Gamma_{2,+}$ lie on opposite sides of any line in the family, then the analog of (2.27) becomes

$$\begin{aligned}2G(\theta,p) &= \int_{-\infty}^a \exp\left\{-\int_t^a \mu_{ns}ds\right\}f_+(y)dt \\ &+ \int_{-\infty}^a \exp\left\{-\int_{-\infty}^t \mu_{ns}ds\right\}f_-(y)dt,\ p \le p_0(\theta), \\ 2G(\theta,p) &= \int_{-\infty}^b \exp\left\{-\int_t^b \mu_{ns}ds\right\}f_+(y)dt \\ &+ \int_{-\infty}^b \exp\left\{-\int_{-\infty}^t \mu_{ns}ds\right\}f_-(y)dt,\ p \ge p_0(\theta),\end{aligned} \qquad (2.30)$$

where the functions f_+ and f_- are defined by (2.16) with f replaced by f_{ns}, and we have assumed without loss of generality that $f_{ns}(p\Theta + t\Theta^{\perp}) \equiv \mu_{ns}(p\Theta + t\Theta^{\perp}) \equiv 0$ if $t \ge a(\theta,p), p \le p_0(\theta)$, or $t \ge b(\theta,p), p \ge p_0(\theta)$, provided that $(\Theta,p) \in V$. Equations (2.25) and (2.26) still hold and we have $WF(g_{ns}) \subset WF(\mu)$. Combining g_{sm} and g_{ns}, we get $WF(g_{\chi}) \subset WF(\mu)$.

Case IV: $(\Theta_0,p_0) \in Y$. Let V be an open rectangle, $(\Theta_0,p_0) \in V = \Omega \times P$. Let χ and g_{χ} be the same as above. We will show that

$$WF(g_{\chi}) \subset E_V := \{(x,\Theta) \in \mathbb{R}^2 \times S^1 : (\Theta,\Theta\cdot x) \in \overline{V}\}. \qquad (2.31)$$

Here and in what follows the overbar denotes closure. Consider the integral with respect to σ in (2.6):

$$H(x,\theta,p) := \int_0^{\infty} \sigma^2 e^{-i\sigma(\Theta\cdot x - p)}d\sigma,\ p = \Theta\cdot y. \qquad (2.32)$$

Using equation (22) in [4, p. 360], we find

$$H(x,\theta,p) := 2i(\Theta\cdot x-p)^{-3} - \pi\delta''(\Theta\cdot x-p). \tag{2.33}$$

Clearly, $\text{singsupp} H = \{(x,\theta,p) : \Theta\cdot x = p\}$. Moreover, for a test function $\varphi\in C_0^\infty(\mathbb{R}^2)$ we get

$$\int_{\mathbb{R}^2} H(x,\theta,p)\varphi(x)e^{i\eta x}dx = \int_0^\infty \sigma^2 e^{i\sigma p}\tilde{\varphi}(\eta-\sigma\Theta)d\sigma. \tag{2.34}$$

If $\eta=\lambda\alpha, \alpha\in S^1, \alpha\neq\Theta$, then the right side of (2.34) is $o(\lambda^{-N}), \lambda\to\infty$, for any $N=1,2,\dots$. Pick a point $(x^{(0)},\alpha)\in\mathbb{R}^2\times S^1$ such that $(\alpha,\alpha\cdot x^{(0)})\notin\overline{V}$. By the preceding argument, if $\alpha\notin\overline{\Omega}$, then $(x^{(0)},\alpha)\notin WF(g_\chi)$. Suppose now that $\alpha\in\overline{\Omega}$. By the same token, we may assume without loss of generality that the set $\overline{\Omega}$ is as small as we like. Condition $(\alpha,\alpha\cdot x^{(0)})\notin\overline{V}$ implies that $\alpha\cdot x^{(0)}\notin\overline{P}$. Since $\overline{\Omega}\ni\alpha$ can be taken small, there exists a neighborhood U of $x^{(0)}$ such that $\Theta\cdot x\notin\overline{P}$ for any $x\in U$ and $\Theta\in\overline{\Omega}$. This means that $\chi(\Theta,\Theta\cdot y)=0$ whenever $\Theta\in\Omega, x\in U$, and $y\in\mathbb{R}^2$ are such that $\Theta\cdot(x-y)=0$. Using this fact and substituting (2.32) and (2.33) into (2.6), we see that $g_\chi\in C^\infty(U)$. The proof of (2.31) is complete.

End of the proof: Using the results of the four preceding cases we will finish the proof of the theorem. The set Υ defined in (2.3) is bounded and closed, hence it is compact. Pick a finite covering of Υ by open rectangles $\Upsilon\subset\cup_{j=1}^J V_j$, and let $\{V_1,\dots,V_M\}, M>J$, be a covering of $\widehat{S\cup\Gamma}$ (recall that $\Upsilon\subset\widehat{S\cup\Gamma}$). We may assume without loss of generality that the rectangles $V_j, j=J+1,\dots,M$, are sufficiently small: $\Upsilon\cap V_j=\varnothing$ and one of the first three cases occurs inside V_j – either $\hat\Gamma\cap V_j=\varnothing$, or $\hat\Gamma\cap V_j$ is smooth and $\hat S\cap V_j=\varnothing$, or $\hat\Gamma\cap V_j=\hat S\cap V_j$ is smooth. Let χ_j be a partition of unity over $\widehat{S\cup\Gamma}$, subordinate to the covering $\{V_1,\dots,V_M\}$. Denote $\chi_{M+1}=\eta-\sum_{j=1}^M\chi_j$, where $\eta\in C_0^\infty(S^1\times\mathbb{R})$ and $\eta(\Theta,p)=1$ if the line $\Theta\cdot x=p$ intersects $\text{supp} f$. Clearly, $(2\pi)^2\tilde f_\Lambda^{(\Phi)}=\sum_{j=1}^{M+1}g_{\chi_j}$. Using the result of Case IV,

$$WF(g_{\chi_j})\subset E_{V_j} := \{(x,\Theta)\in\mathbb{R}^2\times S^1 : (\Theta,\Theta\cdot x)\in\overline{V_j}\},\ 1\le j\le J.$$

Using the results of Cases I–III, $WF(g_{\chi_j})\subset WF(f)\cup WF(\mu), J+1\le j\le M$. By Lemma 3.2, $g_{\chi_{M+1}}\in C^\infty(\mathbb{R}^2)$. We showed that $WF(\tilde f_\Lambda^{(\Phi)})\subset WF(f)\cup WF(\mu)\cup\left(\cup_{j=1}^J E_{V_j}\right)$. Since $\Upsilon=\bigcap\left(\cup_j\overline{V_j}\right)$, where the intersection is taken over all finite open coverings that contain Υ (this property holds even if the coverings consist only of rectangles), we see that $E(f,\mu)=\bigcap\left(\cup_j E_{V_j}\right)$. The proof of the theorem is complete. □

3. AUXILIARY LEMMAS

Lemma 3.1. *Let $\mathcal{C}$ be a curve. Let $(\Theta_0,p_0)\in\hat{\mathcal{C}}$ be a point such that locally $\hat{\mathcal{C}}$ is a subset of a curve $\Pi\subset S^1\times\mathbb{R}$, which is smooth at $(\Theta_0,p_0)\in\Pi$. Let $x^{(0)}\in\mathcal{C}$ be a point where the line $\Theta_0\cdot x=p_0$ is tangent to $\mathcal{C}$. Then either $\mathcal{C}$ is smooth in a neighborhood of $x^{(0)}\in\mathcal{C}$ and has positive curvature, or $\mathcal{C}$ is a (possibly empty) union of smooth curve segments in a punctured neighborhood of $x^{(0)}$. The curve segments share common endpoint $x^{(0)}$, do not otherwise intersect, and the limiting normals to $\mathcal{C}$ at $x^{(0)}$ are outside of Ω. Moreover, in each case the point $x^{(0)}$ is unique, $\hat{\mathcal{C}}\cap V=\Pi\cap V$ for some open rectangle $V:=\Omega\times(p_0-\epsilon,p_0+\epsilon), \Omega\subset S^1$, and the equation of $\hat{\mathcal{C}}$ is given by $p=p(\theta)$ for some $p(\theta)\in C^\infty(\Omega)$.*

Proof: Suppose first that $\mathcal{C}$ is not smooth at $x^{(0)}$. From the definition, the local equation of $\hat{\mathcal{C}}$ is given by $p(\theta) = x^{(0)} \cdot \Theta$, and all the assertions of the lemma are immediate. Clearly, $p \in C^\infty$. Moreover, $\mathcal{C}$ is smooth in a punctured neighborhood of $x^{(0)}$, because otherwise we would be able to find a sequence of points $(\Theta_k, p_k) \in \hat{\mathcal{C}}$ such that $(\Theta_k, p_k) \to (\Theta_0, p_0), k \to \infty$, and $(\Theta_k, p_k) \notin \Pi$, which contradicts the assumption $\hat{\mathcal{C}} \subset \Pi$ near (Θ_0, p_0). In a similar fashion, if one of the limiting normals to $\mathcal{C}$ at $x^{(0)}$ would belong to Ω or there would exist another point $\tilde{x}^{(0)}$ such that $\tilde{x}^{(0)} \cdot \Theta_0 = p_0$, then $\hat{\mathcal{C}}$ would be self-intersecting at (Θ_0, p_0).

Suppose now that $\mathcal{C}$ is smooth near $x^{(0)}$. Let us show that $\hat{\mathcal{C}}$ and Π coincide in a neighborhood of (Θ_0, p_0). If $\mathcal{C}$ contains a straight line segment through $x^{(0)}$, then looking at the endpoints of the maximal line segment which is contained in $\mathcal{C}$ and passes through $x^{(0)}$, we conclude that $\hat{\mathcal{C}}$ is self-intersecting or has a corner at (Θ_0, p_0), which contradicts the assumption that $\hat{\mathcal{C}}$ is a subset of a C^∞ curve. Using the same argument and taking into account that the map $\mathcal{C} \to \hat{\mathcal{C}}$ is continuous, we conclude that there exists an open $U \ni x^{(0)}$ such that $\mathcal{C}$ does not coincide with a line segment on any interval inside U. Therefore, given any $x \in \mathcal{C} \cap U$, $\mathcal{C}$ always contains a segment with positive curvature which is located as close to x as we like. This implies that $\hat{\mathcal{C}}$ and Π coincide near (Θ_0, p_0). Indeed, let us trace the image of a point under the map $\mathcal{C} \to \hat{\mathcal{C}} \subset \Pi$ as the point traverses the curve segment $\mathcal{C} \cap U$ in one direction. Clearly, the image of the point cannot pause on an open subset of $\mathcal{C} \cap U$ (i.e., a segment of $\mathcal{C} \cap U$ cannot be mapped to a point in Π), because the segment contains a subsegment with positive curvature, which cannot be mapped into a point. Similarly, if the image of the point ever changes direction, we conclude that two different segments of $\mathcal{C} \cap U$ are mapped into the same segment of Π. Again, we easily establish a contradiction.

Our argument proves that there is an open rectangle $V := \Omega \times (p_0 - \epsilon, p_0 + \epsilon), \Omega \subset S^1$, such that $(\Theta_0, p_0) \in \hat{\mathcal{C}} \cap V = \Pi \cap V$. Therefore, $\hat{\mathcal{C}}$ is smooth at (Θ_0, p_0). Let $\mathcal{C}_V \subset \mathcal{C}$ be a segment of $\mathcal{C}$ such that its dual coincides with $\hat{\mathcal{C}} \cap V$ (cf. (2.7)). We will show that the curvature of $\mathcal{C}_V$ never vanishes. Even though the argument is sufficiently elementary, we present it here for the sake of completeness.

Introduce a coordinate system with the origin at $x^{(0)}$, the x_2-axis of which is along Θ_0. Let $x_2 = g(x_1)$ be the local equation of $\mathcal{C}$ in the new coordinate system. By assumption, g is C^∞ near $x_1 = 0$. Let us suppose that the local equation of $\mathcal{C}$ can be written in the form $p = p(\theta)$, where $p(\theta)$ is C^∞ near $\theta = \pi/2$. We have to show that $g''(0) \neq 0$. Suppose $g''(0) = 0$. Since $\mathcal{C}_V$ is the envelope of the family of lines $\Theta \cdot x = p, (\Theta, p) \in \hat{\mathcal{C}} \cap V$, we have in the new coordinate system:

$$x_1 \cos\theta + g(x_1)\sin\theta = p(\theta), \tag{3.1}$$

$$g'(x_1)\sin\theta + \cos\theta = 0. \tag{3.2}$$

Assuming $\theta = \theta(x_1)$ and differentiating (3.2) with respect to x_1 we get

$$\theta'(x_1) = \frac{g''(x_1)}{(g'(x_1))^2 + 1}. \tag{3.3}$$

By the implicit function theorem, $\theta(x_1)$ is C^∞ near $x_1 = 0$. Moreover, the assumption $g''(0) = 0$ together with (3.3) yields $\theta'(0) = 0$. Differentiating (3.1) with respect to x_1 and using (3.2), we find

$$\theta'(x_1)(g(x_1)\cos\theta - x_1 \sin\theta) = \theta'(x_1)p'(\theta). \tag{3.4}$$

By what was said above, $g''(x_1) \neq 0$ on open intervals as close to $x_1 = 0$ as we like. In view of (3.3), the same is true for $\theta'(x_1)$. By continuity, we get from (3.4):

$$g(x_1)\cos\theta - x_1 \sin\theta = p'(\theta),\ \theta = \theta(x_1), \tag{3.5}$$

for x_1 near 0. Differentiating the last equation with respect to x_1 and using (3.1), (3.2), we find:

$$-\sin\theta(1+(g')^2) = \theta'(x_1)(p''+p). \tag{3.6}$$

Taking the limit $x_1 \to 0$ (that is, $\theta \to \pi/2$), we see that the left side is bounded away from zero, while the right side goes to zero. This contradiction proves that $g''(0) \neq 0$. Clearly, the point $x^{(0)}$ is unique.

If $\mathcal{C}$ is smooth but cannot be written in the form $p = p(\theta)$ with $p(\theta) \in C^\infty$ near $\theta = \pi/2$, we conclude that the local equation of $\mathcal{C}$ is $\theta = \theta(p)$, where $\theta \in C^\infty$ near $p = 0$ and $\theta'(0) = 0$. As we have already seen (cf. (3.3)), θ is a C^∞ function of x_1. Therefore, rewriting (3.1) as follows

$$x_1 \cos\theta(x_1) + g(x_1)\sin\theta(x_1) = p, \tag{3.7}$$

we see that p is also a C^∞ function of x_1. Similarly to (3.4) we obtain

$$\theta'_p p'_{x_1}(g(x_1)\cos\theta - x_1\sin\theta) = p'_{x_1}, \tag{3.8}$$

where $\theta = \theta(p(x_1))$ and the subscripts indicate the variables with respect to which the corresponding derivatives are evaluated. Equations (3.7) and (3.8) imply that $p(0) = p'_{x_1}(0) = 0$. However, $p(x_1)$ cannot be identically zero near $x_1 = 0$. Indeed, if this is the case, writing (3.1) as $x_1\cos\theta(p(x_1)) + g(x_1)\sin\theta(p(x_1)) = p(x_1)$, we see that $g(x_1) \equiv 0$ near $x_1 = 0$, which leads to a contradiction with the smoothness assumption. Thus, $p'_{x_1} \not\equiv 0$, and as before, canceling $p(x_1)$ in (3.8) and taking $x_1 \to 0$ leads to a contradiction. This argument implies that $\theta'(p) \neq 0$ and the local equation of $\mathcal{C}$ can always be written in the form $p = p(\theta)$ with $p \in C^\infty$. □

Lemma 3.2. *Let f and μ be as in Theorem 2.1. Suppose an open rectangle $V = \Omega \times P$ is chosen so that any line $\Theta \cdot x = p, (\Theta,p) \in V$, is transversal to Γ and S. Let $\chi \in C_0^\infty(V)$. Then*

$$g(x) := \int_0^\infty \int_\Omega \int_{\mathbb{R}^2} \chi(\Theta, \Theta\cdot y) b(y,\theta) f(y) e^{-i\sigma\Theta\cdot(x-y)} dy d\theta \sigma^2 d\sigma \in C^\infty(\mathbb{R}^2). \tag{3.9}$$

Proof: Define the function

$$I(\sigma,\theta) := \int_{\mathbb{R}^2} \chi(\Theta, \Theta\cdot y) b(y,\theta) f(y) e^{i\sigma\Theta\cdot y} dy. \tag{3.10}$$

Clearly, it suffices to show that $I(\sigma,\theta) \in C^\infty([0,\infty)\times\Omega)$ and $I(\sigma,\theta) = o(\sigma^{-N})$, $\sigma \to \infty$, for all $N = 1,2,\ldots$. Writing $y = p\Theta + t\Theta^\perp$, we have

$$\begin{aligned} I(\sigma,\theta) &:= \int_{-\infty}^{\infty} \chi(\Theta,p) G(\theta,p) e^{i\sigma p} dp, \\ G(\theta,p) &= \int_{-\infty}^{\infty} b(p\Theta + t\Theta^\perp, \theta) f(p\Theta + t\Theta^\perp) dt. \end{aligned} \tag{3.11}$$

Let $t_1(\theta,p),\dots,t_J(\theta,p)$ be the points of intersection of the line $L_{\theta,p} := \{x = p\Theta + t\Theta^\perp, t \in \mathbb{R}\}$ and $\Gamma \cup S$ (if $L_{\theta,p} \cap (\Gamma \cup S) = \varnothing$, the assertion of the lemma is trivial). By assumption, $L_{\theta,p}$ is transversal to $\Gamma \cup S$. Therefore, the implicit function theorem yields that $t_j(\theta,p) \in C^\infty(V), j = 1,\dots,J$. In what follows we will always assume that $(\theta,p) \in V$. We have

$$G(\theta,p) = \left(\int_{-\infty}^{t_1(\theta,p)} + \sum_{j=1}^{J-1}\int_{t_j(\theta,p)}^{t_{j+1}(\theta,p)} + \int_{t_J(\theta,p)}^{\infty}\right) b(p\Theta + t\Theta^\perp, \theta) f(p\Theta + t\Theta^\perp)dt. \tag{3.12}$$

Consider, for example, the interval $[t_j, t_{j+1}]$. We have using the definition of $b(y,\theta)$ (cf. (1.4)):

$$\int_{t_j}^{t_{j+1}} b(p\Theta + t\Theta^\perp, \theta) f(p\Theta + t\Theta^\perp)dt = \int_{t_j}^{t_{j+1}} \frac{1}{2}\left\{\exp(-F_\mu(p\Theta + t\Theta^\perp, \Theta)) + \exp(-F_\mu(p\Theta + t\Theta^\perp, -\Theta))\right\} \times f(p\Theta + t\Theta^\perp)dt, \tag{3.13}$$

where $F_\mu(y,\Theta)$ is the fan beam transform of μ:

$$F_\mu(y,\Theta) = \int_0^\infty \mu(y + s\Theta^\perp)ds. \tag{3.14}$$

One has

$$F_\mu(p\Theta + t\Theta^\perp, \Theta) = \left(\int_t^{t_{j+1}} + \sum_{m=j+1}^{J-1}\int_{t_m}^{t_{m+1}} + \int_{t_J}^{\infty}\right)\mu(p\Theta + s\Theta^\perp)ds, \quad t_j \le t \le t_{j+1}. \tag{3.15}$$

By construction, μ is C^∞ on the intervals $[t, t_{j+1}], [t_m, t_{m+1}], j+1 \le m \le J-1$, and $[t_J, \infty)$. Therefore, $F_\mu(p\Theta + t\Theta^\perp, \Theta)$ is smooth provided that $t \in [t_j, t_{j+1}]$. In a similar fashion one shows that $F_\mu(p\Theta + t\Theta^\perp, -\Theta)$ is smooth. By construction, $f(p\Theta + t\Theta^\perp)$ is also C^∞ on the interval $[t_j, t_{j+1}]$. This implies that the integral in (3.13) defines a C^∞ function of (θ,p). Therefore, the function $G(\theta,p)$ is C^∞. The smoothness of $I(\sigma,\theta)$ is now obvious. By assumption, $\chi(\theta,p)$ is compactly supported. Integrating by parts in (3.11) we see that $I(\sigma,\theta) = o(\sigma^{-N}), \sigma \to \infty$, for all $N = 1,2,\dots$. The lemma is proved. □

Lemma 3.3. *Let f and μ be as in Theorem 2.1. Consider the function g_χ defined by (2.22), where Ψ_1 admits either expansion (2.21) or (2.26). Then $WF(g_\chi) \subset WF(\mu)$.*

Proof: Using property (2.21) (or, (2.26)), and integrating in (2.22) with respect to θ, we obtain

$$WF(g_\chi) \subset \{(x,\Theta) \in \mathbb{R}^2 \times \Omega : \frac{\partial}{\partial\theta}(p_0(\theta) - \Theta\cdot x) = 0, p_0(\theta) - \Theta\cdot x = 0\}. \tag{3.16}$$

Let $\mathcal{C}$ be the envelope of the family of lines $\Theta\cdot x = p_0(\theta), \Theta \in \Omega$. Clearly, $\mathcal{C} \subset \Gamma$. Suppose first that $\mathcal{C}$ is a smooth curve segment. Using the standard argument from the proof of the involutivity of the Legendre transformation (see, e.g. [1], Section 14), we conclude that the set defined on the right side of (3.16) is precisely the intersection of the conormal bundle of

$\mathcal{C}, N^*\mathcal{C}$, with $\mathbb{R}^2 \times \Omega$. If $\mathcal{C} = \{x^{(0)}\}$, then $p_0(\theta) - \Theta \cdot x^{(0)} \equiv 0, \Theta \in \Omega$, and we immediately conclude that $WF(g_\chi) \subset x^{(0)} \times \Omega$. Let $\mathcal{Q}$ denote the set on the right side of (3.16). To finish the proof we note that if $(x^{(0)}, \Theta_0) \in \mathcal{Q}$ and $(x^{(0)}, \Theta_0) \notin WF(\mu)$, that is μ is smooth across $\mathcal{C}$ at $x^{(0)}$, then all the coefficients $c_k(\theta)$ (cf. (2.21) and (2.26)) vanish with all the derivatives at $\theta = \theta_0$. Therefore, $(x^{(0)}, \Theta_0) \notin WF(g_\chi)$. Using the well-known fact that under assumptions (2.1), (2.2), we have $WF(\mu) \subset N^*\Gamma$, we finish the proof. □

REFERENCES

1. V. I. Arnold. *Mathematical Methods of Classical Mechanics*. Springer-Verlag, New York, 1989.
2. S. Deans. *The Radon Transform and Some of Its Applications*. Wiley, New York, 1983.
3. A. Faridani. Results, old and new, in computed tomography. In G. Chavent, G. Papanicolaou, P. Sacks, and W. Symes, editors, *The IMA Volumes in Mathematics and Its Applications*. Springer-Verlag. (to appear).
4. I. Gelfand and G. Shilov. *Generalized Functions. Volume 1: Properties and Operations*. Academic Press, New York, 1964.
5. A. Katsevich. Analysis of artifacts in local tomography with non-smooth attenuation. (submitted).
6. A. Katsevich. Local tomography with non-smooth attenuation. *Transactions of the American Mathematical Society*. (to appear).
7. A. Katsevich. Local tomography for the generalized Radon transform. *SIAM Journal on Applied Mathematics*, 57(4):1128–1162, 1997.
8. P. Kuchment, K. Lancaster, and L. Mogilevskaya. On local tomography. *Inverse Problems*, 11:571–589, 1995.
9. A. Ramm and A. Katsevich. *The Radon Transform and Local Tomography*. CRC Press, Boca Raton, Florida, 1996.
10. A. Ramm and A. Zaslavsky. Reconstructing singularities of a function given its Radon transform. *Math. and Comput. Modelling*, 18(1):109–138, 1993.
11. A. Ramm and A. Zaslavsky. Singularities of the Radon transform. *Bull. Amer. Math. Soc.*, 25:109–115, 1993.

6

INVERSE PROBLEMS OF DETERMINING NONLINEAR TERMS IN ORDINARY DIFFERENTIAL EQUATIONS

Yutaka Kamimura

Tokyo University of Fisheries
Konan 4-5-7, Minato-ku
Tokyo 108, Japan

1. INTRODUCTION

We study two inverse problems to determine unknown nonlinear terms in nonlinear Sturm–Liouville problems from their spectral information. The first problem, which we discuss in Section 2, is:

Problem 1.1. *Determine a nonlinear term f of the boundary value problem*

$$\begin{cases} u'' + [\lambda - q(x)]u = f(u), & 0 \leq x \leq \pi/2, \quad ' = \frac{d}{dx} \\ u'(0) = u(\pi/2) = 0. \end{cases} \tag{1.1}$$

from its first bifurcating branch.

The second problem, which we discuss in Section 3, is:

Problem 1.2. *Given functions $a(\lambda)$, $b(\lambda)$ on the interval $[0, \Lambda]$, find a function $f(u)$ so that the (overspecified) boundary value problem*

$$\begin{cases} u''(x,\lambda) = \lambda f'(u(x,\lambda)), & 0 \leq x \leq 1, \\ u(0,\lambda) = 0, \quad u'(0,\lambda) = a(\lambda), \quad u(1,\lambda) = b(\lambda), \end{cases} \tag{1.2}$$

admits a solution $u(x,\lambda)$ for each $\lambda \in [0,\Lambda]$.

Our main goal here is to show that a method based upon the use of the implicit function theorem in appropriate Banach space setting is effective commonly to the above two problems. By the method, the problems are reduced to solving integral equations of the form

$$\int_0^1 \Phi(\sigma) g(x\sigma) d\sigma = G(x), \quad (G \text{ given}) \tag{1.3}$$

which are solved by means of the Mellin transform and the Paley–Wiener theorem.

Inverse Problems, Tomography, and Image Processing, edited by Ramm,
Plenum Press, New York, 1998

2. INVERSE BIFURCATION PROBLEM

In (1.1) we assume that $q(x) \in C[0, \pi/2]$ and that $f(u) \in C^1(\mathbb{R}), f(0) = f'(0) = 0$. Then, as is seen from general theorems (see e.g., [1, 10, 11]) in bifurcation theory, the first bifurcating branch bifurcates at the point $(\lambda_1, 0)$ from the trivial solution $u(x) \equiv 0$. Here λ_1 denotes the first eigenvalue of

$$\begin{cases} u'' + [\lambda - q(x)]u = 0, & 0 \le x \le \pi/2, \\ u'(0) = u(\pi/2) = 0. \end{cases} \tag{2.1}$$

Let Γ denote the correspondence which assigns to the nonlinear term f its first bifurcating branch. It is then of interest what the image of Γ is, and moreover, whether Γ is injective or not. From this point of view the author established in the former work [5] a local existence result for Problem 1.1 in the case $q(x) \equiv 0$. In this particular case the relationship between the nonlinear term and the first bifurcating branch is characterized by an integral condition, and the local invertibility of the correspondence Γ is equivalent to the solvability of Abel's integral equation. This analysis leads to the question: what kind of integral equation appears in the analysis of Problem 1.1 if $q(x) \equiv 0$ is replaced by more general $q(x)$. The investigation concerning Problem 1.1 is motivated by this question.

Precisely speaking, the first bifurcating branch is defined as the set

$$\begin{aligned} \Gamma(f) := \{(\lambda, h) \in \mathbb{R}^2 \mid & \text{ for } (\lambda, h) \text{ there exists a solution } u \\ & \text{of (1.1) such that (i) } u(x) \neq 0 \text{ for any } x \in [0, \pi/2); \\ & \text{(ii) } u(0) = h\} \cup \{(\lambda_1, 0)\} \end{aligned}$$

and our problem can be formulated as follows:
Given curve γ, determine a function f such that $\Gamma(f) = \gamma$.

In order to give an answer to the above problem we introduce the following two function spaces. Let $0 < \alpha < 1/2$. The first space is that for the nonlinear term f:

$$\begin{aligned} X := \{ & f(h) \in C^1(\mathbb{R}) | f(0) = f'(0) = 0, \\ & ||f||_X := \sup_{h,k \in \mathbb{R}, h \neq k} \frac{|(1+|k|^\alpha) f'(k) - (1+|h|^\alpha) f'(h)|}{|k-h|^\alpha} < \infty\}. \end{aligned}$$

The second space is that for the difference $\mu(h)$ between the first bifurcating branch and the straight line $\lambda = \lambda_1$:

$$\begin{aligned} Y := \{ & \mu(h) \in C(\mathbb{R}) | h\mu'(h) \in C(\mathbb{R}), \mu(0) = 0, \\ & ||\mu||_Y := \sup_{h \in \mathbb{R}} |\mu(h)| + \\ & \sup_{h,k \in \mathbb{R}, h \neq k} \frac{||k|^{3/2}(1+|k|^\alpha)\mu'(k) - |h|^{3/2}(1+|h|^\alpha)\mu'(h)|}{|k-h|^{\alpha+1/2}} < \infty\}. \end{aligned}$$

The space X and Y are Banach spaces, which are modifications of the Hölder spaces $C^{1,\alpha}$ and $C^{1,\alpha+1/2}$, respectively.

Let $v(x)$ be the first eigenfunction of (2.1) normalized by the condition $v(0) = 1$ and we assume that

(A1) $v''(0) < 0$.

(A2) $v'(x) < 0 \quad \text{for} \quad 0 < x \leq \pi/2.$

(A3) $v''(x)v(x) \leq 2v'(x)^2 \quad \text{for} \quad 0 \leq x < \pi/2.$

We note that that if $\max_{0 \leq x \leq \pi/2} q(x) < \lambda_1$ then (A1)–(A3) hold. For other sufficient conditions for (A1)–(A3) we refer to [4, Remark 4.8].

With the notation and assumption we can state the following local existence result:

Theorem 2.1 (see [4]). *Let $q(x) \in C^2[0,\pi/2]$ and assume that (A1)–(A3) hold. Then, given $\lambda(h)$ with $||\lambda(h) - \lambda_1||_Y$ sufficiently small, there exists a function $f \in X$ such that $\Gamma(f) = \{(\lambda(h),h) | h \in \mathbb{R}\}$.*

We briefly describe the basic idea of the proof of Theorem 2.1. Let $(f,\mu) \in X \times Y$ be sufficiently small, let $u(h,x;f,\mu)$ be the solution of

$$\begin{cases} u'' + [(\lambda_1 + \mu(h)) - q(x)]u = f(u), \\ u(0) = h, u'(0) = 0, \end{cases} \tag{2.2}$$

and set

$$F(f,\mu)(h) := h^{-1}u(h,\pi/2;f,\mu).$$

Clearly $F(0,0) = 0$. Moreover $(\lambda_1 + \mu(h),h) \in \Gamma(f)$ if and only if $F(f,\mu) = 0$. $F(f,\mu)$ is a C^1-mapping of an open neighborhood of $(0,0)$ in $X \times Y$ to Y and the Fréchet derivative $F_f(0,0)$ at $(0,0)$ with respect to f is given in the form

$$(F_f(0,0)g)(h) = -\frac{1}{hv'(\pi/2)} \int_0^{\pi/2} v(\theta) g(hv(\theta)) d\theta.$$

If we can show that the linear integral equation $F_f(0,0)g = \phi$, where $\phi(h)$ is a given function in Y, has a unique solution g in X then we can apply the implicit function theorem (see e.g., [10, Theorem 2.7.2]) to find the nonlinear term f whose first bifurcating branch coincides with $\lambda(h) = \lambda_1 + \mu(h)$. By the substitution $v(\theta) =: \sigma$, the equation $F_f(0,0)g(h) = \phi(h)$ becomes the following equation of the form (1.3):

$$\int_0^1 -\frac{\sigma}{v'(v^{-1}(\sigma))} g(h\sigma) d\sigma = -v'(\pi/2)h\phi(h), \tag{2.3}$$

where v^{-1} denotes the inverse function of $v(x)$ and we use the variable h instead of x in (1.3).

The equation (1.3) can be rewritten in the form of a Volterra integral equation of the first kind

$$\int_0^x \Phi(\tau/x) g(\tau) d\tau = xG(x).$$

However this can not be handled by the standard method (see e.g., [12, Section 41]) of reduction to a Volterra integral equation of the second kind, because the integral kernel is singular at $x = 0$. In what follows we shall outline the basic idea of solving (1.3).

We first note that the operator J_Φ defined by

$$J_\Phi g(x) := \int_0^1 \Phi(\sigma) g(x\sigma) d\sigma$$

satisfies the relation $J_\Phi J_\Psi = J_{\Phi*\Psi}$, where

$$(\Phi * \Psi)(\sigma) = \int_0^1 \Phi(\sigma/\tau)\Psi(\tau)\frac{d\tau}{\tau}. \tag{2.4}$$

Hence, if there exists a function Ψ satisfying

$$(\Psi * \Phi)(\sigma) = \sigma^{\epsilon-1} \quad (\epsilon > 0), \tag{2.5}$$

then (1.3) can be solved as

$$\begin{aligned} g(x) &= x^{1-\epsilon}\frac{d}{dx}\left(x^\epsilon \int_0^1 \sigma^{\epsilon-1} g(x\sigma)d\sigma\right) \\ &= x^{1-\epsilon}\frac{d}{dx}\left(x^\epsilon J_{\Psi*\Phi} g(x)\right) \\ &= x^{1-\epsilon}\frac{d}{dx}\left(x^\epsilon J_\Psi G(x)\right). \end{aligned} \tag{2.6}$$

Thus solving (1.3) is reduced to finding Ψ which satisfies (2.5). The integral (2.4) is a convolution associated with the integral transform

$$\mathcal{K}[\Phi](z) := \int_0^1 \Phi(\sigma)\sigma^z d\sigma.$$

In other words we have the following convolution formula:

$$\mathcal{K}[\Phi * \Psi] = \mathcal{K}[\Phi]\mathcal{K}[\Psi].$$

Accordingly (2.5) is rewritten as $\mathcal{K}[\Psi](z)\mathcal{K}[\Phi](z) = (z+\epsilon)^{-1}$. We observe that the integral transform $\mathcal{K}$ may be connected with the Mellin transform $\mathcal{M}$ by the relation

$$\mathcal{K}[\Phi](z) = \int_0^\infty \sigma\tilde{\Phi}(\sigma)\sigma^{z-1}d\sigma = \mathcal{M}[\sigma\tilde{\Phi}(\sigma)](z),$$

where $\tilde{\Phi}(\sigma)$ is the extension of $\Phi(\sigma)$ defined by $\tilde{\Phi}(\sigma) = 0$ for $\sigma > 1$. It follows from this observation and the Paley–Wiener theorem that if

$$\mathcal{K}[\Phi](z) \neq 0 \quad \text{in the right half plane } \mathrm{Re}(z \geq 0, \tag{2.7}$$

then the function

$$\Psi(\sigma) := \mathcal{K}^{-1}\left[\frac{1}{(z+\epsilon)\mathcal{K}[\Phi](z)}\right] \tag{2.8}$$

is well defined as a function on the interval $[0, 1]$ and satisfies (2.5). This is a way to solve the integral equation (1.3).

Under the assumptions (A1)–(A3) the function $\Psi(\sigma) = -\dfrac{\sigma}{v'(v^{-1}(\sigma))}$ satisfies the condition (2.7). Hence, by the way mentioned above, we can show that the equation (2.3), with $\phi(h) \in Y$, has a unique solution g in X. We have sketched the proof of Theorem 2.1. For the details of the proof we refer to [4].

Concerning the uniqueness we have the following:

Theorem 2.2 (see [8]). *The function f in Theorem 2.1 is unique in X. In particular, if the first bifurcating branch is the straight line $\lambda(h) \equiv \lambda_1$ then $f = 0$.*

Theorems 2.1 and 2.2 imply that the nonlinear term f is determined locally from the first bifurcating branch and hence that the first bifurcating branch controls other (the nth) bifurcating branches. This is not necessarily true for the second bifurcating branch. Actually in the case $q \equiv 0$ there exist infinitely many nonlinear terms realizing the straight line as the second bifurcating branch. For this fact we refer to [6].

In applications the problem remains: *how to reconstruct the nonlinear term from the first bifurcating branch.* We conclude this section with an observation concerning this problem. We first remark that the nonlinear term f can be expressed in terms of $\mu(h)$ *approximately* as

$$f \sim -F_f(0,0)^{-1}F_\mu(0,0)\mu,$$

if μ is small. We call $f_a := -F_f(0,0)^{-1}F_\mu(0,0)\mu$ the *approximate nonlinear term* corresponding to $\mu(h)$. In view of (2.3), (2.6) the inverse $F_f(0,0)^{-1}$ is given by the formula

$$F_f(0,0)^{-1}\phi(h) = -v'(\pi/2)h^{1-\epsilon}\frac{d}{dh}(h^\epsilon J_\Psi(h\phi(h))),$$

where Ψ is a function defined by (2.8). Moreover $F_\mu(0,0)$ can be computed as

$$F_\mu(0,0)\mu = v'(\pi/2)^{-1}c\mu,$$

where c is a constant defined by $c := \int_0^{\pi/2} v(x)^2dx$. Therefore the approximate nonlinear term corresponding to $\mu(h)$ can be explicitly computed by the formula

$$f_a(h) = ch^{1-\epsilon}\frac{d}{dh}(h^\epsilon J_\Psi(h\mu(h))), \tag{2.9}$$

because $\Psi(\sigma)$ is determined from $\Phi(\sigma) = -\frac{\sigma}{v'(v^{-1}(\sigma))}$ via (2.8). As an example we consider the case

$$q(x) := -m\kappa^2\ell(x)^{2(m-1)}, \tag{2.10}$$

where $m \geq 1$, $\kappa := (m\pi)^{-1}B(1/2m, 1/2)$ ($B(\cdot,\cdot)$ denotes the beta function), and $\ell(x)$ is a function defined by

$$\int_{\ell(x)}^1 (1-t^{2m})^{-1/2}dt = \kappa x.$$

Then the first eigenvalue λ_1 and the first eigenfunction $v(x)$ of (2.1) are calculated as $\lambda_1 = 0, v(x) = \ell(x)$. It is easy to see that $v(x)$ satisfies the assumptions (A1)–(A3). Moreover we have $\Phi(\sigma) = \kappa^{-1}\sigma(1-\sigma^{2m})^{-1/2}$. Hence, taking $\epsilon = 2$ in (2.8), $\Psi(\sigma)$ is computed as

$$\begin{aligned}\Psi(\sigma) &= \mathcal{K}^{-1}\left[\frac{2m\kappa}{(z+2)B((z+2)/2m,1/2)}\right]\\ &= (\kappa/\pi)\mathcal{K}^{-1}[B((z+m+2)/2m,1/2)]\\ &= (2m\kappa/\pi)\sigma^{m+1}(1-\sigma^{2m})^{-1/2}.\end{aligned}$$

Thus, by means of (2.9) with $\epsilon = 2$, we arrive at

$$f_a(h) = (2mc\kappa/\pi)h \int_0^1 \frac{\sigma^{m+2}}{(1-\sigma^{2m})^{1/2}} \left\{\sigma^{-2}(\sigma^3\mu)'\right\}(h\sigma)d\sigma.$$

For the potential $q(x)$ given in (2.10) the approximate nonlinear term can be computed by this formula. In the cases $m = 1$ (potential free case) and $m = 2$ (Lamé's equation) the reader may refer to [4, Section 5], where the approximate nonlinear term corresponding to $\mu(h) = h^a e^{-h}$ ($a > 0$) is written down in terms of the first Humbert function.

3. PROBLEM OF DENISOV–LORENZI

Problem 1.2 was studied by Lorenzi [9], under the assumption

$$a(\lambda) \in C^2[0,\Lambda], a(0) = 0, a'(\lambda) > 0 \text{ for any } \lambda \in [0,\Lambda]; \tag{3.1}$$

$$b(\lambda) \in C^2[0,\Lambda], \quad b(0) = 0, \quad b'(\lambda) > 0 \text{ for any } \lambda \in [0,\Lambda]. \tag{3.2}$$

Problems closely related to that above were treated by Denisov [2] and Denisov–Lorenzi [3].

Obviously we may assume that $f(0) = 0$ without loss of generality. The following, local existence theorem is an improvement of [9, Theorem 0.1].

Theorem 3.1 (see [7]). *Let $a(\lambda)$ and $b(\lambda)$ satisfy the conditions (3.1) and (3.2) respectively, and assume that $a'(0) < b'(0)$. Then there exist a number $\Lambda' \in (0,\Lambda]$ and a positive (except at $u = 0$) function $f(u) \in C^1[0, b(\Lambda')]$ such that (1.2) admits a solution $u(x,\lambda)$ for each $\lambda \in [0,\Lambda']$.*

We briefly describe the basic idea of the proof of Theorem 3.1. We first note that, in the case $f(u) \geq 0$, Problem 1.2 is equivalent to finding a positive (except at $t = 0$) solution of the nonlinear integral equation

$$\int_0^{b(\lambda)} \frac{dt}{(a(\lambda)^2 + 2\lambda f(t))^{1/2}} = 1, \quad \lambda \in (0,\Lambda]. \tag{3.3}$$

Let us fix a function $b(\lambda)$ satisfying (3.2) and set

$$F(f,a)(\lambda) := \int_0^{b(\lambda)} \frac{dt}{(a(\lambda)^2 + 2\lambda f(t))^{1/2}} - 1.$$

If, for $b'(0) > k > 0$, we define functions $f_0(t)$ and $a_0(t)$ by

$$f_0(t) := 2kt, \quad a_0(t) := b(\lambda) - k\lambda,$$

then we obtain $F(f_0, a_0) = 0$. We define Banach spaces X, Y, Z by

$$\begin{aligned}
X &:= \{f \in C^1[0, b(\Lambda)], | f(0) = 0\}, \\
Y &:= \{a \in C^2[0,\Lambda], | a(0) = 0\}, \\
Z &:= \{\phi \in C^2(0,\Lambda], | \phi(\lambda), \lambda\phi'(\lambda), \lambda^2\phi''(\lambda) \in C[0,\Lambda]\}.
\end{aligned}$$

Then $F(f,a)$ is a C^1-mapping of an open neighborhood of (f_0,a_0) in $X\times Y$ to Z and the Fréchet derivative $F_f(f_0,a_0)$ at (f_0,a_0) with respect to f is given in the form

$$(F_f(f_0,a_0)g)(\lambda) = -\lambda\int_0^{b(\lambda)} \frac{g(t)}{(a_0(\lambda)^2+4k\lambda t)^{3/2}}dt$$
$$= -\frac{b(\lambda)}{\lambda^2}\int_0^1 \frac{g(b(\lambda)\sigma)}{(\lambda^{-2}a_0(\lambda)^2+4k\lambda^{-1}b(\lambda)\sigma)^{3/2}}d\sigma.$$

If we can show that the linear integral equation $F_f(f_0,a_0)g=\phi$, where ϕ is a given function in Z, has a unique solution g in X then we can apply the implicit function theorem mentioned in Section 2 to see that, for $a(\lambda)$ near $a_0(\lambda)$, there exists a solution $f\in X$ of (3.3).

For small λ, the operator $F_f(f_0,a_0)$ can be approximated by an operator L defined by

$$(Lg)(\lambda) := -\frac{b(\lambda)}{\lambda^2}\int_0^1 \frac{g(b(\lambda)\sigma)}{(a_0'(0)^2+4kb'(0)\sigma)^{3/2}}d\sigma$$
$$= -\frac{b(\lambda)}{\lambda^2}a_0'(0)^{-3}\int_0^1 \frac{g(b(\lambda)\sigma)}{(1+c\sigma)^{3/2}}d\sigma,$$

where $c := 4kb'(0)/a_0'(0)^3$. Namely, in the case when Λ is sufficiently small, the residual $R := F_f(f_0,a_0)-L$ is so small that, if L is an isomorphism from X onto Y then $F_f(f_0,a_0)$ is also so with the inverse

$$F_f(f_0,a_0)^{-1} = L^{-1}(I+RL^{-1})^{-1}.$$

Thus our task becomes to solve the integral equation $Lg=\phi$, where ϕ is given in Z. Changing the variables via $x=b(\lambda)$ this integral equation is written as

$$\int_0^1 \frac{1}{(1+c\sigma)^{3/2}}g(x\sigma)d\sigma = G(x) \quad \left(:= -a_0'(0)^3\frac{\lambda^2}{b(\lambda)}\phi(\lambda)\right), \tag{3.4}$$

The method of solving (1.3), which is explained in Section 2, is applicable to the differential form of (3.4), because $\Phi(\sigma) := \frac{\sigma}{(1+c\sigma)^{3/2}}$ with $c>0$ satisfies the condition (2.7). In this way we can prove that, for $a(\lambda)$ near $a_0(\lambda)$, there exists a solution $f\in X$ of (3.3). This is the core of the proof of Theorem 3.1. For the details of the proof we refer to [7]. We wish to emphasize that the method explained above is very similar to that used in the proof of Theorem 2.1.

Concerning the uniqueness for Problem 1.2, we have the following:

Theorem 3.2 (see [7]). *Let $a(\lambda)$ and $b(\lambda)$ satisfy conditions (3.1) and (3.2) respectively, and assume that $a'(0) < b'(0)$. If positive (except at $u=0$) functions $f_1(u), f_2(u) \in C^1[0,b(\Lambda)]$ are solutions of Problem 1.2 then $f_1(u)=f_2(u)$ for any $u\in[0,b(\Lambda)]$.*

REFERENCES

1. M. G. Crandall and P. H. Rabinowitz, "Bifurcation from simple eigenvalues," *J. Funct. Anal.*, **8**, 321–340 (1971).
2. A. M. Denisov, "Inverse problems for nonlinear differential equations," *Dokl. Akad. Nauk.*, **307**, 1040–1042 (1989).
3. A. Denisov and A. Lorenzi, "Identification of Nonlinear terms in boundary value problems related to ordinary differential equations," *Differential and Integral Equations*, **5**, 567–579 (1992).

4. K. Iwasaki and Y. Kamimura, "An inverse bifurcation problem and an integral equation of the Abel type," *Inverse Problems*, **13**, 1015–1031 (1997).
5. Y. Kamimura, "An inverse problem in bifurcation theory," *J. Differential Equations*, **106**, 10–26 (1993).
6. Y. Kamimura, "An inverse problem in bifurcation theory, II," *J. Math. Soc. Japan*, **46**, 89–110 (1994).
7. Y. Kamimura, "An inverse problem of determining a nonlinear term in an ordinary differential equation," *Differential and Integral Equations*, (in press).
8. Y. Kamimura, "Uniqueness of nonlinearities realizing the first bifurcating branch," (submitted 1997).
9. A. Lorenzi, "An inverse spectral problem for a nonlinear ordinary differential equation," *Applicable Analysis*, **46**, 129–143 (1992).
10. L. Nirenberg, *Topics in Nonlinear Functional Analysis*, Courant Institute of mathematical Sciences, (1974).
11. P. H. Rabinowitz, "Nonlinear Sturm–Liouville problems for second order ordinary differential equations," *Comm. Pure Appl. Math.*, **23**, 939–961 (1970).
12. K. Yosida, *Lectures on Differential and Integral Equations*, Interscience, New York, (1960).

7

COMPLEX DAUBECHIES WAVELETS: FILTERS DESIGN AND APPLICATIONS

J.-M. Lina

Centre de Recherches Mathématiques
Univ. de Montréal
C. P. 6128 Succ. Centre-Ville
Montréal, Québec, H3C 3J7, Canada
Atlantic Nuclear Services Ltd.
Fredericton, New Brunswick, E3B 5C8, Canada
E-mail: `lina@crm.umontreal.ca`

ABSTRACT

The first part of this work describes the full set of Daubechies Wavelets with a particular emphasis on symmetric (and complex) orthonormal bases. Some properties of the associated complex scaling functions are presented in a second part. The third and last part describes a multiscale image enhancement algorithm using the phase of the complex multiresolution representation of the 2 dimension signals.

1. INTRODUCTION: THE ORTHONORMAL DYADIC WAVELET BASES

We consider orthonormal bases of $L^2(\mathbb{R})$ of the form

$$\psi_{j,k}(x) = 2^{\frac{j}{2}}\,\psi(2^j x - k) \tag{1.1}$$

where j and k are integer. In most applications, the discrete wavelets (1.1) are real valued functions. This restriction is mainly due to the immediate and efficient applications of such bases in various aspects of signal processing (regression, nonlinear estimation and compression). Indeed, for $\psi(x)$ sufficiently **regular** and well **localized**, those bases are also unconditional for many important spaces in approximation theory such as Besov spaces. This means that, unlike the Fourier representation in which a crucial role is played by the phase, the norm associated with those spaces can be written in terms of the modulus of the wavelet modes *only*.

Inverse Problems, Tomography, and Image Processing, edited by Ramm,
Plenum Press, New York, 1998

The present work describes the construction and some properties of **Complex Daubechies Wavelets**. The initial motivation is to make possible the **symmetry** of ψ. Let us recall that such a property avoids many artifacts in the wavelet synthesis of 2d signals. Complex valued discrete wavelets raise the question about the *role of the phase* in such wavelet representations. This is the main subject of this paper.

The approach proposed by Daubechies to set up dyadic orthonormal bases will be followed; most of the material presented in this section and the next one will refer to her book [1]. However, for the sake of self-consistency, we summarize here the basic tools of the **multiresolution** approach and illustrate them with the well-known spline examples [2].

The multiresolution analysis of $L^2(\mathbb{R})$ consists in a sequence of closed subspaces $V_j \subset L^2(\mathbb{R})$ such that

$$V_j \subset V_{j+1}, \qquad \bigcap_j V_j = \{0\}, \qquad \overline{\bigcup_j V_j} = L^2(\mathbb{R}), \tag{1.2a}$$

$$f(x) \in V_0 \Leftrightarrow f(x-1) \in V_0, \qquad f(x) \in V_j \Leftrightarrow f(2x) \in V_{j+1} \tag{1.2b}$$

Such a sequence is called **r-regular** if a function $h(x) \in V_0$ exists such that $\{h(x-k), k \in \mathbb{Z}\}$ is a Riesz basis of V_0, *i.e.*, for $f(x) = \sum_k f_k h(x-k)$

$$A\|f\|_2^2 \leq \sum_k |f_k|^2 \leq B\|f\|_2^2, \quad A > 0 \tag{1.3}$$

and

$$|\nabla^q h(x)| \leq C_m(1+|x|)^{-m}, \ \forall m \geq 0 \quad \text{and } 0 \leq q \leq r \tag{1.4}$$

Let us recall that the first property can be fully characterized by $0 < \sigma_h(\omega) < \infty$ where $\sigma_h(\omega)$ is the 2π-periodic function defined by

$$\sigma_h(\omega) = \sum_p |\hat{h}(\omega + 2\pi p)|^2 \tag{1.5}$$

and $\hat{h}(\omega)$ is the Fourier transform of $h(x)$. The second property is more subtle: let us only recall that for orthonormal bases of the form (1.1), it is *impossible* that ψ has exponential decay in both space and frequency. It will be more convenient to control the regularity through the polynomial content of the approximation spaces V_j or, equivalently, the **vanishing moments** of the wavelet associated with (see [1, p. 154]):

$$\int x^l \psi(x) dx = 0, \quad \text{for} \quad l = 0, 1, \ldots, J \tag{1.6}$$

where J is some integer. The **scaling function** φ is the basic ingredient of the construction. Beside the various constraints related to the properties that we want to impose on the approximation spaces V_j, the scaling property of φ implies a fundamental functional equation: since $\varphi \in V_0 \subset V_1$, a sequence of complex-valued coefficients a_k exists such that $\sum a_k = 1$ and

$$\varphi(x) = 2\sum_k a_k \quad \varphi(2x-k) \tag{1.7}$$

Defining the trigonometric polynomial

$$m_0(\omega) = \sum_k a_k e^{ik\omega}, \tag{1.8}$$

Eq. (1.6) can be written as

$$\hat{\varphi}(\omega) = m_0(\frac{\omega}{2})\hat{\varphi}(\frac{\omega}{2}) \tag{1.9}$$

A first theorem establishes the foundations of the orthonormal multiresolution bases: a function $\varphi \in V_0$ with unit integral and satisfying Eq. (1.4) exists such that

$$\sigma_\varphi(\omega) = 1 \tag{1.10}$$

This condition characterizes the **orthonormal basis** $\{\varphi(x-k), k \in \mathbb{Z}\}$ of V_0. Consequently, the set of functions

$$\varphi_{j,k}(x) = 2^{\frac{j}{2}}\varphi(2^j x - k) \tag{1.11}$$

is an orthonormal basis of the space V_j for any integer j. and the orthonormality condition (1.7) is equivalent with

$$|m_0(\omega)|^2 + |m_0(\omega+\pi)|^2 = 1 \tag{1.12}$$

Let us note that Eq. (1.12) *does not* guarantee orthonormality of the basis: extra conditions [3] that are requested on $|m_0(\omega)|$ will be always satisfied in the present work (see [1, p. 182]).

• Example: *The Spline scaling function.* For the sake of illustration and to motivate the forthcoming discussion about *symmetric Daubechies Wavelets*, we consider two well-known wavelet bases both related to the piecewise constant spline:

$$h(x) = sup(1-|x|, 0), \quad i.e., \quad \hat{h}(\omega) = \left(\frac{\sin(\frac{\omega}{2})}{\frac{\omega}{2}}\right)^2 \tag{1.13}$$

The integer translates of $h(x)$ span V_0; they form a Riesz basis:

$$\frac{1}{3} \leq \sigma_h(\omega) = \frac{2+\cos\omega}{3} \leq 1 \tag{1.14}$$

The scaling equation, Eq. (1.7) reads as $h(x) = \frac{1}{2}h(2x-1) + h(x) + \frac{1}{2}h(2x+1)$ and the trigonometric polynomial is

$$m_0(\omega) = \left(\frac{1+e^{i\omega}}{2}\right)^2 e^{-i\omega} \tag{1.15}$$

Writing

$$\sigma_h(\omega) = u(\omega)\overline{u(\omega)} \tag{1.16}$$

the scaling function defined by

$$\hat{\varphi}(\omega) = \frac{\hat{h}(\omega)}{u(\omega)} \tag{1.17}$$

does satisfy the orthonormality condition $\sigma_\varphi(\omega) = 1$. Different **factorizations** of $\sigma_h(\omega)$ define different scaling functions φ through the phase of $u(\omega)$. A first factorization $\sigma_h(\omega) = |u_1(\omega)|^2$ has been proposed by Stromberg [4]:

$$u_1(\omega) = \frac{3+\sqrt{3}}{6}(1+re^{i\omega}), \quad \text{with} \quad r = 2-\sqrt{3} \tag{1.18}$$

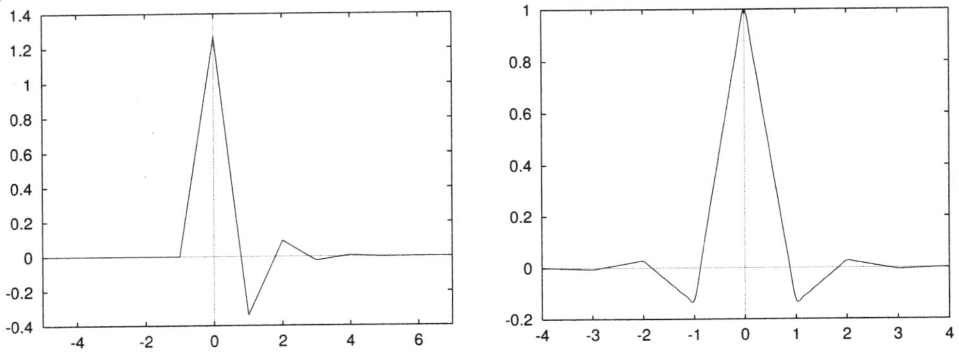

Figure 1. The Stromberg scaling function (left) and the Battle–Lemarié scaling function (right) for the linear spline.

It gives

$$m_0^{(1)}(\omega) = \frac{\hat{\varphi}(2\omega)}{\hat{\varphi}(\omega)} = \left(\frac{1+e^{i\omega}}{2}\right)^2 e^{-2i\omega}\left(\frac{e^{-i\omega}+r}{e^{-2i\omega}+r}\right) \tag{1.19}$$

Later, Battle [5] and Lemarié [5] have considered $\sigma_h(\omega) = |u_2\omega)|^2$ with

$$u_2(\omega) = \sqrt{\frac{2+\cos\omega}{3}} = u_1(\omega)\, e^{i\xi(\omega)} \tag{1.20}$$

$$\cos\xi(\omega) = \frac{3+\sqrt{3}}{2\sqrt{3}}\,\frac{1+r\cos\omega}{\sqrt{2+\cos\omega}}$$

$$\sin\xi(\omega) = \frac{3+\sqrt{3}}{2\sqrt{3}}\,\frac{r\sin\omega}{\sqrt{2+\cos\omega}}$$

leading to $m_0^{(2)}(\omega) = m_0^{(1)}(\omega)e^{i(\xi(\omega)-\xi(2\omega))}$. As illustrated in Fig. 1, the later factorization gives a symmetric scaling function: $\varphi(x) = \varphi(-x)$.

The second basic theorem is: a **wavelet** $\psi \in V_1$ with vanishing integral and satisfying (1.4) exists such that $\{\varphi(x-k), \psi(x-k), k \in \mathbb{Z}\}$ is an **orthonormal basis** of V_1.

Wavelet multiresolution therefore aims to decompose $V_1 = V_0 \oplus W_0$ where W_0 is generated though the integer translates of a function ψ. Since $\psi \in W_0 \subset V_1$, a sequence of complex-valued coefficients b_k exists such that:

$$\psi(x) = 2\sum_k b_k \quad \varphi(2x-k) \tag{1.21}$$

or, defining $m_1(\omega) = \sum_k b_k e^{ik\omega}$,

$$\hat{\psi}(\omega) = m_1(\frac{\omega}{2})\hat{\varphi}(\frac{\omega}{2}) \tag{1.22}$$

It can be shown that $m_1(\omega) = e^{-3i\omega}\overline{m_0(\omega+\pi)}$ is a possible candidate for ensuring the set $\{\psi(x-k), k \in \mathbb{Z}\}$ to be an orthonormal basis of W_0. This results amounts to take $b_k = (-1)^k \overline{a}_{1-k}$ in Eq. (1.13). The orthonormal decomposition of each dyadic approximation space, *i.e.*, $V_{j+1} = V_j \oplus W_j$, defines the **details spaces** W_j generated by the set of orthonormal wavelets

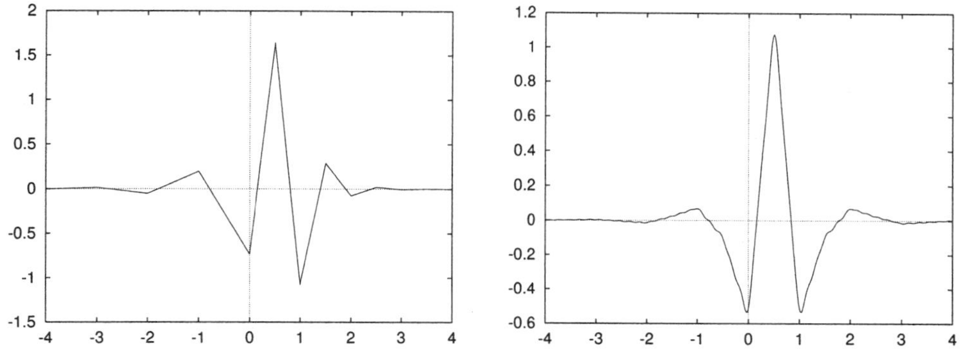

Figure 2. The Stromberg (left) and Battle–Lemarié (right) wavelets.

$\{\psi_{j,k}(x) = 2^{\frac{j}{2}}\psi(2^j x - k)\}$, $k \in \mathbb{Z}$. All together, those functions generated by the translates of all dyadic scaling transforms of ψ make an orthonormal basis of $L^2(\mathbb{R})$.

• Example: *The Spline Wavelets* (cont.). The construction of the wavelet associated to the two scaling functions displayed in Fig. 1 is straightforward: using the previous expression for $m_1(\omega)$, we obtain

$$\hat{\psi}(\omega) = \overline{u(\frac{\omega}{2} + \pi)} e^{-\frac{3}{2}i\omega} \frac{\sin(\omega 4)^4}{\sigma_h(\omega 2)(\omega 4)^2} \tag{1.23}$$

As illustrated in Fig. 2, the factorization $\sigma_h(\omega) = |u_2\omega)|^2$ gives a symmetric wavelet: $\psi(x) = \psi(1-x)$.

Those two examples are illustrating nicely the scope of the forthcoming sections: provided we can select an appropriate phase in $\hat{\psi}$, *i.e.*, in $m_0(\omega)$, a **symmetric wavelet** can be constructed on the multiresolution spaces. The same phase analysis will be carried out in the context of Daubechies wavelets.

Let us make a final comment about the regularity of the multiresolution bases. As mentioned before, a fast frequency decay will be controlled through the number of vanishing moments of ψ or, in an equivalent way, the vanishing of the successive derivatives of $\hat{\psi}$ at $\omega = 0$. Using Eq. (1.22) and the definition of $m_1(\omega)$, the criteria of regularity can be written as

$$\frac{d^l}{d\omega^l} m_0(\omega)_{|\omega=0} = 0, \quad \text{for} \quad l = 0, 1, \ldots, J \tag{1.24}$$

This is the Strang–Fix [6] condition; previous examples illustrate this condition with $J = 2$.

2. DAUBECHIES WAVELETS

Daubechies scaling functions are subject to the following constraints:

1) Compactness of the support of φ: We require that φ (and consequently ψ) has a compact support inside the interval $[-J, J+1]$ for some integer J. This requirement amounts to consider a finite number of terms in the expansion (1.7): $a_k \neq 0$ for $k = -J, -J+1, \ldots, J, J+1$.

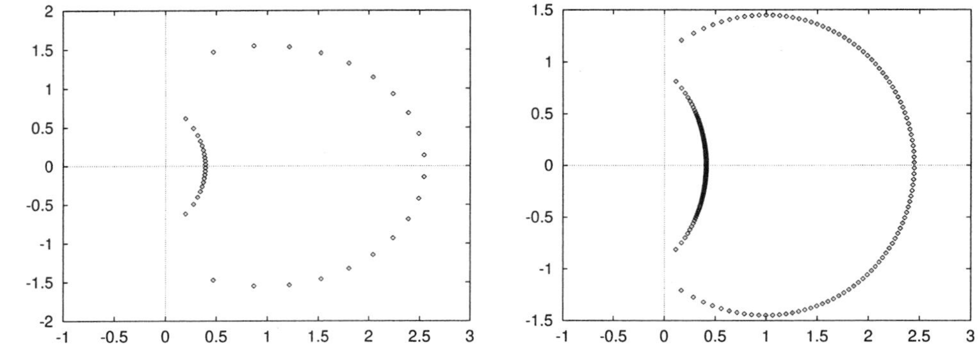

Figure 3. The roots of $p_{12}(z)$ (left) and $p_{100}(z)$ (right).

2) Orthogonality of the $\varphi(x-k)$: Instead of working with $m_0(\omega)$ and solving Eq. (1.12), we define the polynomial

$$F(z) = \sum_{n=-J}^{J+1} a_n z^n, \quad \text{with} \quad F(1) = 1 \tag{2.1}$$

where z is on the unit circle, $|z| = 1$. The orthonormality condition (1.10) (or (1.12)) can be stated through the following equation

$$P(z) - P(-z) = z \tag{2.2}$$

where the polynomial $P(z)$ is defined as

$$P(z) = zF(z)\overline{F(z)} \tag{2.3}$$

3) Strang–Fix condition: To maximize the regularity of the functions generated by the scaling function φ, we require the vanishing of the first J moments of the wavelet. In terms of the polynomial (2.1), the Strang–Fix condition reads as

$$F(-1) = F'(-1) = F''(-1) = \cdots = F^{(J)}(-1) = 0 \tag{2.4}$$

Let us consider the polynomial defined by

$$P_J(z) = \left(\left(\frac{1+z}{2}\right)^{2J+2} p_J(z^{-1})\right) \tag{2.5}$$

where

$$p_J(z) = \sum_{j=0}^{2J} r_j (z+1)^{2J-j}(z-1)^j, \text{ with } \begin{cases} r_{2j} = (-1)^j 2^{-2J} \binom{2J+1}{j}, & j = 0, 1, \ldots, J \\ r_{2j+1} = 0 \end{cases} \tag{2.6}$$

Straightforward algebra shows that $P_J(z)$ does satisfy Eq. (2.2).

The relevance of the polynomial (2.6) in the construction of multiresolution bases relies on the particular relationship between the $2J$ roots of $p_J(z)$. Indeed, we can write the following factorization of $p_J(z)$:

$$p_J(z) = \prod_{k=1}^{J} \left(\frac{z - x_k}{1 - x_k}\right) \prod_{k=1}^{J} \left(\frac{z - \bar{x}_k^{-1}}{1 - \bar{x}_k^{-1}}\right) \tag{2.7}$$

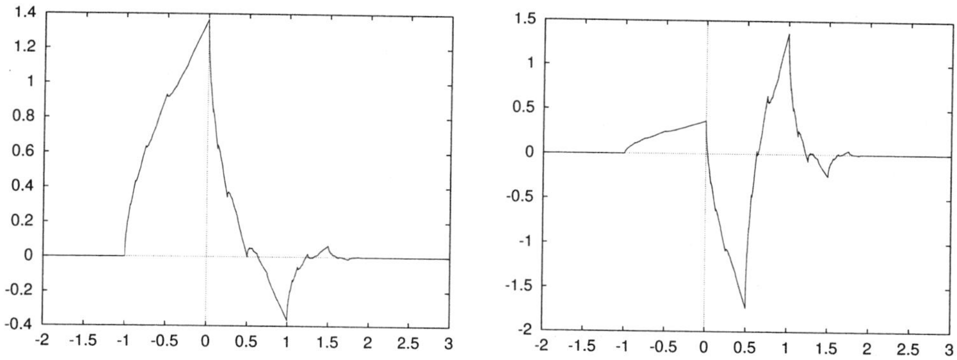

Figure 4. Left: The scaling function φ for J=1. Right: The Daubechies wavelet ψ for J=1.

where $x_{k=1,2,\ldots,J}$ are the J roots inside the unit circle, $|x_k| < 1$, and $\mathrm{Re}(x_k) > \mathrm{Re}(x_{k+1})$ (see Fig. 3). Writing $F(z)$ as

$$F(z) = \left(\frac{1+z}{2}\right)^{1+J} p(z^{-1}) \tag{2.8}$$

the polynomial $p(z)$ is defined through some particular roots of $p_J(z)$ and it is easily found that for *any* subset $R \subset \{1,2,3,\ldots,J\}$ all solutions of the form

$$p(z) = \prod_{m\in R}\left(\frac{z-x_m}{1-x_m}\right)\prod_{n\notin R}\left(\frac{z-\bar{x}_n^{-1}}{1-\bar{x}_n^{-1}}\right) \tag{2.9}$$

factorize $P_J(z) = zF(z)\overline{F}(z)$. Therefore, for any integer J, the trigonometric polynomial given by

$$m_0(\omega) = \left(\frac{1+e^{i\omega}}{2}\right)^{1+J}\prod_{k\in R}\left(\frac{e^{-i\omega}-x_k}{1-x_k}\right)\prod_{k\notin R}\left(\frac{e^{-i\omega}-\bar{x}_k^{-1}}{1-\bar{x}_k^{-1}}\right) \tag{2.10}$$

with any selection R of roots of $p_J(z)$, defines an admissible trigononometric polynomial and thus a compactly supported orthonormal dyadic wavelet basis (with all the material described in Section 1). Let us notice that exchanging R and $\overline{R}$ in Eq. (2.10) corresponds to a complex conjugation (up to some trivial translation) of the coefficient a_k. So, excepted for the Haar case ($J=0$), we obtain 2^{J-1} solutions. In her seminal work [7], Daubechies investigated a subset of this family: she selected R so that the coefficients in the trigonometric expansion $m_0 = \sum_k a_k e^{ik\omega}$ are **real** valued. The usual Daubechies wavelets are thus real valued functions.

• Example $J=1$: The polynomial $p_1(z)$ has two roots $x_1 = r$ (as defined in Eq. (1.18)) and $\bar{x}_1^{-1}$. The unique solution is thus

$$m_0(\omega) = \left(\frac{1+e^{i\omega}}{2}\right)^2\left(\frac{e^{-i\omega}-r}{1-r}\right) \tag{2.11}$$

and corresponds to the well-known *DAUB4* wavelet (see Fig. 4).

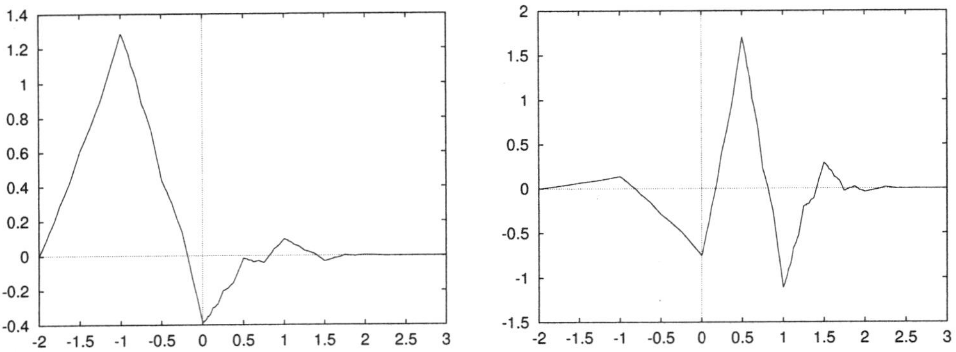

Figure 5. The real scaling function and wavelet (*DAUB6*) for J=2.

• Example $J = 2$: The polynomial $p_2(z)$ has four roots

$$x_1 = \frac{3}{2} - i\sqrt{\frac{5}{12}} - \frac{1}{2}\sqrt{\frac{10}{3} - 2i\sqrt{15}}$$
$$x_2 = \frac{3}{2} - i\sqrt{\frac{5}{12}} + \frac{1}{2}\sqrt{\frac{10}{3} - 2i\sqrt{15}}$$

and $\bar{x}_1^{-1}, \bar{x}_2^{-1}$. Two distinct cases are found: $R = \{1,2\}$ and $R = \{1\}$.

The first case

$$m_0(\omega) = \left(\frac{1+e^{i\omega}}{2}\right)^3 \left(\frac{e^{-i\omega} - x_1}{1 - x_1}\right) \left(\frac{e^{-i\omega} - x_2}{1 - x_2}\right) \tag{2.12}$$

corresponds to the *DAUB6* solution displayed in Fig. 5. The second selection of roots gives

$$m_0(\omega) = \left(\frac{1+e^{i\omega}}{2}\right)^3 \left(\frac{e^{-i\omega} - x_1}{1 - x_1}\right) \left(\frac{e^{-i\omega} - \bar{x}_2^{-1}}{1 - \bar{x}_2^{-1}}\right) \tag{2.13}$$

As anticipated by Lawton (see [1, p. 253]), this solution leads to **symmetric** but **complex-valued** scaling function and wavelet (see Fig. 6).

Such complex solutions exist for any value of J but symmetry is only possible with J **even**. In the next section we will consider a particular family of Daubechies symmetric solutions. Let us however mention the existence of the solution displayed in Fig. 7 for which $J = 6$. Two things must be noted: the functions have a small imaginary part and a real part that bears a close resemblance to the Battle–Lemarié orthogonal basis associated with the quadratic spline (see [1, p. 150]).

3. SYMMETRIC DAUBECHIES WAVELETS

The symmetry condition $\varphi(x) = \varphi(1-x)$ defines a subset of solutions corresponding to the following rule of selection for the roots in Eq. (2.10):

$$k \in R \Longleftrightarrow J - k + 1 \notin R \tag{3.1}$$

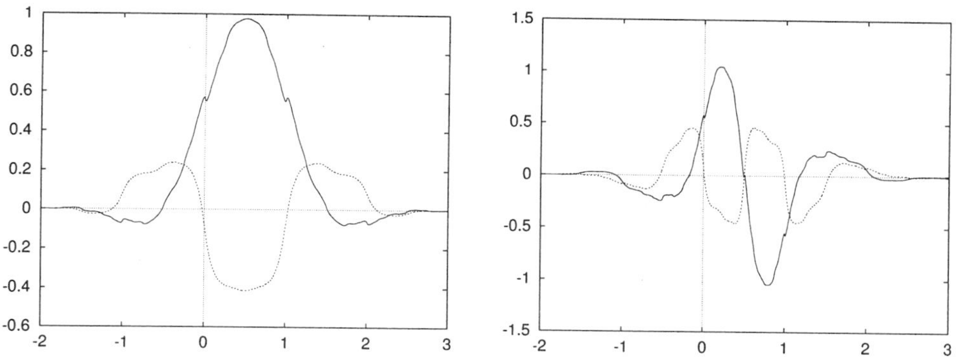

Figure 6. The complex scaling function (left) and wavelet (right) for J=2 (Imaginary part in dashed line).

We first notice that symmetry rules out the "reality" of the scaling function: all the symmetric Daubechies wavelets are complex valued and for any even value of J, $2^{\frac{J-1}{2}}$ distinct solutions exist. In the present work, we consider a particular family of solutions, the so-called SDWJ Daubechies wavelets, that correspond to the following selection of roots:

$$R = \{1, 3, 5, \dots, 2k+1, \dots, J-1\} \tag{3.2}$$

that clearly satisfies the rule (3.1). For $J = 2$, the solution (SDW2) is shown on Fig. 6. Fig. 8 and Fig. 9 display the two complex solutions for $J = 4$. SDW4 corresponds to Fig. 9.

4. THE PHASE OF SDW SCALING FUNCTION

All Symmetric Daubechies Wavelets share the usual properties of the standard *real* Daubechies bases. Writing $\varphi(x) = h(x) + ig(x)$, we investigate the relationship between the real functions h and g.

Using the Fourier representation, we consider the ratio

$$r(w) = i\frac{\hat{g}(\omega)}{\hat{h}(\omega)} \tag{4.1}$$

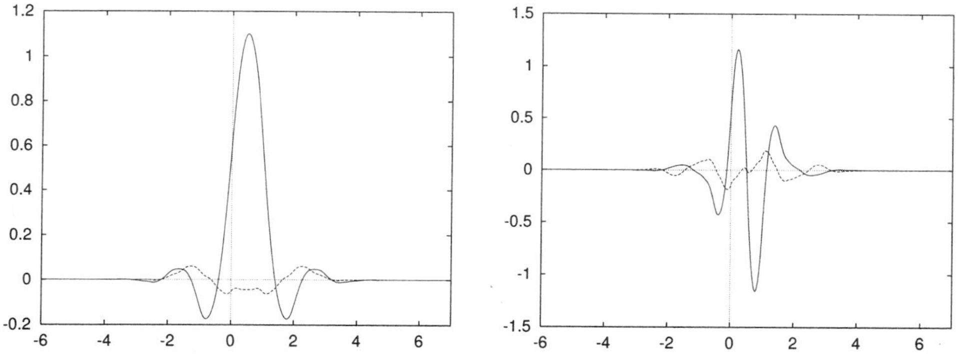

Figure 7. A complex scaling function (left) and wavelet (right) for J=6 (Imaginary part in dashed line).

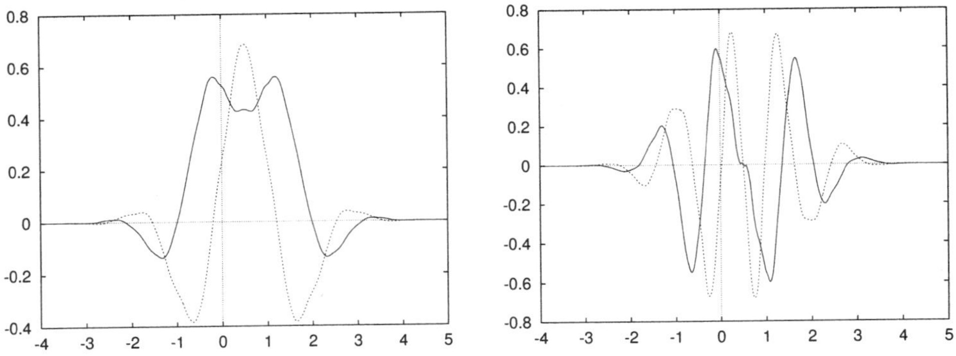

Figure 8. Complex scaling function (left) and wavelet (right) for J= 4 (Imaginary part in dashed line).

This quantity is singular at $\omega = 2\pi$ and real-valued, because of the symmetry. On Fig. 10, we plot the numerical computation of $r(\omega)$ in Log–Log scale for $J = 2,4,6$ and 8. As seen on this figure, the complex scaling function is well approximated by the expression

$$\varphi(x) \simeq (1 + i\alpha\partial_x^2)\,h(x) \tag{4.2}$$

This approximation is accurately verified on the frequency domain defined by the sampling rate of the analyzed signal. In other words, this identity is verified in the interval $[0, \pi]$ (with a sampling step renormalized to unity) when they are written in the Fourier representation.

For $J > 10$, higher derivative terms in $g(x)$ become non negligible. Let us note that $h(x)$ is further endowed with interesting vanishing moments:

$$\int dx\,h(x) = 1 \quad \text{and} \quad \int dx\,h(x)\,(x - \frac{1}{2})^m = 0 \quad \text{for} \quad m = 1,2 \text{ and } 3 \tag{4.3}$$

In the early age of the Daubechies wavelets, the introduction of vanishing moments for the scaling function led to the construction of the well-known *coiflets*. The parameter α in Eq. (4.2) can be directly computed from the filters coefficients a_k by using the first non vanishing momentum of $\varphi(x)$: writing

$$\gamma_i = \int \bar{\varphi}(x)\,x^i dx, \tag{4.4}$$

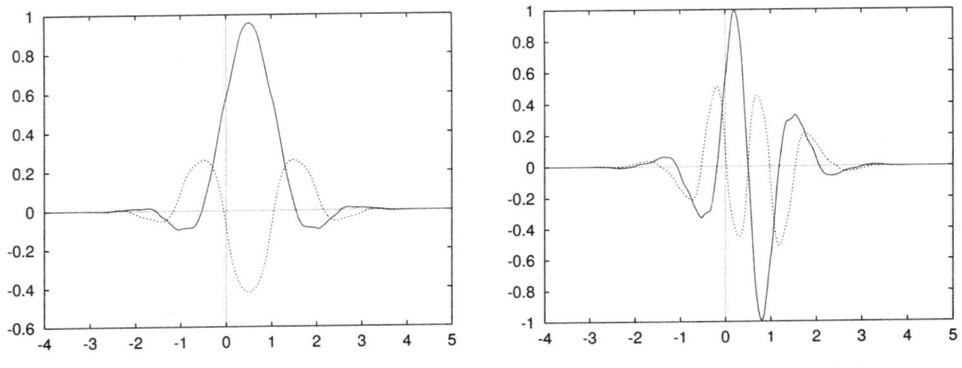

Figure 9. SDW4: scaling function (left) and wavelet (right) (Imaginary part in dashed line).

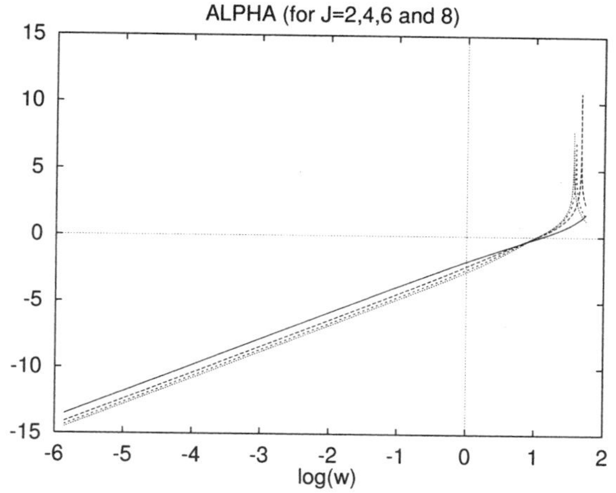

Figure 10. Left: $r(\omega)$; log-log scale. The slope of the straight lines is 2

we have

$$\gamma_i = \frac{1}{2^i - 1} \sum_{j=0}^{i-1} m_{i-j} \gamma_j, \quad \text{with} \quad m_k = \sum_{n=-J}^{J+1} n^k \bar{a}_n \quad \text{and} \quad \gamma_0 = 1 \tag{4.5}$$

Straightforward integrations by part lead to

$$\alpha = -\frac{1}{2} \Im(\gamma_2) \tag{4.6}$$

For $J = 2$ and 4, α is respectively equal to -0.164 and -0.089. We observe that Fig. 6 and Fig. 9 are consistent with Eq. (4.2).

5. THE PROJECTIONS ONTO V_J AND W_J

The discrete multiresolution analysis of f consists in the computation of the coefficients of the expansion

$$f(x) = \sum_k c_k^{j_0} \varphi_{j_0,k}(x) + \sum_{j=j_0}^{\infty} \sum_k d_k^j \psi_{j,k}(x) \tag{5.1}$$

where j_0 is a given scale (low resolution). In practice, the sum over j (the details at finest scales) is finite and f is projected onto some approximation space $V_{j_{max}}$:

$$P_{V_{j_{max}}} f(x) = \sum_k c_k^{j_{max}} \varphi_{j_{max},k}(x) \tag{5.2}$$

The coefficients in the expansion (5.1) and (5.2) are computed through the orthogonal projection of the field over the multiresolution basis:

$$c_k^j = \langle \varphi_{j,k} | f \rangle, \qquad d_k^j = \langle \psi_{j,k} | f \rangle \tag{5.3}$$

Starting with $P_{V_{jmax}}f$, the wavelet coefficients are computed with the *fast wavelet decomposition algorithm* $\mathcal{W}$ composed with the low-pass projection $V_j \to V_{j-1}$ and the high-pass projection $V_j \to W_{j-1}$:

$$c_n^{j-1} = \sqrt{2}\sum_k \bar{a}_{k-2n} c_k^j, \qquad \text{and} \qquad d_n^{j-1} = \sqrt{2}\sum_k \bar{b}_{k-2n} c_k^j \tag{5.4}$$

Conversely, any elements of V_{j-1} and of W_{j-1} can combine to give a unique vector in V_j; this reconstruction (denoted by $\mathcal{W}^{-1}$) is expressed by the inverse fast wavelet transform:

$$c_n^j = \sqrt{2}\sum_k a_{n-2k} c_k^{j-1} + \sqrt{2}\sum_k b_{n-2k} d_k^{j-1} \tag{5.5}$$

In most applications, the signal to be analyzed is real valued: the complex wavelet representation provides a redundant description of the signal. Eq. (4.2) helps in interpreting this redundancy since, using the Taylor expansion of a one dimensional field, we can estimate the real and imaginary parts of the coefficients c_k^j as

$$\begin{cases} \mathrm{Re}(c_k^j) \simeq 2^{\frac{-j}{2}} f(x_{j,k}) \\ \Im(c_k^j) \simeq \frac{\alpha}{2^{\frac{3}{2}j+1}} f''(x_{j,k}) \end{cases} \qquad \text{with} \quad x_{j,k} = \frac{2k+1}{2^{j+1}}. \tag{5.6}$$

Let us consider the estimate of the finest scale approximation of f, *i.e.*, $P_{V_{jmax}}(f)$, given a sampled function f_k. A crude approximation is simply given by $c_k^{jmax} = 2^{\frac{-j}{2}} f_k$. Denoting by $\mathrm{Re}_j \subset V_j$ the set of all function in V_j with *real* valued modes; this approximation is nothing but the orthogonal projection (denoted by $P_{\mathrm{Re}_{jmax}}$) of f onto Re_{jmax}. This corresponds to the "Mallat's initial conditions" for the fast wavelet transform. A more accurate estimate of $P_{V_{jmax}}(f)$ is obtained by using the operator

$$P_{V_{jmax}} \approx \mathcal{W} P_{\mathrm{Re}_{jmax+1}} \mathcal{W}^{-1} P_{\mathrm{Re}_{jmax}} \tag{5.7}$$

This projection gives a non trivial imaginary part for the c_k^{jmax}. As expected, they correspond to the Laplacian of the estimated real part. This is nicely illustrated in the 2d example displayed in Fig. 11.

6. MULTI-SCALE EDGE ENHANCEMENT

The bi-dimensional multiresolution analysis is built from the product of two multiresolution spaces V_i. The scaling function $\varphi(x)\varphi(y)$ generates V_0 and, complemented with three wavelets $\Psi^0(x,y) = \psi(x)\psi(y)$, $\Psi^1(x,y) = \psi(x)\varphi(y)$, $\Psi^2(x,y) = \varphi(x)\psi(y)$, it spans V_1. The functions are complex-valued. In particular, we have

$$\Phi(x,y) = \varphi(x)\varphi(y) = \Theta(x,y) + i\Psi(x,y) \tag{6.1}$$

and expansions (5.1) and (5.2) now generalize in two dimensions as

$$P_{V_{jmax}} I(x,y) = \sum_{m,n} c_{m,n}^{jmax} \Phi_{jmax,m,n}(x,y) \tag{6.2}$$

$$= \sum_{k_1,k_2} c_{k_1,k_2}^{j_0} \Phi_{j_0,k_1,k_2}(x,y) + \sum_{i=0}^{2} \sum_{j=j_0}^{jmax-1} \sum_{k_1,k_2} d_{j,k_1,k_2}^i \Psi_{j,k_1,k_2}^i(x,y) \tag{6.3}$$

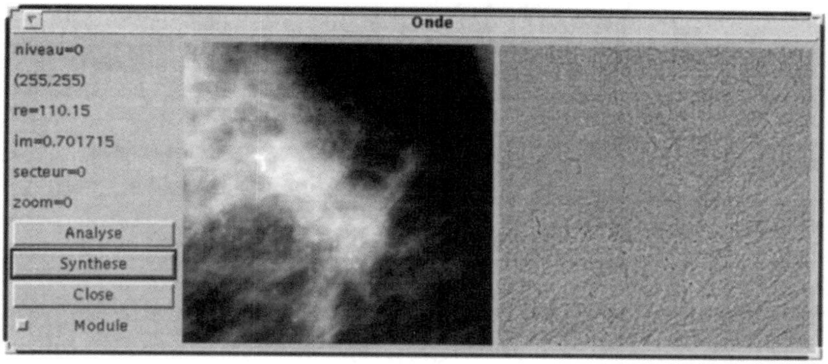

Figure 11. Projection onto V_{jmax} (The original image I is the lower image in Fig. 13); real part (left) and imaginary part (right) of $P_{V_{jmax}} I$.

where $\Phi_{j,k_1,k_2}(x,y) = 2^j\Phi(2^jx - k_1, 2^jy - k_2)$ and $\Psi^i_{j,k_1,k_2}(x,y) = 2^j\Psi^i(2^jx - k_1, 2^jy - k_2)$ span the spaces V_j and W^i_j respectively such that $V_{j+1} = V_j \oplus W^0_j \oplus W^1_j \oplus W^2_j$. In the sequel, we denote by $\mathcal{W}^N$ the N-levels wavelet transform

$$\{c^{j_{max}}_{m,n}\} \xrightarrow{\mathcal{W}^N} \{c^{j_{max}-N}_{m,n}, \mathbf{d}_{j_{max}-N,m,n}, \mathbf{d}_{j_{max}-2,m,n}, \ldots \mathbf{d}_{j_{max}-1,m,n}\}$$

where $\mathbf{d} = (d^0, d^1, d^2)$. Fig. 11 shows an example of the projection $P_{V_{jmax}}(I)$ (as defined by Eq. (5.7)) for a specific detail within a mammography. Fig. 12 displays the modulus of the complex wavelet coefficients (and the $c^{j0}_{k_1,k_2}$'s in the upper left corner).

The real and imaginary parts of the scaling function are

$$\begin{cases} \Theta(x,y) = h(x)h(y) - g(x)g(y) \simeq G(x,y) \\ \Psi(x,y) = h(x)g(y) + g(x)h(y) \simeq \alpha \triangle G(x,y) \end{cases} \tag{6.4}$$

where $G(x,y)$ denotes the real smoothing kernel $h(x)h(y)$. On one hand, the real part of the 2-d scaling function is close (because $\alpha^2 << 1$) to the smoothing kernel $G(x,y)$ while, on the other hand, the imaginary part is proportional to the Laplacian of $G(x,y)$: $\Psi(x,y)$ is thus the "Marr wavelet" [8] associated with $\Theta(x,y) \simeq G(x,y)$.

Since the real and imaginary parts of the wavelet transform coefficients of some *real* image correspond to the convolution of the original field with the real part and the imaginary part of $\Phi_{j,m,n}(x,y)$ respectively, we then have access to the (multiscaled) smoothed Laplacian of the image:

$$\begin{cases} h^j_{k_1,k_2} = \mathrm{Re}(c^j_{k_1,k_2}) = 2^jI(x,y) * G(2^jx - k_1, 2^jy - k_2) \\ g^j_{k_1,k_2} = \Im(c^j_{k_1,k_2}) = -\frac{\alpha}{2^j}\Delta I(x,y) * G(2^jx - k_1, 2^jy - k_2) \end{cases} \tag{6.5}$$

The simultaneous presence of a smoothing kernel and its Laplacian in the complex scaling function can be exploited to define some elementary operations on the wavelet coefficients. In other words, we use this information to synthesize a *new* image that corresponds to some prescribed operation. A typical example is de-noising; this application is among the most successful applications of wavelets. Here, we investigate the *edge enhancement*.

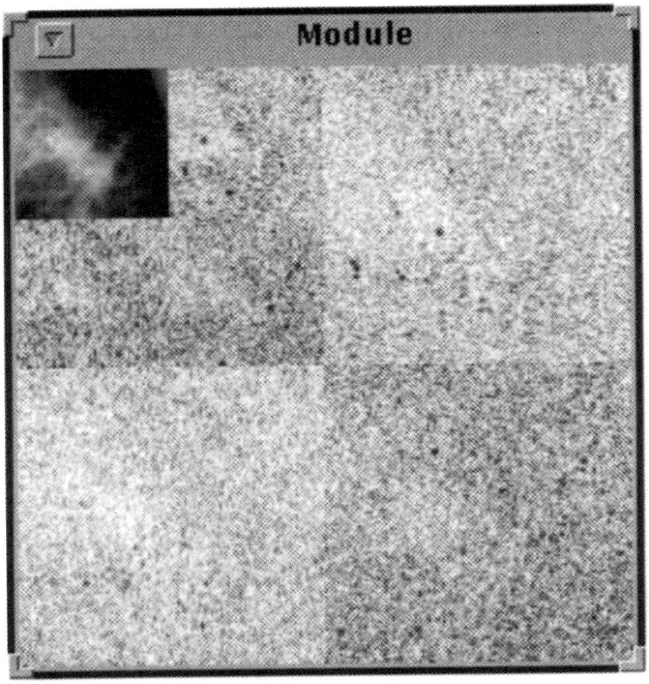

Figure 12. Modulus of the complex wavelet coefficients (SDW4, N=2).

Let us consider the sharpening operator, $I \to \tilde{I} = I - \rho \triangle I$. It can be implemented at any scale $j \leq j_{max}$ through

$$c^j_{m,n} \to \mathcal{S}_j(c^j_{m,n}) = c^j_{m,n} + \frac{\rho_j}{2^{2(j_{max}-j)}\alpha} g^j_{m,n} \tag{6.6}$$

where ρ_j is a small parameter. Eq. (6.6) defines an operator in V_j: to map it on the wavelet coefficients, we consider a *modified wavelet decomposition* operator, $\tilde{\mathcal{W}}_j$, defined by

$$\tilde{\mathcal{W}}_j = \mathcal{W}\mathcal{S}_j \tag{6.7}$$

The N-levels sharpening operator is then defined by

$$\mathcal{S} = \mathcal{W}^{-N}\tilde{\mathcal{W}}_N\tilde{\mathcal{W}}_{N-1}\dots\tilde{\mathcal{W}}_1 \tag{6.8}$$

Fig. 13 shows an example of such a processing with *SDW*4 and $N = 3$. In comparison with the original image (bottom:low-resolution, low-contrast mammographic image), the local contrast has been improved significantly. Let us mention that other efficient multiscale sharpening transformations have been proposed in the recent past [9]. The main difference here in the present work is the orthogonality property of the SDW transform and the use of the phase of a complex basis. We recall that the SDW bases are not derived from a representation that allows specific enhancements. On the contrary, we have shown that the Laplacian was inherent to this particular orthogonal basis.

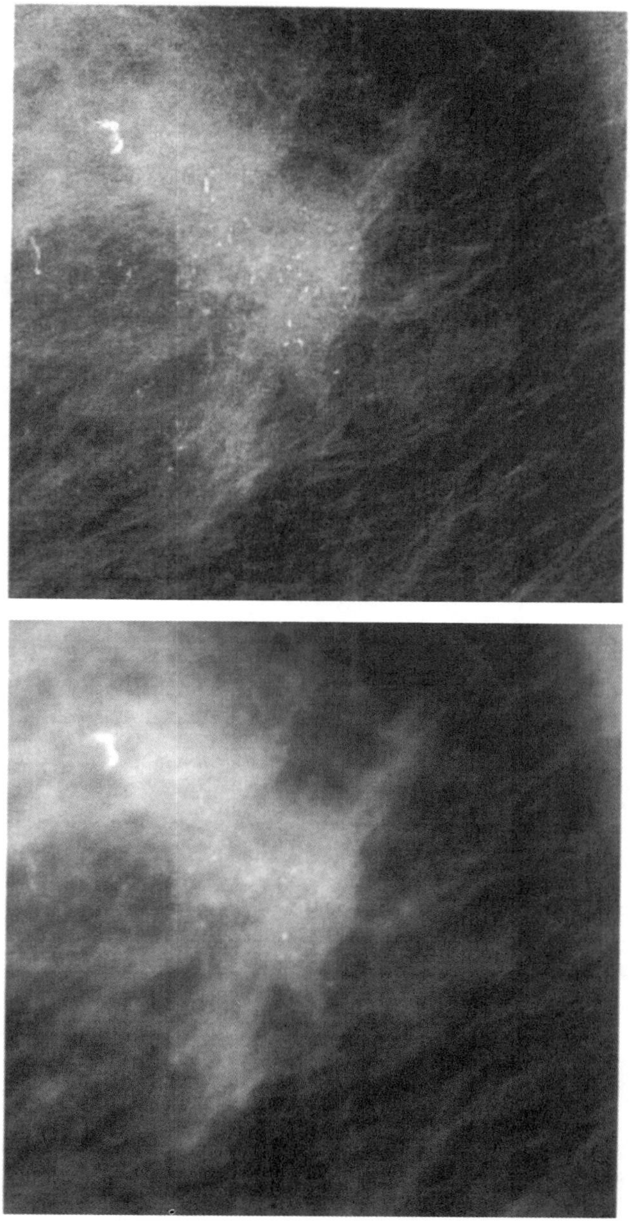

Figure 13. Image Enhancement: The test image (bottom) is a region of a digitized mammography. The upper image has been synthesized using $\mathcal{S}$ with SDW4 and N=3.

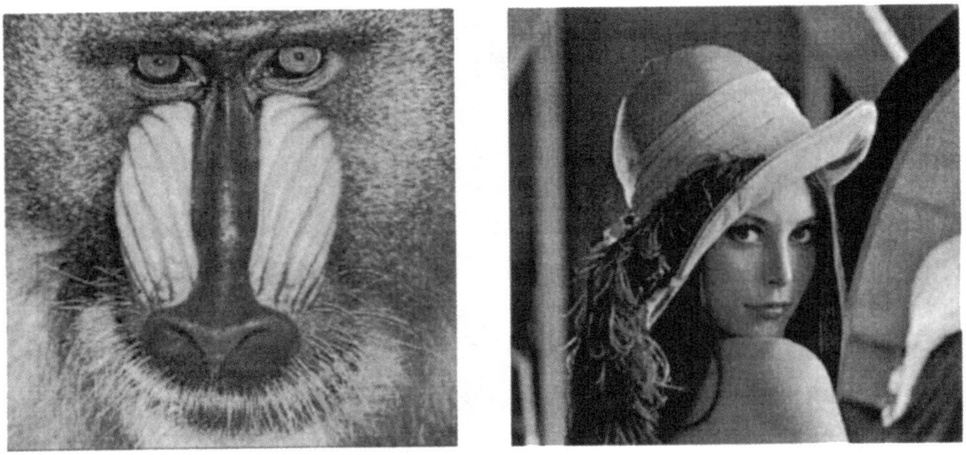

Figure 14. Original images: A (left) and B (right).

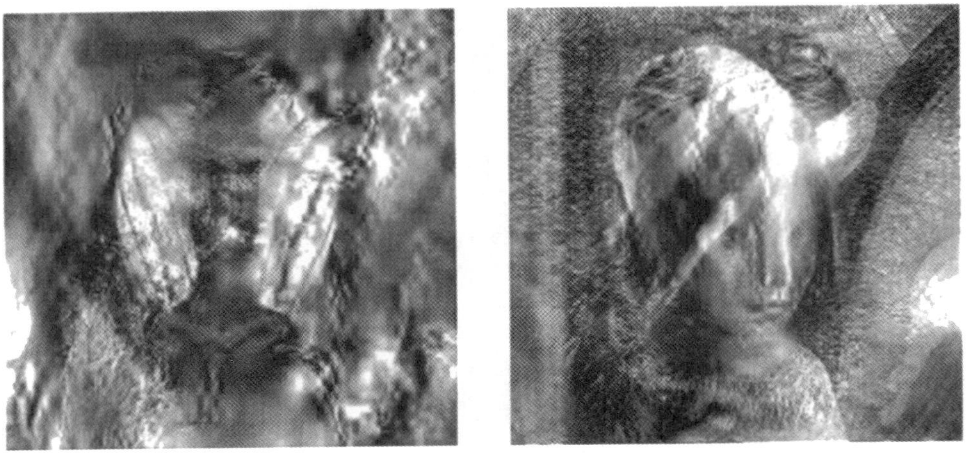

Figure 15. Left (respectively right): wavelet synthesis with the phases of $\mathcal{W}$(A) (resp. B) and modulus of $\mathcal{W}$(B) (resp. A). (SDW4 and 5 levels).

7. CONCLUSION

Investigation of the full set of Daubechies wavelets has shown the existence of a huge subset of complex valued multiresolution analyses. Beside the importance of symmetry endowed by some of those bases, we unveil interesting properties of the phase of the scaling function, as in Eq. (4.2). It is worth mentioning that a similar result is also valid for complex wavelets. The "role of the phase" [11] is certainly most intriguing problem in the present context of unconditional bases. First, superiority of multiwavelets on standard wavelets in some applications may be extended to complex wavelets in view of the obvious relationship of complex wavelets and multiwavelets. Second, we can reproduce the famous experiment of "restoration of signal from the phase only" [12]. Let us recall that the issue of the role of the phase in signals is a standard problem in the Fourier representation. Since complex Daubechies wavelets are not analytic, there is not direct equivalence between the Fourier and wavelets as to the meaning and the role of the phase. However, similar observations are possible. For instance, if we consider two signals, say A and B as the two images displayed in Fig. 14, we can synthesize two images by permuting the modulus of the wavelet coefficients of A and B. As shown in Fig. 15, an image can be mostly recognized from its wavelet phases. Such a result also exists in Fourier [11] and various works have described how to restore the initial image from the phase only [13]. Using a different constraint to do so, the same restoration with alternate projections onto convex sets can be designed within the complex multiresolution framework [14]. Setting $P_{V_0}I$ as initial condition, this iterative algorithm reconstructs the details of the image but the noise: empirically at least, the phase of wavelet coefficients seems to be sensitive to the coherent (both in space and scale) structures present in the signals. The role of the modulus of the coefficient is better understood: robust estimation algorithms based on amplitude shrinkage have been designed for removing noise [15,16]. The module somehow weights the information contained in the phase. We must recall here the particular role of the modulus of the coefficients for computing the norm in Besov spaces [15]. The enhancement algorithm discussed at the end of this paper illustrates this point nicely. We modify the information of the initial image by changing mostly the phase of wavelet coefficients. Let us remark that the modulus of coefficients are "monitoring" the smoothness of the signal: a more adaptive sharpening operator with robustness against noise is presently under investigation. Complex scaling functions also raise the important problem of the local regularity of multi-self-similar functions. As illustrated by Eq. (4.2), the real and imaginary part of *SDW*'s scaling functions hold quite different regularities. Further mathematical investigations of this interesting point are currently pursued.

The author wants to thank B. Goulard and P. Turcotte for providing precious advise and help. This work was supported in part by the Natural Sciences and Engineering Research Council (NSERC) of Canada.

REFERENCES

1. I. Daubechies, *Ten lectures on Wavelets*, SIAM, CBMS Series, 1992.
2. C. Chui, *An Introduction to Wavelets*, Academic Press, New York, 1992.
3. A. Cohen, *Ondelettes, analyses multirésolutions et filtres miroir en quadrature*, Ann. Inst. H. Poicaré, An. non linéaire, 7, p. 439, 1990.
4. J. Stromberg, "A modified Franklin system and higher order spline systems on $\mathbb{R}^n$ as unconditional bases for Hardy spaces," Conf. in honor of A. Zygmund, Vol. II, Wadsworth math. series, p. 475, (1982).

5. G. Battle, "A block spin construction of ondelettes. Part I: Lemarié functions," Comm. Math. Phys., 110, p. 601 (1987); P. G. Lemarié, "Une nouvelle base d'ondelettes de $L^2(\mathbb{R}^n)$," J. de Math. Pures et Appl., 67, p. 227, (1988).
6. G. Fix and G. Strang, *Fourier Analysis of the finite element method in Ritz–Galerkin theory*, Stud. Appl. Math., 48, p. 265, 1969.
7. I. Daubechies, "Orthonormal bases of compactly supported wavelets," Comm. Pure Appl. Math., vol.41, p. 909–996, 1988.
8. D. Marr and E. Hildreth, "Theory of edge detection," Proc. Royal So. London, vol.207, p. 187–217, 1980.
9. A. F. Laine, S. Schuler, J. Fan and W. Huda, "Mammographic Feature Enhancement by Multiscale Analysis," IEEE Transactions on Medical Imaging vol. 13, pp. 725–740, 1994; J. Lu, D. M. Healy Jr. and J. B. Weaver, "Contrast Enhancement of Medical Images Using Multiscale Edge Representation," SPIE vol. 2242 Wavelet Applications, pp. 711–719, 1994; L. Gagnon,
10. M. Lina and B. Goulard, "Sharpening Enhancement of Digitalized Mammograms with Complex Symmetric Daubechies Wavelets," 17th IEEE and EMBS Conf., Montreal, Sept. 1995.
11. A. V. Oppenheim and J. S. Li, "The importance of phase in signals," Proc. IEEE, vol.69, p. 529–541, 1981.
12. M. Hayes, "The reconstruction of a multidimensional sequence from the phase or magnitude of its Fourier transform," IEEE Trans. ASSP, vol.30, p. 140–154, 1982.
13. A. Levi and H. Stark, "Signal restoration from phase by projections onto convex sets," J. Opt. soc. Am., vol.73, p. 810–822, 1983.
14. J.-M. Lina and P. Drouilly, "The Importance of the Phase of the Symmetric Daubechies Wavelets Representation of Signals," Proc. IWISP'96, Mertzios et al. ed., Elsevier, p. 61, 1996; P. Drouilly, M. Sc Thesis, Physics Dept and CRM, Univ. of Montreal, 1996.
15. R. De Vore and B. J. Lucier, "Fast wavelet techniques for near-optimal image processing," Proc. 1992 IEEE Military Commun. Conf., IEEE Communications Soc., NY 1992.
16. D. Donoho and I. Johnstone, "Adapting to unknown smoothness via wavelet shrinkage," to be published in J. Amer. Statist. Assoc., 1995 (and reference therein).

8

EDGE-PRESERVING REGULARIZATION FOR QUANTITATIVE RECONSTRUCTION ALGORITHMS IN MICROWAVE IMAGING

Pierre Lobel,[1]* Christian Pichot,[1] Laure Blanc-Féraud,[2] and Michel Barlaud[2]

[1]Laboratoire d'Electronique
Antennes et Télécommunications
Université de Nice-Sophia Antipolis/CNRS
Bât 4, 250 rue Albert Einstein, 06560 Valbonne (France)
[2]Laboratoire d'Informatique
Signaux et Systèmes de Sophia Antipolis
Université de Nice-Sophia Antipolis/CNRS
Bât 4, 250 rue Albert Einstein, 06560 Valbonne (France)

1. INTRODUCTION

The inverse scattering problem in microwave imaging is considered in this paper. It involves the reconstruction of the complex contrast profile of an inhomogeneous object. This object is illuminated by several excitations of an incident electromagnetic wave, and the values of the scattered field are then measured on a set of receivers. From these data, the complex contrast profile of the object can be reconstructed. But this problem is nonlinear and ill-posed in the sense of Hadamard [1]: the existence, uniqueness and stability of the solution is not simultaneously ensured. The first algorithms used to solve this problem belong to the so-called "qualitative reconstruction algorithms" or spectral methods such as diffraction tomography [2, 3]. They involve the use of backpropagation techniques and allow quasi-real time or very fast computation, but their limitations [4] have stimulated the development of spatial iterative methods or so-called "quantitative reconstruction algorithms" [5–12]. These methods are more sophisticated and need more computations but provide solutions with a better spatial resolution. In general, they involve the iterative minimization of a cost functional.

Two different methods are proposed in this paper. The first one linearizes the cost functional by using a Newton–Kantorovich (NK) algorithm [7]. This method also needs a Tikhonov (TK) regularization procedure to converge, and is delicate to bring into operation with noisy data [13]. In the second method, starting from the integral representation of the

*Current address: Fachbereich 9 Mathematik, Saarlandes University, Geb. 38, Zi. 103, Postf. 151150, D-66041 Saarbruecken (Germany

Inverse Problems, Tomography, and Image Processing, edited by Ramm,
Plenum Press, New York, 1998

electric field, and applying a moment method solution, we deal with a unique nonlinear relation between the scattered field and the contrast. The resulting cost functional is minimized using a Conjugate Gradient (CG) method [12].

However, working with strongly noisy data or trying to reconstruct objects with large contrast values, can degrade the quality of the reconstruction and in some cases, can prevent the convergence of the algorithms. The knowledge of the direct problem is not sufficient to determine a satisfactory solution. Consequently, a new Edge-Preserving (EP) regularization scheme is proposed by adding *a priori* information to the solution and modeling the object to be reconstructed with homogeneous areas separated by borderlike discontinuities. This regularization procedure was successfully applied to the CG algorithm and the enhancement has been demonstrated both from noisy synthetic data [15], and from the experimental data known as the *Ipswich data* [14–16]*. We propose in this paper to apply the EP regularization on the NK method and then to illustrate the enhancement throughout a reconstruction obtained from synthetic noisy data. The influence of the regularization parameters on the solution is also shown and finally, we discuss the choice of the regularization parameters.

2. THE FORWARD PROBLEM

The cylindrical object characterized by a complex contrast $c(r)$ (r is a position vector), is contained in a bounded region $\mathcal{D}$ and illuminated successively by L different incident TM plane waves e_l^I, $l \in [1,L]$. The M receivers are located in the domain $\mathcal{S}$ in the far-field region. For each excitation l, and for $r \in \mathcal{D}$, the forward scattering problem may be formulated as the following domain integral equation

$$\begin{aligned} e_l(r) &= e_l^I(r) + \int_{\mathcal{D}} k_0^2 c(r') e_l(r') G(r-r') dr', \; r \in \mathcal{D} \\ &= e_l^I(r) + G^{\mathcal{D}} c e_l(r), \; r \in \mathcal{D}, \end{aligned} \tag{2.1}$$

and integral representation for the scattered field

$$\begin{aligned} e_l^{\mathcal{S}}(s_{lm}) &= \int_{\mathcal{D}} k_0^2 c(r') e_l(r') G(s_{lm}-r') dr', \; s_{lm} \in \mathcal{S} \\ &= G^{\mathcal{S}} c e_l(s_{lm}), \; s_{lm} \in \mathcal{S}, \end{aligned} \tag{2.2}$$

where s_{lm} is the position vector of each receiver and for each excitation, k_0 is the wavenumber of the background medium and $G^{\mathcal{D}}$ and $G^{\mathcal{S}}$ are two integral operators mapping respectively $L^2(\mathcal{D})$ into itself, and $L^2(\mathcal{D})$ into $L^2(\mathcal{S})$ (the notation $L^2(\cdot)$ represents the square integrable functions in $\cdot$). The operators $G^{\mathcal{D}}$ and $G^{\mathcal{S}}$ both involve the 2D free space Green's function

$$G(r-r') = \frac{i}{4} H_0^{(1)}\left(k_0|r-r'|\right). \tag{2.3}$$

The direct problem is solved using the method of moment (MoM) with pulse basis functions and point matching, which transforms the integral equations (2.1) and (2.2), into the

*Measured data provided by Rome Laboratory, Electromagnetics & Reliability Directorate, 31 Grenier Street, Hanscom AFB, MA 01731-3010.

following matrix equations

$$\begin{cases} E^I &= \left(I - G^{\mathcal{D}} C\right) E \\ E^{\mathcal{S}} &= G^{\mathcal{S}} C E \end{cases} \tag{2.4}$$

where the rectangular image (or test domain) containing the region $\mathcal{D}$ is discretized into $N = N_{lin} \times N_{col}$ elementary square cells. Let us denote c to be the $N_{lin} \times N_{col}$ contrast matrix and $C = \text{diag}(c)$ the $N \times N$ diagonal matrix associated with c. The matrix system (2.4) can be also formulated as a nonlinear equation in C [12]

$$E^{\mathcal{S}} = G^{\mathcal{S}} C \left(I - G^{\mathcal{D}} C\right)^{-1} E^I = G^{\mathcal{S}} C \mathcal{L}(C) E^I = \mathcal{F}(C) \tag{2.5}$$

3. THE FORWARD PROBLEM

3.1. The Newton–Kantorovich (NK) Algorithm

The matrix system to be solved is strongly nonlinear and ill-posed. The Newton–Kantorovich method builds up an iterative solution of the inverse problem, by solving successively the direct problem and a local linear inverse problem [7, 17, 18]. At each iteration, an estimate of the complex contrast function c is given by

$$c^{i+1} = \Delta c + c^i, \tag{3.1}$$

where Δc is an update correction obtained by solving in the least squares sense, the linearized forward problem

$$D \Delta c = e^{\mathcal{S}} - \mathcal{F}(c^i) = \Delta e^{\mathcal{S}}, \tag{3.2}$$

where $e^{\mathcal{S}}$ represents the measured data vector*, and the matrix D is a linearized version of the nonlinear operator relating the scattered field to the contrast function c,

$$D = \frac{\partial \mathcal{F}(c^i)}{\partial c^i}, \tag{3.3}$$

The scattered field vector $\mathcal{F}(c^i)$ is calculated through the forward problem solver, with a previous estimate of c. Unfortunately, the problem of finding the solution of equation (3.2) is ill-posed and needs some regularization. For this, we use a Tikhonov (TK) regularization procedure and minimize the functional

$$J_{NK}(c) = \left\| \Delta e^{\mathcal{S}} - D \Delta c \right\|_{\mathcal{S}}^2 + \lambda \left\| R \Delta c \right\|_{\mathcal{D}}^2, \tag{3.4}$$

where R is the regularization matrix and λ a regularization parameter, chosen according to an empirical formula [7] or with the General Cross Validation method [13, 19]. Two regularization operators R have already been used: an identity operator and a gradient-by-zone operator. The gradient-by-zone operator is based, first, on the assumption that the object is composed of homogeneous zones of arbitrary geometry, separated by borderlike discontinuities, and second, on the notion of neighborhood for each elementary cell of the image [20].

*For sake of simplicity, we note the fields with lower-case letters when they have to be used as vectors and in upper-case letters when they have to used as matrices.

3.2. The Conjugate Gradient (CG) Algorithm

The CG method minimizes the functional obtained from (2.5) and applied for each excitation l [12]

$$J_{CG}(C) = \sum_{l=1}^{L} \|\rho_l(C)\|_{\mathcal{S}}^2, \tag{3.5}$$

where

$$\rho_l(C) = e_l^{\mathcal{S}} - \mathcal{F}_l(C). \tag{3.6}$$

A conjugate gradient method is then used to minimize (3.5), with the iterative procedure

$$c^{i+1} = c^i + \alpha^i p^i, \tag{3.7}$$

where p^i is the update direction and α^i is a complex parameter (weight factor). The value of α^i is found, using a first order approximation and minimizing $J_{CG}(C^{i+1})$ according to α^i. Three different update directions p^i have been studied. First, *the backpropagation of the error*, using the adjoint (or conjugate transpose) operator $G^{\mathcal{S}^*}$ of $G^{\mathcal{S}}$. Second, *the gradient direction*, and finally *the Polak–Ribière conjugate gradient direction* [21]. As the third gives better results in terms of convergence and stability than the other directions, we choose to use it in all our experiments.

3.3. Discussion on NK and Gradient Algorithms

We want to present the NK and gradient algorithms using terminology which reveals their similarities and differences.

For the NK method, if we minimize (3.2) in the least squares sense, we obtain

$$D^* D \Delta c = D^* \Delta e^{\mathcal{S}}, \tag{3.8}$$

where the matrix D is defined in (3.3). To first order approximation, D takes the following form:

$$D = \begin{pmatrix} D_1 \\ D_2 \\ \vdots \\ D_L \end{pmatrix}, \tag{3.9}$$

with

$$D_l = G^{\mathcal{S}} \left(I - CG^{\mathcal{D}}\right)^{-1} e_l, \ \forall l \in [1, L]. \tag{3.10}$$

So, the iterative sequence for the NK algorithm without any regularization using (3.1), (3.2) and (3.8) is

$$c^{i+1} = c^i - (D^* D)^{-1} D^* (\mathcal{F}(c^i) - e^{\mathcal{S}}) \tag{3.11}$$

For the gradient method, the iterative sequence from (3.7) is [12]

$$c^{i+1} = c^i - 2\alpha^i D^*(\mathcal{F}(c^i) - e^{\mathcal{S}}) \tag{3.12}$$

We can obtain these 2 expressions from the general definitions of the NK and gradient methods

- Newton–Kantorovich

$$c^{i+1} = c^i - H^{-1}\nabla J(c^i), \tag{3.13}$$

where H is the Hessian of J ($H = \frac{\partial}{\partial c^i}\nabla J(c^i)$)

- Gradient method

$$c^{i+1} = c^i - \alpha^i \nabla J(c^i), \tag{3.14}$$

by setting $J = J_{CG}$ (see eq. (3.5)), which implies that the gradient of J is

$$\nabla J(c^i) = 2D^*(\mathcal{F}(c^i) - e^{\mathcal{S}}), \tag{3.15}$$

and the Hessian is

$$H = \frac{\partial}{\partial c^i}\left[2D^*(\mathcal{F}(c^i) - e^{\mathcal{S}})\right] \approx 2D^*D \tag{3.16}$$

As the Hessian is generally ill-conditioned for the cases we have studied, the NK method cannot be used without any regularization procedure (see eq. (3.4)).

4. THE EDGE-PRESERVING (EP) REGULARIZATION

4.1. Description of the Method

For highly contrasted objects, and/or with noisy data, the ill-posedness of the inverse scattering problem becomes more severe. Some *a priori* information is needed in order to reconstruct a stable solution. We choose a piecewise constant solution. From general point of view, the additional information takes the form of the following regularization term in the cost functional

$$\lambda \int_{\mathcal{D}} \varphi(|\nabla c(r)|)dr, \tag{4.1}$$

where λ is the regularization parameter fixing the influence of the regularization term above the data term, and φ is a real function, defined on $[0,+\infty[$, and called the regularizing function. Choosing $\varphi(t) = t^2$, yields to the well-known Tikhonov (TK) regularization, which produces oversmooth solutions, while choosing $\varphi(t) = t$, yields to the Total Variation criterion [22,23]. We propose to use a φ function defined in order to perform an isotropic smoothing in the homogeneous areas of the image (corresponding to small gradients), while preserving edges (corresponding to high gradients) [15,24–29]. From a study of the derivative of (4.1) given by

$$-\nabla\cdot\left(\frac{\varphi'(|\nabla c(r)|)}{|\nabla c(r)|}\nabla c(r)\right), \tag{4.2}$$

it is found that three main conditions for the function $\frac{\varphi'(t)}{t}$ must be satisfied [27,29,30]

1. $\lim_{t\to 0}\frac{\varphi'(t)}{t} = M < \infty$: isotropic smoothing in homogeneous areas.

2. $\lim_{t\to\infty}\frac{\varphi'(t)}{t} = 0$: preservation of edges.

3. $\frac{\varphi'(t)}{t}$ strictly decreasing: to avoid instabilities in the reconstruction algorithm.

Several φ functions have been proposed in the literature [24–27], and we used the *Hebert and Leahy* φ_{HL} function [25] for computing the reconstructions presented in this paper. φ_{HL} is defined by

$$\varphi_{HL}(t) = \log(1+t^2) \tag{4.3}$$

This function is non convex and fits well for peacewise constant profile objects.

4.2. Application to the CG Algorithm

The cost functional (3.5) becomes after introducing the EP regularization

$$J_{CG}^{EP}(C) = \sum_{l=1}^{L}\|\rho_l(C)\|^2 + \sum_{p=1}^{N_{lin}}\sum_{q=1}^{N_{col}}\lambda_R^2\,\varphi\left(\frac{1}{\delta_R}\|\mathrm{Re}(\nabla c)_{p,q}\|\right) + \sum_{p=1}^{N_{lin}}\sum_{q=1}^{N_{col}}\lambda_I^2\,\varphi\left(\frac{1}{\delta_I}\|\Im(\nabla c)_{p,q}\|\right) \tag{4.4}$$

Dealing with the reconstruction of a complex matrix, we consider the real and imaginary parts of the contrast as independent in the regularization scheme. In fact, there is no link in the structure between the real and imaginary parts of the permittivity. Thus, the edge-preserving regularization term is applied separately on the real and imaginary parts of the contrast. The weighting parameters λ_R and λ_I fix the influence of the regularization term versus the difference between the scattered field and the data, and the parameters δ_R and δ_I fix the threshold level on the gradient norm above which a discontinuity is preserved and under which it is smoothed.

The regularization terms are non quadratic in c, and in order to avoid additional instabilities an new formulation of the cost functional is proposed in [15], with a half-quadratic regularization term. An alternate minimization is then performed both on c and an edge variable b which map the edges of the image.

4.3. Application to the NK Algorithm

As defined in (3.4), the NK method involves the minimization of a cost functional with respect to Δc. So in order to apply this kind of regularization to the NK method, we must introduce an additional hypothesis.

Hypothesis. *Starting the NK iteration from an initial guess with constant value, the evolution of the contrast between two successive iterations will be homogeneous in each piecewise constant zone of the contrast.*

Based on this hypothesis, we can now introduce the EP regularization in the NK method, with respect to Δc.

$$J_{NK}^{EP}(\Delta c) = \left\|\Delta e^{\mathcal{S}} - D.\Delta c\right\|_{\mathcal{S}}^{2} + \sum_{p=1}^{N_{lin}}\sum_{q=1}^{N_{col}} \lambda_R^2\, \varphi\left(\frac{1}{\delta_R}\left\|\mathrm{Re}\left[\nabla(\Delta c)\right]_{p,q}\right\|\right) + \sum_{p=1}^{N_{lin}}\sum_{q=1}^{N_{col}} \lambda_I^2\, \varphi\left(\frac{1}{\delta_I}\left\|\Im\left[\nabla(\Delta c)\right]_{p,q}\right\|\right) \quad (4.5)$$

In order to minimize this cost functional, we apply a conjugate gradient algorithm (with a Polak–Ribière descent direction [21]) on Δc.

5. NUMERICAL AND EXPERIMENTAL RESULTS

5.1. Reconstruction from Numerical Data (NK+EP)

We have tested the NK+EP algorithm with a synthetic square cylinder (surrounded by 13 receivers), of complex permittivity 1.8 surrounded by free space. The domain $\mathcal{D}$ is discretized into 13×13 subsquares of 2 mm^2. This object is illuminated by an incident wave of 2.45 GHz under 13 view angles. We corrupt the scattered data with Gaussian noise of about 10% of the maximum value of the scattered field. In Fig. 1 we show the reconstructions obtained with the CG algorithm (without any regularization), and with the NK algorithm (with TK and EP regularizations).

The reconstruction obtained with the NK+EP algorithm is enhanced with regard to the reconstruction obtained with the NK+TK algorithm. The CG algorithm also gives a good solution. The convergence of these 3 methods is shown in Fig. 2. We can see that the NK+TK method diverges very rapidly while the EP regularization gives a more stable convergence. But we also wish to emphasize the fact that for the NK+TK method, we did not use in these experiments a regularization parameter calculated using the cross validation method [13].

5.2. Reconstruction from Experimental Data (CG+EP)

The scattered fields were collected for six incident angles $\theta_I \in \{0°, 60°, 120°, 180°, 240°, 300°\}$, over an observation sector $\theta_I + 180° \leq \theta_S \leq \theta_I + 355°$, with a sample spacing $\Delta\theta_S = 0.5°$ [14]. The known dielectric target is a lossless polystyrene square cylinder with $\epsilon_r = 1.03$ and side equal to 11.2 cm. We use a domain $\mathcal{D}$ divided into 29×29 subsquares of 5.3×5.3 mm^2. Using *a priori* information about the geometry of the target, we symmetrize

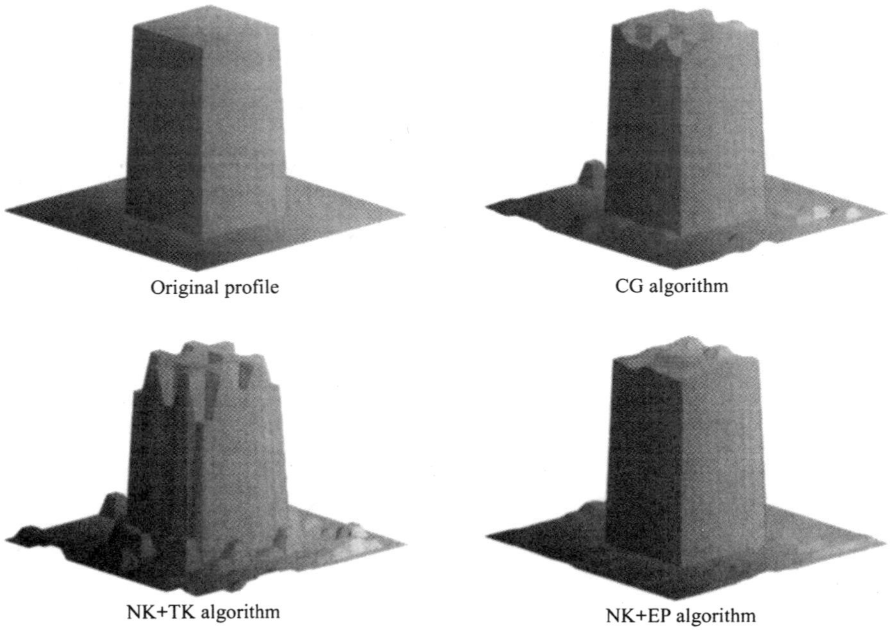

Figure 1. Reconstructions from noisy corrupted synthetic data using NK algorithm with EP regularization

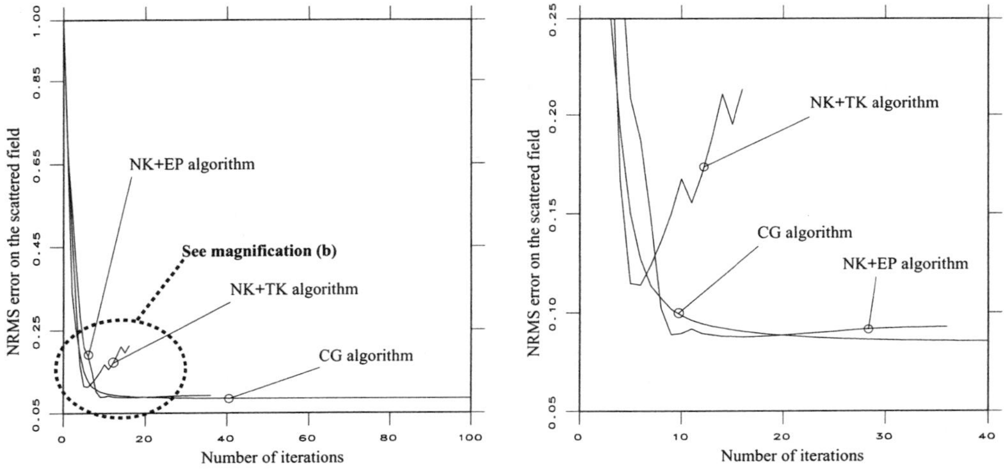

(a) Comparisons of the convergence for different reconstruction algorithms GC, NK+TK et NK+EP

(b) Magnification for the 3 algorithms

Figure 2. Convergences of the 3 algorithms

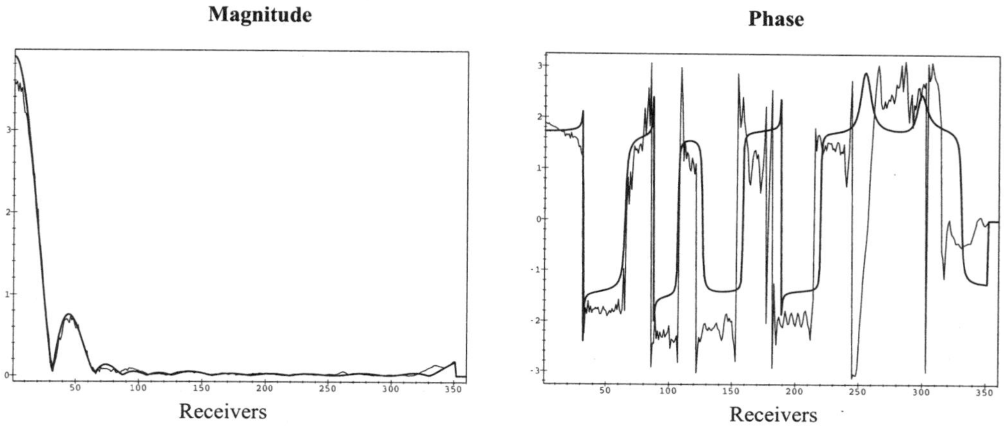
Magnitude
Phase
Receivers
Receivers

Figure 3. Comparison between a cross section of the measured scattered field and the simulated one

the object during the iterative reconstruction. We show in Fig. 3 a comparison between a cross section of the measured scattered field and the simulated one. We can see that the error in the phase is severe.

A comparative study has been made on results obtained without any regularization, with a Tikhonov regularization and with our EP regularization scheme (Fig. 4). In these different results, no initial guess was used, i.e., the starting value is zero contrast and the iterative process is stopped at the same degree of convergence. The reconstruction without regularization shows a blurred profile with a rough shape. The use of Tikhonov regularization smoothes the profile and the edges are not preserved. The new regularization scheme improves the performance of the conjugate gradient algorithm: the edges are clearly preserved while the homogeneous areas are smoothed (the average value found for the permittivity of the polystyrene is 1.029).

5.3. Influence of the Regularization Parameters

In order to illustrate the influence of the EP regularization parameters (λ and δ), we reconstruct with the CG+EP method a synthetic object shown in Fig. 5. The computed scattered field is corrupted with Gaussian noise of about 10% of the maximum value of the scattered field.

In Fig. 6, we can see the influence of choosing small and high values for the λ (λ_R and λ_I) and δ (δ_R and δ_I) parameters.

From these results, it appears that a proper choice of the parameters is crucial in the

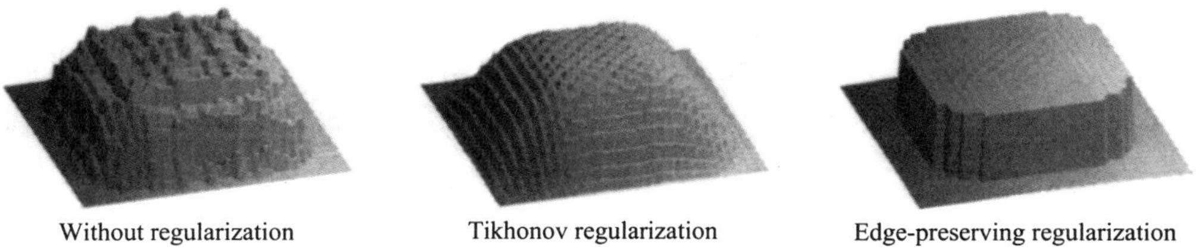
Without regularization
Tikhonov regularization
Edge-preserving regularization

Figure 4. Reconstructions of a polystyrene square cylinder using CG algorithm with EP regularization

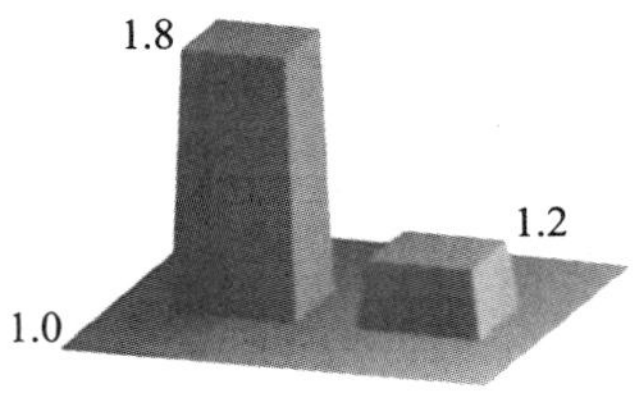

Figure 5. Original profile

regularization scheme. Choosing values which are too small or too high can lead respectively to rough or oversmoothed solutions (the peak at 1.2 has completely disappeared in Fig. 6-a). Thus, when high values of λ are chosen, the regularization term will constrain the solution to be smoothed (especially if the initial guess of the iterative reconstruction algorithm has the value of zero-contrast). Choosing high values of δ leads to high threshold levels (small or medium variations in the image are smoothed), while choosing small values of δ leads to small threshold levels (small variations such as noise peaks are detected and preserved instead of being smoothed).

From our experience, a reasonable initial estimate for the choice of the λ parameters must be such that the weight of the regularization term is half the weight of the data term. A reasonable initial estimate for the δ parameters is half the smallest variation in contrast in the object to be reconstructed. Of course, these values for the λ and δ parameters need to be adjusted for each reconstruction.

6. CONCLUSION

An Edge-Preserving regularization procedure is proposed and applied on two quantitative reconstruction algorithms (Newton–Kantorovich and Conjugate Gradient) in order to solve an

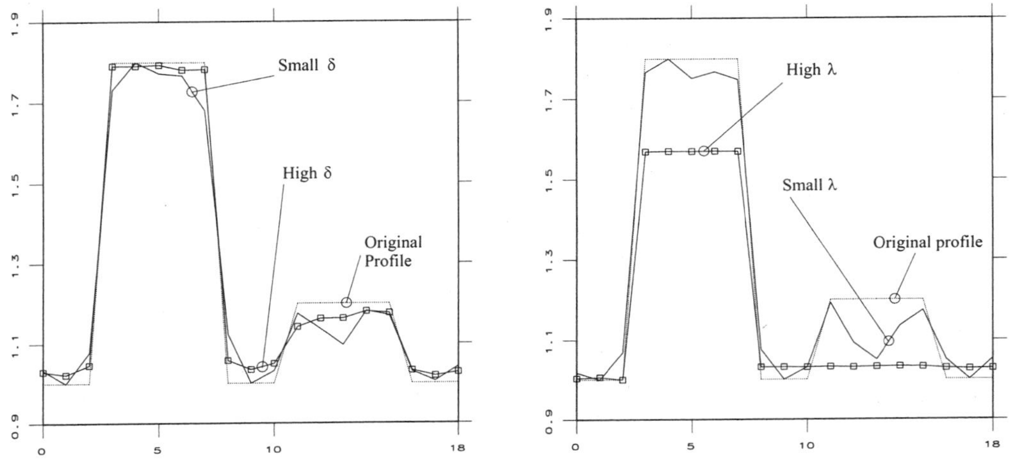

(a) Influence of the λ parameters

(b) Influence of the δ parameters

Figure 6. Influence of the regularization parameters

inverse scattering problem in microwave tomography. The two procedures have been compared using both synthetic and experimental data. Results obtained with the NK+EP method are very promising as well as with the CG+EP method which gives good reconstructions also. Finally, the influence of the EP regularization parameters on the solution have been demonstrated.

REFERENCES

1. J. Hadamard, *Lectures on Cauchy's Problem in Linear Partial Differential Equations*, Yale University Press, New Haven, 1923.
2. J. Devaney, "A computer simulation study of diffraction tomography," *IEEE Trans. on Biomedical Engineering*, **BME-30**, 1983, pp. 377–386.
3. Ch. Pichot, L. Jofre, G. Peronnet, and J. Ch. Bolomey, "Active microwave imaging of inhomogeneous bodies," *IEEE Trans. on Antennas and Propagation*, **AP-33**, 1985, pp. 416–425.
4. J. Ch. Bolomey, Ch. Pichot, and G. Gaboriaud, "Planar microwave imaging camera for biomedical applications: Critical and prospective analysis of reconstruction algorithms," *Radio Science*, **26**, 2, 1991, pp. 541–549.
5. W. C. Chew and Y. M. Wang, "Reconstruction of two-dimensional permittivity distribution using the distorded Born iterative method," *IEEE Trans. on Medical Imaging*, **MI-9**, 2, 1990, pp. 218–225.
6. T. M. Habashy, M. L. Oristaglio, and M. L. de Hoop, "Simultaneous nonlinear reconstruction of two-dimensional problems in tomography," *J. Comput. Appl. Math.*, **4**, 1990, pp. 1101–1118.
7. N. Joachimowicz, Ch. Pichot, and J. P. Hugonin, "Inverse scattering: an iterative numerical method for electromagnetic imaging," *IEEE Trans. on Antennas and Propagation*, **AP-39**, 1991, pp. 1742–1751.
8. R. E. Kleinman and P. M. van den Berg, "A modified gradient method for two-dimensional problems in tomography," *J. Comput. Appl. Math.*, **42**, 1992, pp. 17–35.
9. R. E. Kleinman and P. M. van den Berg, "An extended range-modified gradient technique for profile inversion," *Radio Science*, **28**, 5, 1993, pp. 877–884.
10. H. Harada, D. J. N. Wall, and T. Takenaka, "Conjugate gradient method applied to inverse scattering problem," *IEEE Trans. on Antennas and Propagation*, **AP-43**, 8, 1995, pp. 784–792.
11. K. Belkebir, R. Kleinman, and Ch. Pichot, "Microwave Imaging - Location and Shape Reconstruction from Multifrequency Scattering Data," *IEEE Trans. on Microwave Theory and Techniques*, **MTT-45**, 1997, pp. 469–476.
12. P. Lobel, R. Kleinman, Ch. Pichot, L. Blanc-Féraud, and M. Barlaud, "Conjugate gradient method for solving inverse scattering with experimental data," *IEEE Antennas & Propagation Magazine*, **38**, 3, 1996, pp. 48–51.
13. A. Franchois and Ch. Pichot, "Microwave Imaging - Complex Permittivity Reconstruction with a Levenberg–Marquardt Method," *IEEE Trans. on Antennas and Propagation*, **AP-45**, 2, 1997, pp. 203–215.
14. P. Lobel, Ch. Pichot, L. Blanc-Féraud, and M. Barlaud, "Conjugate Gradient Algorithm With Edge-Preserving Regularization for Image Reconstruction from Experimental Data," in *IEEE AP-S/URSI International Symposium*, Baltimore, Maryland, USA, 1996, vol. 1, pp. 644–647.
15. P. Lobel, L. Blanc-Féraud, Ch. Pichot, and M. Barlaud, "A new regularization scheme for inverse scattering," *Inverse Problems*, **13**, 1997, pp. 403–410.
16. P. Lobel, Ch. Pichot, L. Blanc-Féraud, and M. Barlaud, "Conjugate Gradient Algorithm with Edge-Preserving Regularization for Image Reconstruction from Ipswich Data for Mystery Objects." *IEEE Antennas & Propagation Magazine*, **39**, 2, 1997, pp. 12–14.
17. A. Roger, "Newton-kantorovitch algorithm applied to an electromagnetic inverse problem," *IEEE Trans. on Antennas and Propagation*, **AP-29**, 2, 1981, pp. 232–238.
18. J. P. Hugonin, N. Joachimowicz, and Ch. Pichot, "Quantitative reconstruction of complex permittivity distributions by means of microwave tomography," in *Inverse Methods in Action*, P. C. Sabatier Ed., pp. 302–311. Springer-Verlag, Berlin, 1990.
19. A. Franchois and Ch. Pichot, "Generalized cross validation applied to a Newton-type algorithm for microwave tomography," in *Proc. Inverse Problems in Scattering and Imaging*, M. A. Fiddy Ed., San Diego, 1992, pp. 232–240.
20. Ch. Pichot, P. Lobel, L. Blanc-Féraud, M. Barlaud, K. Belkebir, J. M. Elissalt, and J. M. Geffrin, "Gradient and Gauss–Newton Methods for Microwave Tomography," in *Inverse Problems in Medical Imaging and Nondestructive Testing*. H. W. Engl, A. K. Louis, W. Rundell (Eds.), Springer-Verlag, Wien, 1997, pp. 168–187.
21. E. Polak and G. Ribière, "Note sur la convergence de méthodes de directions conjuguées," *Revue Française d'Informatique et de Recherche Opérationnelle*, **R1**, 16, 1969, pp. 35–43.
22. R. Acar and C. R. Vogel, "Analysis of bounded variation penalty methods for ill-posed problems," *Inverse Problems*, **10**, 6, 1994, pp. 1217–1229.

23. P. M. van den Berg and R. E. Kleinman, "A total variation enhanced modified gradient algorithm for profile reconstruction," *Inverse Problems*, **11**, 1995, pp. L5–L10.
24. S. Geman and D. E. Mc Clure, "Bayesian image analysis: an application to single photon emission tomography," in *Proc. Statist. Comput. Sect.*, Washington DC, 1985, Amer. Statist. Assoc., pp. 12–18.
25. T. Hebert and R. Leahy, "A generalized EM algorithm for 3-D Bayesian reconstruction from Poisson data using Gibbs priors," *IEEE Trans. on Medical Imaging*, **MI-8**, 2, 1989, pp. 194–202.
26. P. Perona and J. Malik, "Scale-space and edge detection using anisotropic diffusion," *IEEE Trans. on Pattern Analysis and Machine Intelligence*, **PAMI-12**, 7, 1990, pp. 629–639.
27. P. Charbonnier, L. Blanc-Féraud, G. Aubert, and M. Barlaud, "Deterministic Edge-Preserving Regularization in Computed Imaging," *IEEE Trans. on Image Processing*, **IP-6**, 2, 1997, pp. 298–311.
28. S. Geman and G. Reynolds, "Constrained restoration and the recovery of discontinuities," *IEEE Trans. on Pattern Analysis and Machine Intelligence*, **PAMI-14**, 3, 1992, pp. 367–383.
29. L. Blanc-Féraud, P. Charbonnier, G. Aubert, and M. Barlaud, "Nonlinear image processing: Modeling and fast algorithm for regularization with edge detection," in *Proc. IEEE-ICIP*, Washington, USA, 1995, pp. 474–477.
30. G. Aubert and L. Lazaroaia, "A variational method in image recovery," Research Note 423, Laboratoire Jean-Alexandre Dieudonné, 1995. To appear in *SIAM Journal of Num. Anal.* (November 1997).

9

ON S. SAITOH'S CHARACTERIZATION OF THE RANGE OF LINEAR TRANSFORMS

A. G. Ramm

Department of Mathematics
Kansas State University
Manhattan, KS, 66506-2602, USA

ABSTRACT

It is shown that the characterization of the range of linear transforms, given by S. Saitoh, is not a solution of the characterization problem.

1. INTRODUCTION

Let E be an abstract set whose elements we call points, let $T \subset \mathbb{R}^n$ be a domain and $H = L^2(T, dm)$, where dm is a finite measure on T. Define linear map

$$L\mathfrak{F} := f(p) := \int_T \overline{h(t,p)}\mathfrak{F}(t)dm(t) := (\mathfrak{F}, h(\cdot,p)) \tag{1.1}$$

where $h(t,p)$ is an element of H for any $p \in E$. The problem of characterization of the range of L consists of describing the set $\{L\mathfrak{F}\}_{\forall \mathfrak{F} \in H}$ in terms of some standard norms, such as the norms of the Sobolev spaces or Hölder spaces, for example.

In numerous publications (see [1,2] and references therein) S. Saitoh claims that he has solved the characterization of the range of L for nearly arbitrary kernel $h(t,p)$. Let us assume for simplicity that L is *injective*. Then S. Saitoh gives the following characterization of the range $R(L)$ of L ([1, p. 82], [2, p. 52]):

$R(L)$ consists of those and only those $f(p)$ which belong to the Hilbert space H_K with the reproducing kernel

$$K(p,q) := \int_T h(t,q)\overline{h(t,p)}dm(t) := Lh(\cdot,q). \tag{1.2}$$

The inner product in H_K is defined in [1, p. 84] by the formula

$$(f,g)_{H_K} = (L\mathfrak{F}, LG)_{H_K} := (\mathfrak{F}, G)_H, \tag{1.3}$$

Inverse Problems, Tomography, and Image Processing, edited by Ramm,
Plenum Press, New York, 1998

where $f := L\mathcal{F}$, $g := LG$. Equation (1.3) implies

$$||f||_{H_K} := ||\mathcal{F}||_H, \tag{1.4}$$

which means that L is an isometry. Since L is injective and its range is the whole space H_K by definition, the operator L is an isomorphism of H onto H_K. Note that (1.2) is the reproducing kernel for H_K because, by (1.2) and (1.3),

$$(f(p), K(p,q))_{H_K} = (\mathcal{F}, h(\cdot,q))_H = f(p).$$

If $A(p,q)$ is the kernel, possibly distributional, of the operator inverse to the one, defined by the kernel $K(p,q)$ in $L^2(E)$, then the inner product in the Hilbert space H_K is given by the formula

$$(f,g)_{H_K} := (Af,g)_{L^2(E)} = \int_E \int_E A(p,q) f(p) \overline{g(q)} dp dq. \tag{1.3'}$$

Therefore, in general, the space H_K is not realizable as $L^2(E, d\mu)$ space, while in [1] and [2] it is assumed that H_K is an $L^2(E, d\mu)$ space for some measure $d\mu$. Such an assumption means that the kernel $A(p,q) = a(p)\delta(p-q)$, where $a(p)$ is the density of the measure $d\mu$, this measure is assumed to be absolutely continuous, and $\delta(p-q)$ is the delta-function.

Moreover, equations (1.1), (1.3) and (1.3') imply:

$$\int_E \int_E A(p,q) \overline{h(t,p)} h(s,q) dp dq = \frac{\delta(t-s)}{a(t)}, \tag{1.3''}$$

where we assume that the measure $dm(t) = a(t)dt$ is absolutely continuous. This shows that the assumptions in [1,2] are of very special nature and are not satisfied for an arbitrary linear transforms of the form (1.1). The meaning of these assumptions is not discussed in [1,2].

In [3, p. 50] it is shown that if $R(x,y)$ is a continuous in $D \times D$ kernel, where $D \subset \mathbb{R}^n$, A is the operator in $H := L^2(D)$ with the kernel $R(x,y)$, and $(Au,u) := (Au,u)_{L^2(D)} > 0$ for all $u \not\equiv 0$, then the Hilbert space H_+ with the inner product $(u,u)_+ := (Au,u)$ has reproducing kernel $K(x,y)$, which is the kernel of the operator A^{-1}. The space $H_+ \subset H$ has the norm $||u||_+ := ||A^{1/2}u||$, where $||\cdot||$ is the $H-$norm. Therefore, the characterization of the range of the operator $A^{1/2}$ in this setting is equivalent to the characterization of the norm of the space H_+ in terms of some standard norms. In [3], for some class of the kernels $R(x,y)$, the characterization of the range of the operator A is given in terms of the Sobolev spaces.

In addition to the above characterization of $R(L)$, S. Saitoh gives an inversion formula:

$$\mathcal{F}(t) = \lim_{N\to\infty} \int_{E_N} f(p) h(t,p) d\mu(p). \tag{1.5}$$

Here he assumes that the sets E_N satisfy the following conditions:

a) $E_N \subset E_{N+1} \subset \dots$,

b) $\bigcup_1^\infty E_N = E$,

c) $\sup_N \int_{E_N} K(p,p) d\mu(p) < \infty$, $d\mu$ is an σ-finite measure and $H_K \subset L^2(E, d\mu)$.

The aim of this note is to argue that the characterization of $R(L)$ proposed by S. Saitoh and formulated above formula (1.2), is not a solution to the interesting and important problem of the characterization of $R(L)$.

In my view, it is not possible to solve non-trivially the characterization problem for "all linear integral transforms." Each kernel $h(t,p)$ yields a problem.

It is true (and trivial) that the set $\{L\mathfrak{F}\}_{\forall \mathfrak{F}\in H}$ equipped with the norm $||L\mathfrak{F}||_{H_K} := ||\mathfrak{F}||_H$, is a Banach space (complete linear normed space).

However, this observation does not solve the characterization problem because the description of the norm in H_K in terms of any standard norms, such as Sobolev, Hölder, etc., is not given.

2. AN EXAMPLE

As an example, consider $H = L^2(-1,1)$, $dm = dt$,

$$L\mathfrak{F} = \int_{-1}^{1} e^{-(x-t)^2}\mathfrak{F}(t)dt := f(x), \tag{2.1}$$

and let $E = (-1,1)$. One can write the reproducing kernel for H_K by formula (1.2):

$$K(x,y) = \int_{-1}^{1} e^{-[(x-t)^2+(t-y)^2]}dt, \tag{2.2}$$

but it is impossible using S. Saitoh's result to characterize H_K in terms of the commonly used norms: given a function $\varphi(x) \in C^\infty(-1,1)$, one cannot tell, using S. Saitoh's result, whether $\varphi \in H_K$ or not.

One can characterize the range of L in this particular example using a different approach: define $g(x) := \exp(x^2)f(x)$ and $h(t) := \exp(-t^2)\mathfrak{F}(t)$, and write (2.1) as

$$L_1 h := \int_{-1}^{1} e^{2xt}h(t)dt = g(x). \tag{2.3}$$

One can characterize the range of L_1 using the Paley-Wiener theorem, and there is one-to-one correspondence between the range of L and the range of L_1, so one characterize the range of L as well. This range consists of (the restrictions to the interval [-1,1] of) entire functions with the specific growth rate, and cannot be described in terms of the standard norms mentioned above.

Another example is the transform $L\mathfrak{F} := \int_{-1}^{1}\exp(-itp)\mathfrak{F}(t)dt$. Here $H := L^2(-1,1)$, $dm = dt$, $T = E = (-1,1)$, $K(p,q) = 2\frac{\sin(q-p)}{q-p}$. In this example the Paley-Wiener theorem gives a complete description of $R(L)$ as the set of restrictions to $(-1,1)$ of the values of entire functions of exponential type 1 which are square integrable over the real axis. On the other hand, $R(L)$ in this example cannot be described in terms of the Sobolev or Hölder norms, and the description of the space H_K, corresponding in this example to the kernel $2\frac{\sin(q-p)}{q-p}$, requires the knowledge of $R(L)$.

By definition (1.3), one can write:

$$(f,g)_{H_K} = (L^*L\mathfrak{F}, G)_H = (\mathfrak{F}, G)_H. \tag{2.4}$$

Equation (2.4) implies that $L^*L = I_H$, where L^* is the adjoint operator to L and I_H is the identity operator in H. Since L is boundedly invertible, one has:

$$L^* = L^{-1}, \tag{2.5}$$

which is essentially the inversion formula described by S. Saitoh in [1,2], in a more complicated way. The operator $L : H \to H_K$ has the adjoint $L^* : H_K \to H$, and the inverse $L^{-1} : H_K \to H$, so (2.5) can be considered as an inversion formula as long as H_K is realized as a functional Hilbert space $L^2(E, d\mu)$, which is the assumption in [1,2]. Such an assumption, made by S. Saitoh [2, p. 56], is equivalent to assuming that the inversion formulas are valid, i.e.,

$$(h(t,p), h(s,p))_{H_K} = \frac{\delta(t-s)}{a(s)}, \tag{2.6}$$

where $dm = a(s)ds$, and it is assumed here that $a(s) > 0$ is a continuous function. The assumption that H_K is realized as $L^2(E, d\mu)$ space is a very restrictive assumption: it means that the reproducing kernel of H_K is a distribution with support on the diagonal $x = y$ (cf. (1.3") and (2.6)).

If one assumes that the inner product in H_K is given by $(f, g)_{H_K} := (Af, g)_H$, where $A > 0$ is a linear positive operator on $\mathcal{H} = L^2(E)$ with the kernel $A(x,y)$, then the reproducing kernel in H_K is the kernel $A^{-1}(x,y)$ of the operator A^{-1}. Indeed, if the kernel of A^{-1} is $K(x,y)$, then

$$(K(x,y), g)_{H_K} = (AK, g)_{\mathcal{H}} = AA^{-1}g = g(x). \tag{2.7}$$

Note that in this argument we use the kernel of the identity operator in $\mathcal{H}$, which is $\delta(x-y)$, a distribution, not an element of $\mathcal{H}$. This distribution is well defined as the kernel of the identity operator by the formula $(\delta(x-y), f)_{\mathcal{H}} := f(x)$. The value of f at a point is not defined, and f is considered as an equivalence class of functions.

Therefore an effective description of the norm in H_K, that is, a characterization of this norm in terms of some standard norms, is equivalent to the solution of the problem of the characterization of the range of L in Saitoh's setting. In [1] and [2] such an effective description of the norm in H_K is not given, and therefore the characterization of $R(L)$ problem is not solved for general linear integral transforms.

REFERENCES

1. Saitoh, S., "Theory of reproducing kernels and applications," in: *Pitman Research Notes N189*, Longman, New York (1988).
2. ———, "One approach to some general integral transforms and its applications," *Integr. Transforms and Special Functions* **3**, No. 1, 49–84 (1995).
3. Ramm, A.G., *Random Fields Estimation Theory*, Longman/Wiley, New York (1990).

10

WAVELET MODELLING OF CLINICAL MAGNETIC RESONANCE TOMOGRAPHY: AN ENSEMBLE QUANTUM COMPUTING APPROACH

Walter Schempp

Lehrstuhl für Mathematik I
University of Siegen

Mensch, streck deine Vernunft hierher, diese Dinge zu begreiffen! — Johann Keppler (1571–1630)

There is nothing that nuclear spins will not do for you, as long as you treat them as human beings. — Erwin Louis Hahn (1949)

Die Philosophie ist Konstruktivismus, und der Konstruktivismus besitzt zwei komplementäre Aspekte, die sich wesensmäßig voneinander unterscheiden: Begriffe erschaffen und eine Ebene entwerfen. Die Begriffe sind gleichsam die mannigfachen Wellen, die sich heben und senken, die Immanenzebene aber ist die eine Welle, von der sie auf— und abgewickelt werden. Die Ebene ist es, die den Zusammenschluß der Begriffe mit stets wachsenden Verbindungen garantiert, und es sind die Begriffe, die die Besiedelung der Ebene in einer stets neuen, stets variablen Krümmung gewährleisten.

Die Immanenzebene ist eine Blätterung. Sie ist gleichsam ein Schnitt durch das Chaos und wirkt wie ein Sieb. Das Chaos ist durch die Unmöglichkeit eines Bezugs zwischen zwei Bestimmungen gekennzeichnet. Indem sie einen Schnitt durch das Chaos legt, appelliert die Immanenzebene an eine Schöpfung von Begriffen. — Gilles Deleuze und Félix Guattari (1991)

The link between different energetic strata represented by symmetry groups is best sought in some appropriate Lie group transform. And since it is not possible to correlate events directly across energy gaps, the observer always being on one side of the gap, one may try to correlate the geometric patterns they form in each stratum as a result of the interactions they are subjected to and of the laws they obey, rather than in terms of the interactions themselves. — George L. Farre (1996)

Inverse Problems, Tomography, and Image Processing, edited by Ramm,
Plenum Press, New York, 1998

ABSTRACT

Phase coherent wideband signal wavelets form a unified basis of the multichannel reconstructive analysis–synthesis filter bank of high resolution synthetic aperture radar (SAR) imaging and clinical MRI. The construction of unitary bank filters is performed by the Kepplerian quadrature detection strategy of physical astronomy which allows for the stroboscopic and synchronous cross-sectional filtering of phase histories in contiguous local frequency encoding subband multichannels relative to the rotating coordinate frame of quadrature reference. The Kepplerian quadrature detection strategy and the associated unitary filter bank construction take place in symplectic affine planes which are immersed into the three-dimensional compact super-encoding projective space. They are implemented in the quadrature format of a phase-splitting network by Fourier analysis of the Heisenberg nilpotent Lie group G. The action of G admits a matrix coordinatization by transvections. In terms of projective geometry, the longitudinal dilations jointly with the transvections of the G-action generate the group of homologies. The tomographic slices, frequency selected by the MRI scanner system, are identified with the projectively immersed, symplectic affine leaves $\mathcal{O}_\nu\,(\nu \neq 0)$ of the canonical coadjoint orbit foliation of G, on which the projective cohomologies linearly act.

The paper leads from Keppler to Heisenberg in order to demonstrate the tight control which Lie group theory exercises over the non-invasive MRI modality via the geometric quantization strategy. For the first time, it allows for a visualization of the canonical coadjoint orbit foliation associated to the coadjoint G-action in the dual vector space $\mathrm{Lie}(G)^\star$ of the Heisenberg Lie algebra $\mathrm{Lie}(G)$. Its leaves $\mathcal{O}_\nu\,(\nu \neq 0)$ are a stack of energetic strata forming a fibration of tomographic slices which carry the associated bundle of $\mathcal{C}^\star$-algebras. In addition, the paper offers the foliated three-dimensional super-encoding projective space $\mathbf{P}(\mathbf{R} \times \mathrm{Lie}(G)^\star)$ as the natural frame of the Lauterbur subband encoding technique of spectral localization by directional derivatives, or linear magnetic field gradients. In the projective split, $\mathbf{R}$ denotes the event line. The three-dimensional real projective space $\mathbf{P}(\mathbf{R} \times \mathrm{Lie}(G)^\star)$ represents the frame for the line geometric implementation of the Larmor equation for the magnetic spin precession. The energetic coordinate frames of the energetic strata are performed via the de Rham cohomology associated to the L^2-sections of the homogeneous line bundle of transvections over the projectively immersed, natural symplectic affine structure of the flat coadjoint orbit leaves $\mathcal{O}_\nu\,(\nu \neq 0)$ of G, and their rotational curvature forms. Tomographic slice selection from the canonical coadjoint orbit foliation in projective space, readout procedure, and phase encoding linear gradients operating on the L^2-sections of a homogeneous hologram line bundle perform the basic MRI functions and are refocused in every repetition period. The refocusing procedures by spatial rewinder gradients and phase conjugation flip depend on Fourier analysis of the metaplectic group pointwise attached to the one-dimensional center C of G as a group of dynamical symmetries specific for the selected energetic stratum. Each point ν of the line $\hat{C} - \{0\}$ with the origin removed corresponds to the distinguished closed exterior differential 2-form $\omega_\nu = \omega_1$ generated cohomologically by the rotational curvature form of the planar coadjoint orbit $\mathcal{O}_\nu \hookrightarrow \mathrm{Lie}(G)^\star\,(\nu \neq 0)$ of G which is immersed as a linear symplectic affine variety into the foliated three-dimensional super-encoding projective space $\mathbf{P}(\mathbf{R} \times \mathrm{Lie}(G)^\star)$. Similar to the refocusing procedures by spatial rewinder gradients, the rephasing procedure of spin echoes by phase conjugation flip depends upon the fact that the normal subgroup $\mathbf{GO}^+(2,\mathbf{R})$ of direct linear similitudes has index two in the non-abelian group $\mathbf{GO}(2,\mathbf{R})$ of all linear similitudes of the symplectic affine plane $\mathbf{R} \oplus \mathbf{R}$.

The fascinating aspects of electronic engineering concerned with the implementation of the dynamical symmetries inherent to the semi-classical approach to clinical magnetic resonance tomography by large scale integrated (LSI) microcircuit technology are also indicated. Once greater understanding has been gained in the quantized calculus foundations of MRI, and the dynamical system approach to the Lauterbur subband encoding technique of spectral localization by linear magnetic field gradients operating on the L^2-sections of a homogeneous hologram line bundle, it will be possible to design new wavelet packets of spin excitation profiles with the desired contrast resolution capability.

Magnetic resonance imaging (MRI) is an important example of an initially purely academic idea, the spin echo response phenomenon of nuclear magnetic resonance, being turned to the benefit of humankind. The speed with which clinical MRI systems spread throughout the world was phenomenal. Although originally a topic of considerable controversy, MRI has become a vital technique in the clinical assessment of morphologic, pathologic, and functional changes, and its complete or, at least, partial displacement of other clinical imaging modalities such as X-ray computed tomography (CT) scanning, is expected.

MRI has been called the most important development in medical diagnosis since the discovery of the X-ray 100 years ago. The physical principles of MRI and X-ray CT, however, are completely different [26, 31, 51]. Due to the phase information utilized by coherent tomography, the MRI modality actually is closer to radar imaging and microwave holography than to X-ray CT. Nuclear magnetic resonance spectroscopy provides direct and incontrovertible evidence of quantization of energy, and nowhere is this more simply illustrated than in magnetic resonance experiments. Nuclear spins can be manipulated in myriad different ways in order to extract information about molecular structure and molecular motion. The moment of birth of the temporal magnetic resonance phenomenon was marked by Bloch's *dynamical* approach. The great Felix Bloch (1905–1983), the first graduate student and former assistant to Werner Heisenberg in Leipzig [69], outlined the nuclear induction experiment in his source paper of 1946 as follows [25]:

> "The first successful experiments to detect magnetic resonance by electromagnetic efects have been carried out recently and independently at the physics laboratories of Harvard and Stanford Universities. The considerations upon which our work was based have several features in common with the two experiments, previously mentioned, but differ rather essentially in others. In the first place, the radiofrequency field is deliberately chosen large enough so as to cause at resonance a considerable change of orientation of the nuclear moments. In the second place, this change is not observed by its relatively small reaction upon the driving circuit, but by directly observing the induced electromotive force in a coil, due to the precession of the nuclear moments around the constant field and in a direction perpendicular both to this field and the applied r-f field. This appearance of a magnetic induction at right angles to the r-f field is an effect which is of specifically nuclear origin and it is the main characteristic feature of our experiment. In essence, the observed perpendicular nuclear induction indicates a rotation of the total oscillating field around the constant magnetic field."

> "Not only a weak r-f field, acting at resonance over very many Larmor periods, can produce an appreciable nuclear change of orientation, but also a strong field pulse, acting over only a few periods. Once the nuclear moments have been turned into an angle with the constant field, they will continue to precess around it and likewise cause a nuclear induction to occur at an instant when the driving pulse has already disappeared. It seems perfectly feasible to receive thus an induced nuclear signal of radiofrequency well above the thermal noise of a narrow band receiver. It is true that, due to the broadening of the Larmor frequency

by internuclear fields or other causes, this signal can last only a comparatively short time, but for normal fields it will still contain many Larmor periods, i.e., it will be essentially monochromatic. The main difference between this proposed experiment and the one which we have actually carried out lies in the fact that it would observe by induction the free nuclear precession while we have studied the forced precession impressed upon the nuclei by the applied r-f field. The existence of a resultant macroscopic moment of the nuclei within the sample under investigation is a common prerequisite for all electromagnetic experiments with nuclear moments. It is in fact a change of orientation of this macroscopic moment which causes the observed effects, and irrespective of the changes of orientation of the individual nuclei which might be induced by a r-f field, their moments would always cancel each other, if they did so initially, and thus escape observation."

The aforementioned experiment at Harvard was performed by Edward M. Purcell who shared the Nobel Award in Physics with Bloch in 1952. The methods of nuclear magnetic resonance spectroscopy in condensed matter due to Bloch and Purcell are not only of high intellectual beauty, they also place an analytic method of high efficacy in the hands of scientists.

Purcell was recruited by the MIT Radiation Laboratory to help in the development of radar. A radar system employs a directional antenna that radiates energy within a narrow beam in a known direction. In terms of projective geometry, the direction is represented by a point at infinity ∞ of the embedding three-dimensional projective space. The radar antenna senses the echo response scattered by the target, and the receiver collects the spread energy. It amplifies the return and translates its energy band to the intermediate frequency of the radar. The intermediate frequency signal wavelet is operated on linearly by the predetection filter. Finally, the output of the predection filtering is coherently detected and analyzed by a linear phase-sensitive correlation processor configuration. Because a large part of the information about the target is in the phase of the image rather than in the intensity, the image phase could not be analyzed if radar were designed as an incoherent imaging system [12, 61].

One unique feature of the synthetic aperture radar (SAR) imaging modality is that its spatial resolution capability is independent of the platform altitude over the subplatform nadir track. This result of SAR system identification follows from the fact that the SAR image is formed by transmitting synchronously the phase histories in parallel, including the differential time delays in contiguous local frequency encoding subband multichannels of wideband radar, none of which is a function of the range from the radar sensor to the scene. It is this unique capability which allows the acquisition of high resolution images from satellite altitude as long as the received echo response has sufficient strength above the noise level [57].

The Kepplerian quadrature detection strategy is quite flexible. It is derived from the quadrature conchoid trajectory construction which is best understood in the projectively immersed, symplectic flat of planetary orbit, and the second fundamental law of planetary motion analysis [76]. To perform orbit localization via the control of the transvectional action by longitudinal dilations, the symplectic affine plane is immersed into the three-dimensional compact super-encoding projective space. According to the classification of homologies of real projective spaces, each homology induces a dilation or a transvection, and therefore allows for detection of elliptical planetary orbits as quadrics avoiding the projective plane at infinity of the embedding three-dimensional projective space. Remarkably, the quadrature conchoid trajectory construction seems to have almost escaped notice in literature so that it is actually no surprise that Keppler is not recognized as one of the founders, along with Desargues, of projective geometry, which is now standard in computer vision and robotics literature. It presents a phase–frequency cycling clockwork displayed in Keppler's greatest book, the Astronomia Nova *αιτιολογητος* seu Physica Coelestis, Tradita Commentariis de Motibus Stellæ Martis

(1609). Keppler was the first astronomer whose analysis reached laws of nature that were physical rather than mathematical or philosophical. Only after he had reduced the observed phenomena to a theory of interactions between material bodies could he see how to synthesize such new and complex relations as elliptical planetary orbits in projective space, or the distance law. The Kepplerian libratory motion analysis [28] turned the helio-centric static system due to Copernicus into a helio-eccentric dynamical system by the moment map of the the second fundamental law. It leads to the symplectic group $\mathbf{Sp}(2,\mathbf{R}) = \mathbf{SL}(2,\mathbf{R})$ which forms the key of the geometric quantization strategy and the quantized calculus.

- The magnetic hypothesis of libratory motion analysis includes the assumption that the magnetic axis of the planet maintains a constant direction, perpendicular to the apsidal line connecting the aphelion and perihelion in the orbital plane through the sun.

- The quadrature conchoid trajectory construction in the projectively immersed, symplectic affine plane of planetary orbit visualizes the moment map which is equivariant for the Hamiltonian action by symplectomorphisms, hence the rotational curvature form of the planetary orbit flat.

It was by shifting the rotating coordinate frame of quadrature reference from the quadrant to the octant phases of the trajectory construction within the projectively immersed, symplectic flat of planetary orbit which led Keppler to the filtering of the famous eccentric anomaly of as much as 8 minutes deviation of the reference frequency cycle. By an application of the area law or alternatively law of conservation of orbital angular momentum to perform resonance matching, he succeeded in the affine reconstruction of the elliptical orbit in projective space from the phase histories of the libratory motion stored in contiguous local frequency encoding multichannels with respect to the rotating coordinate frame of quadrature reference. In this way, the first fundamental law was implied by the second law. The result of his new matched filter bank approach to planetary motion analysis, which anticipated the splitting scheme of the Lauterbur subband encoding principle of wideband signal wavelets for spectral localization, was not only an improvement of nearly two orders of magnitude in the prediction filtering of planetary positions but also showed his way of thinking to have been surprisingly modern from the viewpoint of non-commutative Fourier analysis and semantic filtering.

- In the Kepplerian dynamical system approach, the quadrature conchoid trajectory construction implements a band of locally frequencies in the projectively immersed, symplectic affine plane of the planetary orbit.

- The quadrature format design of the stroboscopic and synchronous system allows for transition from polar coordinates representing the unit circle of the eccentric Kepplerian clockwork to the symplectic coordinates of the phase–frequency cycling clockwork representing the conchoid trajectory of the libratory motion analysis.

- According to the Heisenberg uncertainty principle, the quadrature format design ensures wideband selectivity in phase and local frequency coordinates.

The symplectic format design allows for the stroboscopic and synchronous cross-sectional quadrature filtering of phase histories in contiguous local frequency encoding multichannels relative to the rotating coordinate frame of quadrature reference. It provides the intrinsic implementation in quadrature format of a matched filter bank by orbit stratification in a symplectic affine plane which is immersed into the three-dimensional compact super-encoding projective space. The symplectic affine leaves $\mathcal{O}_\nu\,(\nu \neq 0)$ realize the foliation of rotationally curved planes of immanence or plateaus by their energetic coordinatization. It is remarkable that the canonical foliation of symplectic affine leaves and their rotational curvature forms, parametrized by the *stratigraphic time* of the event line, has been independently rediscovered in the modern philosophy of constructivism and semantic filtering [19]. It places the correspondence principle of early quantum mechanics closer to non-commutative Fourier analysis and hence makes its formulation in the foliated three-dimensional super-encoding projective space

$$\mathbf{P}\,(\mathbf{R} \times \mathrm{Lie}(G)^{\star})$$

of homogeneous *event* line $\mathbf{R}$, canonically associated to the dual vector space $\mathrm{Lie}(G)^{\star}$, more satisfactory for mathematicians. Due to the intrinsic structure of the *projective completion* of the dual of the *affine dual* of each of the tomographic slices $\mathcal{O}_\nu \hookrightarrow \mathrm{Lie}(G)^{\star}\,(\nu \neq 0)$, the foliated projective space $\mathbf{P}\,(\mathbf{R} \times \mathrm{Lie}(G)^{\star})$ is particularly appropriate for radiological imaging applications. The frequency selection from the canonical foliation in projective space, and the transvectional action of the Heisenberg group G provide the frame for the line geometric implementation of the Larmor equation for the magnetic spin precession.

- The geometric quantization strategy assigns to each classical dynamical system for the Hamiltonian action of a connected Lie group a corresponding quantum dynamical system which is an irreducible unitary linear group representation.

It seems significant that connected Lie groups admitting globally square integrable representations play a distinguished role for the geometric quantization strategy.

- The three-dimensional connected Heisenberg two-step nilpotent Lie group G is the basic group of the MRI modality.
- The Lie group G admits a realization by a faithful matrix representation $G \longrightarrow \mathbf{SL}(3,\mathbf{R})$. It acts via the coadjoint action on the foliated three-dimensional super-encoding projective space $\mathbf{P}\,(\mathbf{R} \times \mathrm{Lie}(G)^{\star})$.
- Magnetic resonance tomography is basically a three-dimensional imaging technique represented by the Hopf fibered compact unit sphere $\mathbf{S}_3 \hookrightarrow \mathbf{R}^4$ with antipodes identified.

Adopting the point of view of constructivistic philosophy, the symplectic affine leaves form the domain of human thinking, so that the plane of incidence appears to be an appropriate territory for neurofunctional imaging and recording the planar neuronal excitation profile of cognitive function. The development of neurofunctional MRI in humans offers potential for clinical applications in which cerebral function as well as cerebral morphology are examined [14, 65, 80].

An application of the procedure of quadrature filtering of phase histories in contiguous local frequency encoding multichannels is of considerable ancestry and leads to the landmark observation of the earliest SAR pioneer, Carl A. Wiley, that motion is the solution of the high resolution radar imagery and phased array antenna problem of holographic recording in the three-dimensional compact super-encoding projective space.

Whereas the Kepplerian spatiotemporal strategy may be realized in SAR imaging by the range Doppler principle [15, 48, 49], it is the Lauterbur subband encoding principle combined with Sir Peter Mansfield's idea of switching spatial linear magnetic field gradients on a modular basis instead of simultaneously [45], and spatial linear rewinder gradients [73] which takes place in clinical MRI. Given the implicit role of the nuclear spin position in determining the Larmor precession spectrum under the influence of spatial linear magnetic field gradients, it is remarkable that 23 years elapsed after Erwin L. Hahn's original nuclear magnetic spin echo experiment in 1950 before Paul C. Lauterbur used this spatial signature in magnetic resonance tomography to acquire structural information from a heterogeneous sample [51]. The concurrent development of the Lauterbur subband encoding technique of spectral localization by linear magnetic field gradients was influential in that it ran counter to the widespread dogma that meaningful Larmor precession spectra could not be obtained from complex heterogeneous organizations such as living tissues.

- In clinical MRI, the distribution of protons is scanned, and the contrast between tissues is a function of biophysical parameters such as relaxation times and proton density, and instrumental parameters such as radiofrequency pulse train delays, pulse angles, and excitation profiles.

- Directional derivatives, or linear magnetic field gradients operating on the L^2-sections of a homogeneous hologram line bundle are the source of the spatial encoding in clinical MRI.

The potential of MRI for parameter modulation of the image contrasts between various biological tissues is one of the specificities of the MRI modality, and one of its major strengths (Figure 1). At the time of writing, over 6.000 whole-body MRI scanner systems are available for clinical imaging purposes. In the form of nuclear magnetic resonance spectroscopy, the technique can also be used to study tissue chemistry of biopsy specimens and body fluids by means of smaller scale instruments suitable for more basic research [26]. The spectroscopic applications are of special importance for the study and treatment of Alzheimer disease and associated disorders.

Despite the strong non-linearity of dissipative spin systems, linear response theory holds exactly in MRI processing. Because the spin isochromats are in a position of equilibrium under the ordering influence of the external magnetic flux density, a restoration of the stroboscopically measured phase that preceded each successive radiofrequency pulse needs the application of a spatial linear rewinder gradient of opposite polarity after the data acquisition interval. Arranging for spin echo and anti-echo responses to appear in a tightly time-controlled manner then provides spectral information about the spatial locations inside the spin isochromats. When placed in this context, the importance of the spatiotemporal quantization strategy for the selective wideband excitation of the MRI modality becomes apparent.

- In clinical MRI system identification, the basic objective of the subband splitting scheme is to decompose a wideband signal wavelet into uncorrelated frequency subbands and then to encode independently each subband multichannel for storage or wavelet transmission.

- The Lauterbur subband encoding technique takes advantage of the fact that the Larmor precession frequency y varies affine-linearly with the applied external magnetic flux density. It is based on the control of the transvectional G-action by means of longitudinal dilations.

- The spatial linear rewinder gradients are geared to ensure stability of the phase–frequency coordinates in each repetition interval of the semantic filtering process. They act in conjunction with spin echo pulse sequences as a multichannel transmultiplexer.

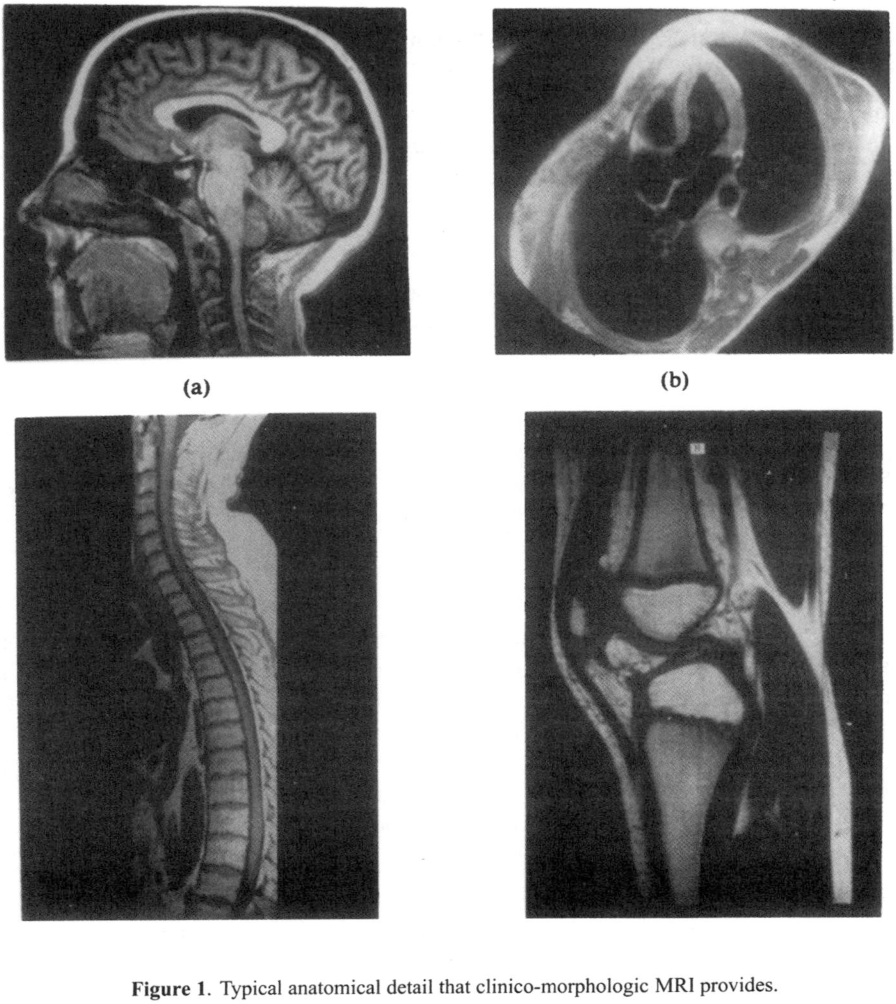

Figure 1. Typical anatomical detail that clinico-morphologic MRI provides.

At the background of the high resolution automated imaging systems, SAR and MRI, lies the unitary construction of a multichannel coherent wavelet reconstructive analysis–synthesis filter bank of matched filter type [17]. Beyond these applications to contiguous local frequency encoding subband multichannels, the Kepplerian quadrature detection strategy leads via the principle of least interaction action of a coplanar two-planet system to the concept of Feynman path integral. The summation over phase histories plays a pivotal role in quantum physics.

Although the origins are deep in the history of science and the chain of misunderstandings of the Kepplerian spatiotemporal quadrature strategy has continued to the present day, an exciting atmosphere of anticipation pervades the field of subband multichannel encoding technique which has not yet become classical. In many ways, the surface of the knowledge obtainable via clinical MRI has been barely scratched. The area is vast, and although today no clinical neurosurgeon or orthopaedic surgeon will operate without having planned his interventional strategies on the basis of MRI scans, frequency selected from the canonical foliation in projective space, the territory is largely unexplored. For the benefit to humankind, however, the developments of this theme are still proceeding at a rapid pace.

As approved by quantum electrodynamics, the geometric quantization strategy allows for a semi-classical approach to the interference pattern of quantum holography [68]. Recall that coadjoint orbits are one of the main sources of symplectic manifolds. The functor Lie(.) from the category of connected, simply connected Lie groups to the category of Lie algebras is an equivalence of categories. The unitary dual $\hat{G}$ of the Heisenberg nilpotent Lie group G consisting of the equivalence classes of irreducible unitary linear representations of G allows for a coadjoint orbit fibration by symplectic flats of incidence $\mathcal{O}_\nu \, (\nu \neq 0)$, spatially located as a stack of tomographic slices in the complement of the plane of foci at infinity $\mathbf{P}\left(\mathbf{R} \times \mathcal{O}_\infty\right)$. The plane at infinity $\mathbf{P}\left(\mathbf{R} \times \mathcal{O}_\infty\right)$ forms the complement of $\mathrm{Lie}(G)^\star$, canonically immersed into the projective completion $\mathbf{P}(\mathbf{R} \times \mathrm{Lie}(G)^\star)$ of the dual vector space $\mathrm{Lie}(G)^\star$ of the real Heisenberg Lie algebra[67,71,72] [67, 71, 72]. This fact is a consequence of the Kirillov homeomorphism

$$\hat{G} \longrightarrow \mathrm{Lie}(G)^\star / \mathrm{CoAd}_G(G),$$

the theorem of Stone–von Neumann of quantum physics, and the Einstein relation. For the dynamical system aspect, it is important to notice that the theorem of Stone–von Neumann assigns to the planar coadjoint orbit $\mathcal{O}_\nu \hookrightarrow \mathbf{P}(\mathbf{R} \times \mathrm{Lie}(G)^\star) \; (\nu \neq 0)$ of G through the driving frequency $\nu \in \hat{C} - \{0\}$ a unique central unitary character χ_ν of non-zero center frequency $\nu \in \mathbf{R}$ and a unique unitary equivalence class of irreducible linear representations of G which are globally square integrable modulo their kernels. As observed earlier, classical dynamical systems seem to be inextricably linked to globally square integrable group representations whenever they occur.

In terms of standard coordinates of semantic filtering, the Heisenberg group [86] consists of the set of unipotent upper triangular matrices

$$G = \left\{ \left(\begin{array}{ccc} 1 & x & z \\ 0 & 1 & y \\ 0 & 0 & 1 \end{array} \right) \middle| \, x, y, z \in \mathbf{R} \right\}$$

under the matrix multiplication law

$$\left(\begin{array}{ccc} 1 & x & z \\ 0 & 1 & y \\ 0 & 0 & 1 \end{array} \right) \cdot \left(\begin{array}{ccc} 1 & x' & z' \\ 0 & 1 & y' \\ 0 & 0 & 1 \end{array} \right) = \left(\begin{array}{ccc} 1 & x+x' & z+z'+x \cdot y' \\ 0 & 1 & y+y' \\ 0 & 0 & 1 \end{array} \right).$$

The form of rank one defining the non-commutative matrix multiplication of G is neither antisymmetric nor non-degenerate. However, it is *cohomologous* to the non-degenerate alternating determinant form, and it suffices to utilize any alternating bilinear form which is cohomologous to this form. The elementary matrices

$$\begin{pmatrix} 1 & x & 0 \\ 0 & 1 & 0 \\ 0 & 0 & 1 \end{pmatrix}, \quad \begin{pmatrix} 1 & 0 & 0 \\ 0 & 1 & y \\ 0 & 0 & 1 \end{pmatrix}, \quad \begin{pmatrix} 1 & 0 & z \\ 0 & 1 & 0 \\ 0 & 0 & 1 \end{pmatrix}$$

represent transvections in a three-dimensional real vector space, which are transformed by longitudinal dilations into the transvections

$$\begin{pmatrix} 1 & ax & 0 \\ 0 & 1 & 0 \\ 0 & 0 & 1 \end{pmatrix}, \quad \begin{pmatrix} 1 & 0 & 0 \\ 0 & 1 & ay \\ 0 & 0 & 1 \end{pmatrix}, \quad \begin{pmatrix} 1 & 0 & a^2z \\ 0 & 1 & 0 \\ 0 & 0 & 1 \end{pmatrix}$$

for $a \neq 0$. The Lebesgue measure $\mathrm{d}x \otimes \mathrm{d}y \otimes \mathrm{d}z$ of the vector space $\mathbf{R}^3$ gives rise to a Haar measure

$$\mathrm{d}x \wedge \mathrm{d}y \wedge \mathrm{d}z$$

of G. If the nilpotent matrices $\{P, Q, I\}$ denote the canonical basis of the three-dimensional real vector space $\mathrm{Lie}(G)$, the linear commutator provides the canonical commutation relations of quantum physics

$$[P, I] = [Q, I] = 0, \quad [P, Q] = I,$$

so that the Jacobi identity

$$[P, [Q, I]] + [Q, [I, P]] + [I, [P, Q]] = 0$$

is trivially satisfied. As a consequence, quantum physics is steeped in symplecticism, owing to the anti-symmetry of the Lie bracket operation occurring in the canonical commutation relations and which characterize $\mathrm{Lie}(G)$.

- The center of $\mathrm{Lie}(G)$ which is given by the one-dimensional commutator ideal

  $$[\mathrm{Lie}(G), \mathrm{Lie}(G)] = \mathrm{Lie}(G)^{[2]} = \mathbf{R}I$$

  is aligned with the direction of the external static magnetic field along the longitudinal axis of the magnet bore.

- The subset $\{P, Q\}$ of the set of nilpotent matrices $\{P, Q, I\}$ forms a symplectic basis of the quotient $\mathrm{Lie}(G)/\mathrm{Lie}(G)^{[2]}$.

The Lie bracket $[\cdot, \cdot]$ which denotes the linear commutator acts as the Poisson bracket $\{\cdot, \cdot\}$ of classical Hamiltonian mechanics on the real vector space $\mathcal{C}^{\infty}_{\mathbf{R}}(\mathbf{R} \oplus \mathbf{R})$ of smooth real-valued functions on the projectively immersed, symplectic affine plane $\mathbf{R} \oplus \mathbf{R}$. For proton densities $p, q \in \mathcal{C}^{\infty}_{\mathbf{R}}(\mathbf{R} \oplus \mathbf{R})$, the Poisson bracket reads

$$\{p, q\} = \frac{\partial p}{\partial y} \frac{\partial q}{\partial x} - \frac{\partial p}{\partial x} \frac{\partial q}{\partial y}.$$

The Poisson bracket is compatible with the Leibniz rule of the derivation $\{r,\cdot\}$. It is given by

$$\{r,pq\} = \{r,p\}q + p\{r,q\}$$

for the pointwise multiplication of functions $r,p,q \in \mathcal{C}^{\infty}_{\mathbf{R}}(\mathbf{R}\oplus\mathbf{R})$. Moreover, it forms a symplectic affine invariant of the plane $\mathbf{R}\oplus\mathbf{R}$. The density differentials

$$\mathrm{d}p = \frac{\partial p}{\partial x}\,\mathrm{d}x + \frac{\partial p}{\partial y}\,\mathrm{d}y, \quad \mathrm{d}q = \frac{\partial q}{\partial x}\,\mathrm{d}x + \frac{\partial q}{\partial y}\,\mathrm{d}y$$

act as symplectic gradients according to the identity

$$\mathrm{d}q \wedge \mathrm{d}p = \{p,q\}\cdot\omega_1$$

for $p,q \in \mathcal{C}^{\infty}_{\mathbf{R}}(\mathbf{R}\oplus\mathbf{R})$, and give rise via contraction to the rotational curvature form

$$\omega_1 = \mathrm{d}x \wedge \mathrm{d}y$$

of the generic coadjoint orbit $\mathcal{O}_1 \hookrightarrow \mathbf{P}(\mathbf{R}\times \mathrm{Lie}(G)^\star)$ of G. Then the integrability condition of the Poincaré lemma reads

$$\mathrm{d}\{p,q\} = \{\mathrm{d}p,\mathrm{d}q\}.$$

The action of the symplectic gradients establishes that the bracket transition

$$\Phi : \{\cdot,\cdot\} \rightsquigarrow [\cdot,\cdot]$$

from Poisson manifolds to symplectic manifolds is at the basis of the Lauterbur subband encoding technique of spectral localization by directional derivatives, which utilizes linear magnetic field gradients operating on the L^2-sections of a homogeneous hologram line bundle. It is the spectral localization which justifies the non-commutative geometric analysis approach to clinical MRI.

The Lie algebra morphism Φ from $\mathcal{C}^{\infty}_{\mathbf{R}}(\mathbf{R}\oplus\mathbf{R})$ endowed with the Poisson bracket of Hamiltonian mechanics, to the real vector space of vector fields on the symplectic affine plane $\mathbf{R}\oplus\mathbf{R}$ with respect to their natural Lie bracket, is given by the symplectically transposed, or alternatively twisted exterior differentiation

$$\Phi = \mathrm{d}^t.$$

It takes the first coordinate function $x = (x,0)$ of the symplectic affine plane $\mathbf{R}\oplus\mathbf{R}$ to $-Q \in \mathrm{Lie}(G)$, and assigns to the second coordinate function $y = \binom{y}{0}$ of the symplectic flat $\mathbf{R}\oplus\mathbf{R}$ the matrix $P \in \mathrm{Lie}(G)$. Thus the canonical commutation relations of quantum physics read in Poisson manifold notation

$$\{x,x\} = \{y,y\} = 0, \quad \{y,x\} = 1.$$

It follows from the identities

$$\Phi(y) = P \qquad \Phi(x) = -Q,$$

which read explicitly on the Lie algebra level

$$\Phi\begin{pmatrix} y \\ 0 \end{pmatrix} = \begin{pmatrix} 0 & 1 & 0 \\ 0 & 0 & 0 \\ 0 & 0 & 0 \end{pmatrix}, \quad \Phi((x,0)) = \begin{pmatrix} 0 & 0 & 0 \\ 0 & 0 & -1 \\ 0 & 0 & 0 \end{pmatrix},$$

that the linear differential forms dy and $-dx$ are the symplectic coordinates relative to the symplectic basis $\{P^\star, Q^\star\}$, dual to the canonical basis $\{P, Q\}$ of the symplectic affine plane $\mathrm{Lie}(G)/\mathrm{Lie}(G)^{[2]}$.

Let $\mathrm{Z}^1(\mathcal{O}_\nu)$ denote the real Lie algebra of the de Rham cocycles of degree 1 of the projectively immersed, affine symplectic plane $\mathcal{O}_\nu\,(\nu \neq 0)$. It follows from the exact sequence

$$\{0\} \longrightarrow \mathbf{R} \longrightarrow \mathcal{C}^\infty_{\mathbf{R}}\left(\mathrm{Lie}(G)/\mathrm{Lie}(G)^{[2]}\right) \xrightarrow{\Phi} \mathrm{Z}^1(\mathcal{O}_\nu) \longrightarrow \{0\}$$

that $\mathcal{C}^\infty_{\mathbf{R}}\left(\mathrm{Lie}(G)/\mathrm{Lie}(G)^{[2]}\right)$ is a one-dimensional central extension of the Lie algebra of vector fields $\mathrm{Z}^1(\mathcal{O}_\nu)$. The exact sequence can be embedded in a de Rham cohomology sequence

$$\begin{aligned} \{0\} \to \mathrm{H}^0\left(\mathrm{Lie}(G)/\mathrm{Lie}(G)^{[2]}\right) &\to \mathcal{C}^\infty_{\mathbf{R}}\left(\mathrm{Lie}(G)/\mathrm{Lie}(G)^{[2]}\right) \\ &\xrightarrow{\Phi} \mathrm{Z}^1(\mathcal{O}_\nu) \to \mathrm{H}^1(\mathcal{O}_\nu) \to \{0\}. \end{aligned}$$

The affine group

$$\mathbf{GA}(\mathbf{R}) \hookrightarrow \mathbf{GL}(2, \mathbf{R})$$

of the real line $\mathbf{R}$, the "$at+b$" group of affine linear transformations of the line $\mathbf{R}$, is generated by the affine dilations of $\mathbf{R}$. It forms a two-dimensional solvable Lie group of matrices

$$\mathbf{GA}(\mathbf{R}) = \left\{ \begin{pmatrix} a & b \\ 0 & 1 \end{pmatrix} \middle| a \neq 0, b \in \mathbf{R} \right\}$$

which represent affine dilations of ratio $a \in \mathbf{R}, a \neq 0$, shift $b \in \mathbf{R}$, and off-set term 1. The operation of $\mathbf{GA}(\mathbf{R})$ on the Hamiltonian action of $\mathrm{Lie}(G)$ by symplectomorphisms on $\mathrm{Z}^1(\mathcal{O}_\nu)$ allows to embed the Lauterbur subband encoding technique of wideband signal wavelets for spectral localization in the coadjoint orbits $\mathcal{O}_\nu\,(\nu \neq 0)$ of G in the foliated projective space $\mathbf{P}(\mathbf{R} \times \mathrm{Lie}(G)^\star)$. Having Damadian's approach to tumor detection in mind[51], in 1971 Lauterbur wrote in his notebook:

> "The distribution of magnetic nuclei, such as protons, and their relaxation times and diffusion coefficients, may be obtained by imposing magnetic field gradients (ideally, a complete set of orthogonal spherical harmonics) on a sample, such as an organism or a manufactured object, and measuring the intensities and relaxation behavior of the resonance as functions of the applied magnetic field. Additional spatial discrimination may be achieved by the application of time-dependent gradient patterns so as to distinguish, for example, protons that lie at the intersection of the zero-field (relative to the main magnetic field) lines of three linear gradients."

> "The experiments proposed above can be done most conveniently and accurately by measurements of the Fourier transform of the pulse response of the system. They should be capable of providing a detailed three-dimensional map of the distributions of particular

classes of nuclei (classified by nuclear species and relaxation times) within a living organism. For example, the distribution of mobile protons in tissues, and the differences in relaxation times that appear to be characteristic of malignant tumors, should be measurable in an intact organism."

In order to do this, complete the basis $\{P^\star, Q^\star\}$ to the basis $\{P^\star, Q^\star, I^\star\}$ of the dual vector space $\mathrm{Lie}(G)^\star$ such that the completed basis forms the dual basis of the canonical basis $\{P, Q, I\}$ of $\mathrm{Lie}(G)$. Different from the saddle-shaped, non-uniform magnetic flux density, chosen to achieve spectral localization by Raymond V. Damadian, the other visionary MRI pioneer [51], the Lauterbur magnetic field gradients are represented by linear differential forms

$$\alpha = \mathrm{d}y, \quad \beta = -\mathrm{d}x$$

imposed on the homogeneous plane spanned as a symplectic affine variety by its symplectic basis $\{P^\star, Q^\star\}$ in $\mathrm{Lie}(G)^\star$. Then the exterior product mapping $\bigwedge^2 \Phi$ generates cohomologically the distinguished closed exterior differential 2-form

$$\omega_\nu = \nu \cdot \alpha \wedge \beta = \nu \cdot \omega_1$$

of

$$\bigwedge^2 (\mathcal{O}_\nu) \cong \mathrm{H}^2(\mathbf{R} \oplus \mathbf{R})$$

as rotational curvature form of $\mathcal{O}_\nu \hookrightarrow \mathbf{P}(\mathbf{R} \times \mathrm{Lie}(G)^\star)$ $(\nu \neq 0)$. It forms a representative of the magnetic moment referred to in Bloch's dynamical approach.

- The bandwidth of the transmitted radiofrequencies controls the width of the tomographic slice, frequency selected from the canonical foliation of symplectic affine leaves $\mathcal{O}_\nu$ $(\nu \neq 0)$ in projective space.

- After tomographic slice selection from the canonical foliation by resonance with the center frequency $\nu \in \hat{C} - \{0\}$, the operation via transport by the morphism

$$\Phi : \mathcal{C}^\infty_{\mathbf{R}} \left(\mathrm{Lie}(G)/\mathrm{Lie}(G)^{[2]} \right) \longrightarrow \mathrm{Z}^1 (\mathcal{O}_\nu)$$

  of the solvable affine Lie group $\mathbf{GA}(\mathbf{R})$ on the spatial linear magnetic field gradients $-\mathrm{d}y$ and $\mathrm{d}x$, respectively, inside the projectively immersed, symplectic affine planes of incidence $\mathcal{O}_\nu$ $(\nu \neq 0)$ is switched in sequence instead of simultaneously.

- Pulsing instead of continuous ramp changes by the action of the solvable affine Lie group $\mathbf{GA}(\mathbf{R})$ allows for sequencing the spatial linear magnetic field gradients.

When the spatial linear magnetic field gradients are removed, the nuclear spins return to the original local frequency of Larmor precession spectrum, but retain the phase shift caused by the phase encoding linear gradient. Most clinical scanner systems use 128, 192, 256, or even 512 incremental phase encoding steps to acquire the signal wavelet data of a scan.

Due to the spin–lattice and spin–spin relaxation phenomena [25,26,73], MRI is basically a slow scan modality. Conventional spin echo imaging methods require long data acquisition times since only one hologram line is collected for each excitation pulse. Fast spin echo imaging, however, markedly reduces scan times. In fast spin echo imaging, the phase encoding linear gradient for each echo in the pulse train is changed so that multiple channel data are acquired within a given repetition time. The excitation profiles can be performed by use of multiwavelets. Each spin echo in the train contributes both spatial resolution and image contrast. Body imaging with fast spin echo benefits from an increased number of excitations to average out respiratory motion and reduce the resultant artifact. Although fast spin echo methods have been employed in neurofunctional MRI and have even shown advantages with respect to selectivity for capillary blood oxygenation level dependent (BOLD) effect, the signal wavelet increases are significantly smaller than for gradient recalled echoes under the condition of good macroscopic magnetic flux density homogeneity.

Recall that each non-trivial transvection represents a non-diagonalizable linear transformation. However, a basis of the underlying vector space may be chosen such that relative to this basis the matrix of the non-trivial transvection has all its entries on the main diagonal equal 1, and all the other matrix entries, with exactly one exception, equal zero. In terms of real projective spaces, the transvections form a normal abelian subgroup of the group of cohomologies which let invariant the foci of the projective plane at infinity $\mathbf{P}(\mathbf{R} \times \mathcal{O}_\infty)$. The projective plane at infinity forms the complement of the image of $\mathrm{Lie}(G)^\star$ under the canonical injection in the projective completion $\mathbf{P}(\mathbf{R} \times \mathrm{Lie}(G)^\star)$ of the real vector space $\mathrm{Lie}(G)^\star$ where $\mathbf{R}$ in the projective split denotes the homogeneous event line. Therefore the linear projective variety $\mathbf{P}(\mathbf{R} \times \mathcal{O}_\infty)$ is canonically immersed into the three-dimensional real projective space $\mathbf{P}(\mathbf{R} \times \mathrm{Lie}(G)^\star)$.

The notion of focus was introduced by Keppler in his book Paralipomena Astronomiae Pars Optica (1604). To complete this book he interrupted his work at the Mars commentaries. Keppler then introduced affine dilations into the quadrature conchoid trajectory construction to achieve elliptical orbits by their operation as homologies on the affine quadric embedded into the projective space and avoiding the projective plane at infinity. Immersion into the three-dimensional compact super-encoding projective space forms a constituent ingredient of his conchoid construction. However, the contributions of Keppler to projective geometry, called 'Perspectiva' at his time, and vision seem to have almost escaped notice in literature, although since about the mid 1980's most of the computer vision and robotics literature discussing geometric invariants has used the language of projective geometry.

- The group of affine dilations and transvections $\mathbf{GA}(\mathrm{Lie}(G)^\star)$ is formed by those cohomologies which transform parallel lines onto parallel lines of the real projective space $\mathbf{P}(\mathbf{R} \times \mathrm{Lie}(G)^\star)$. It is isomorphic to the group of cohomologies consisting of the affine homothetic transformations of the line $\hat{C}$ with the origin removed, transverse to the projective plane of foci at infinity $\mathbf{P}(\mathbf{R} \times \mathcal{O}_\infty)$, and the transvections of the complement of $\mathbf{P}(\mathbf{R} \times \mathcal{O}_\infty)$ in $\mathbf{P}(\mathbf{R} \times \mathrm{Lie}(G)^\star)$.

- The normal subgroup of affine transvections $\mathbf{SA}(\mathrm{Lie}(G)^\star) \hookrightarrow \mathbf{GA}(\mathrm{Lie}(G)^\star)$ is formed by the translations of the additive group of the projective plane of foci at infinity $\mathbf{P}(\mathbf{R} \times \mathcal{O}_\infty)$ in the real projective space $\mathbf{P}(\mathbf{R} \times \mathrm{Lie}(G)^\star)$ canonically associated to the dual vector space $\mathrm{Lie}(G)^\star$.

- The quotient group of the disconnected Lie group of affine dilations and transvections $\mathbf{GA}(\mathrm{Lie}(G)^\star)$ modulo the normal subgroup of affine transvections $\mathbf{SA}(\mathrm{Lie}(G)^\star)$ is isomorphic to the multiplicative group $\mathbf{R} - \{0\}$.

- The normal subgroup of affine transvections $\mathbf{SA}(\mathrm{Lie}(G)^\star)$ has index two in the subgroup of the affine group $\mathbf{GA}(\mathrm{Lie}(G)^\star)$ which is generated by the affine symmetries about an affine plane $\mathcal{O}_\nu (\nu \neq 0)$, canonically immersed into the complement of the projective plane of foci at infinity $\mathbf{P}(\mathbf{R} \times \mathcal{O}_\infty)$ in $\mathbf{P}(\mathbf{R} \times \mathrm{Lie}(G)^\star)$.

Taking into account the transvections with the unipotent upper triangular matrices

$$\exp_G P = \begin{pmatrix} 1 & 1 & 0 \\ 0 & 1 & 0 \\ 0 & 0 & 1 \end{pmatrix}, \quad \exp_G Q = \begin{pmatrix} 1 & 0 & 0 \\ 0 & 1 & 1 \\ 0 & 0 & 1 \end{pmatrix}, \quad \exp_G I = \begin{pmatrix} 1 & 0 & 1 \\ 0 & 1 & 0 \\ 0 & 0 & 1 \end{pmatrix},$$

it becomes obvious that the matrix exponential map

$$\exp_G : \mathrm{Lie}(G) \longrightarrow G,$$

is a diffeomorphism which takes Lebesgue measure on $\mathrm{Lie}(G)$ to Haar measure on G. It shows that G is a connected, simply connected Lie group. The coordinate functions of the transvections which give rise to the Hamiltonian action of G by symplectomorphisms on $\mathrm{Z}^1(\mathcal{O}_\nu)$ now read on the Lie group level

$$\begin{pmatrix} y \\ 1 \end{pmatrix} = \begin{pmatrix} 1 & 1 & 0 \\ 0 & 1 & 0 \\ 0 & 0 & 1 \end{pmatrix}, \qquad (x, 1) = \begin{pmatrix} 1 & 0 & 0 \\ 0 & 1 & -1 \\ 0 & 0 & 1 \end{pmatrix}.$$

The homogeneous hologram line bundle splitting on which the Lauterbur subband encoding is based then is performed by multiplication on the left and right of the column and row vectors, respectively, by the gradient matrices

$$\begin{pmatrix} a & 1 \\ 0 & 1 \end{pmatrix} \in \mathbf{GA}(\mathbf{R}), \quad \begin{pmatrix} a & 0 \\ 1 & 1 \end{pmatrix} \in \mathbf{GA}(\mathbf{R})^t$$

of ratio $a \neq 0$, polarity

$$\operatorname{sgn}\det \begin{pmatrix} a & 1 \\ 0 & 1 \end{pmatrix} = \operatorname{sgn} a,$$

and normalized shift $b = 1$. The associated affine linear transformations are affine dilations of ratio $a \neq 0$. In gradient recalled echo imaging, gradient recalled echoes are formed following a single radiofrequency pulse with the spin echo generated by refocusing spins using rewinder gradient matrices of opposite polarity

$$\begin{pmatrix} -a & 1 \\ 0 & 1 \end{pmatrix} \in \mathbf{GA}(\mathbf{R}), \quad \begin{pmatrix} -a & 0 \\ 1 & 1 \end{pmatrix} \in \mathbf{GA}(\mathbf{R})^t \qquad (a \neq 0),$$

respectively. Indeed, the transition to the frequency domain is performed by the affine wavelet transform on the positive half-line $\mathbf{R}_+$. By structure transportation to the complex Hilbert space $L^2_{\mathbf{C}}(\mathbf{R}_+)$ of transverse sections of square integrable functions of positive energy, the affine wavelet transform is deduced from the spin labelled holomorphic discrete series representation of the special linear group $\mathbf{SL}(2,\mathbf{R})$ over $\mathbf{R}$ onto which the metaplectic group $\mathbf{Mp}(2,\mathbf{R})$ projects with kernel $\mathbf{Z}/2\mathbf{Z}$ as the group of dynamical symmetries [73].

In order to perform the structure transport onto the group of dynamical symmetries, apply the Gram–Schmidt orthonormalization procedure to $\mathbf{R} \oplus \mathbf{R}$ in order to generate the left

Iwasawa topological decomposition of the Lie group $\mathbf{SL}(2,\mathbf{R})$ of quantized calculus. Denote the decomposition by

$$K \cdot \underbrace{A_0 \cdot N_0}\,,$$

where

$$N_0 = [\mathbf{GA}(\mathbf{R}), \mathbf{GA}(\mathbf{R})]$$

is the commutator subgroup of the solvable affine Lie group $\mathbf{GA}(\mathbf{R})$. If $\mathbf{GA}(\mathbf{R})$ is embedded into the projective group $\mathbf{GP}_1(\mathbf{R})$ of the real projective line $\mathbf{P}_1(\mathbf{R}) = \mathbf{P}(\mathbf{R} \times \mathbf{R})$ by letting invariant the point at infinity ∞, N_0 acts smoothly and transitively via bilinear maps on $\mathbf{P}_1(\mathbf{R})$, hence biholomorphically and transitively via homographies or Möbius fractional linear transformations on the open upper complex half-plane, the Poincaré half-plane

$$\mathcal{O}_+ = \{w \in \mathbf{C} \mid \Im w > 0\}.$$

The exterior differential 2-form on $\mathcal{O}_+$ given as

$$\frac{1}{y^2} \cdot \mathrm{d}x \wedge \mathrm{d}y = \frac{i}{2y^2} \cdot \mathrm{d}w \wedge \mathrm{d}\bar{w}$$

is invariant under the action of the group $\mathbf{SL}(2,\mathbf{R})$ by automorphisms of $\mathcal{O}_+$, so that the measure

$$\frac{1}{y^2} \cdot \mathrm{d}x \otimes \mathrm{d}y$$

associated to the Poincaré metric of the open upper complex half-plane $\mathcal{O}_+$, is invariant under the biholomorphic and transitive action of $\mathbf{SL}(2,\mathbf{R})$. The maximal compact, connected component K of the Iwasawa decomposition is isomorphic to the Lie group $\mathbf{SO}(2,\mathbf{R})$ of planar rotations, hence to the reference unit circle $\mathbf{T} \hookrightarrow \mathbf{C}$ of the eccentric Kepplerian clockwork dynamics. Because the stabilizer of the point $w = i \in \mathcal{O}_+$ is given by $\mathbf{SO}(2,\mathbf{R})$, it follows the homogeneous manifold representation

$$\mathcal{O}_+ \cong \mathbf{SL}(2,\mathbf{R})/\mathbf{SO}(2,\mathbf{R}).$$

The special importance of the open upper complex half-plane $\mathcal{O}_+$ for linear magnetic field actions stems from this homogeneous manifold representation which is a special case of the general principle:

Semi-simple real Lie group/maximal compact subgroup $\cong$ symmetric manifold

The orbit of the point $w = ir \in \mathcal{O}_+$ where $r \in]0,1]$ is formed by the circle of center $i\xi \in \mathcal{O}_+$, where the positive real number ξ is given by the Joukowski transform

$$\xi = \frac{1}{2}\left(r + \frac{1}{r}\right)$$

of external magnetic flux density correction, and has the two points $\{ir, \frac{i}{r}\}$ located on the imaginary axis as diametrically opposed points.

- The points $\{ir, \frac{i}{r}\}$ serve as off-center shimming control points of the magnetic flux density in an azimuthal polar plot transverse to the longitudinal axis of the magnet bore.

The solvable component of the left Iwasawa decomposition, the underbraced closed subgroup

$$A_0 \cdot N_0 = \left\{ \left(\begin{array}{cc} a & b \\ 0 & \frac{1}{a} \end{array} \right) \middle| a \neq 0, \quad b \in \mathbf{R} \right\}$$

of $\mathbf{SL}(2,\mathbf{R})$, forms the stabilizer of the point $\infty \in \mathbf{P}_1(\mathbf{R})$. Let $A_0 \cdot N_0 \hookrightarrow \mathbf{SL}(2,\mathbf{R})$ act on the point $w = i \in \mathcal{O}_+$ as follows:

$$\left(\begin{array}{cc} a & b \\ 0 & \frac{1}{a} \end{array} \right) \cdot i = \frac{ai+b}{\frac{1}{a}} = a^2 i + ab \qquad (a \neq 0)$$

Then the solvable affine Lie group $\mathbf{GA}(\mathbf{R})$ acts transitively on the planar coadjoint orbit $\mathcal{O}_+$, and $\mathbf{GA}(\mathbf{R})$ inherits a left Haar measure from one half of the measure of $\mathcal{O}_+$ associated to the Poincaré metric of the open upper complex half-plane. For this action which admits the 1-cocycle

$$\left(\begin{array}{cc} a & b \\ 0 & \frac{1}{a} \end{array} \right) \rightsquigarrow \frac{1}{a^{2m+1}} \qquad (a \neq 0),$$

the functions

$$\mathbf{R}_+ \ni t \rightsquigarrow e^{\pi i w t} t^m \qquad (w \in \mathcal{O}_+)$$

give rise to a total set in the Hilbert space $L^2_{\mathbf{C}}(\mathbf{R}_+)$ of square integrable, complex-valued functions of positive energy, provided $2m \in \mathbf{N}$, $m > 0$.

- The affine wavelet transform is generated by unitary induction from the Pontryagin dual $\hat{K}$ of the maximal compact, connected subgroup K of $\mathbf{SL}(2,\mathbf{R})$.

By inducing the unitary character of order $2m+1$ of the subgroup $K \hookrightarrow \mathbf{SL}(2,\mathbf{R})$, the kernel function attached to the affine wavelet transform of matrix

$$\left(\begin{array}{cc} a & b \\ 0 & 1 \end{array} \right) \in \mathbf{GA}(\mathbf{R})$$

and the spin label of half-integral or integral value

$$m \in \frac{1}{2}\mathbf{N}, \quad m > 0$$

takes for the choice $w = i \in \mathcal{O}_+$ the following form in the transverse line bundle section $L^2_{\mathbf{C}}(\mathbf{R}_+)$:

$$\mathbf{R}_+ \ni t \rightsquigarrow a^{2m+1} e^{2\pi i a b t} e^{-2\pi a^2 t} t^m$$

in order to trivialize in biomedical magnetic resonance spectroscopic imaging the cocycle of the projectivized representation of spin label $2m \in \frac{1}{2}\mathbf{N}$, $m > 0$, the special linear group

$\mathbf{SL}(2,\mathbf{R})$ has to replaced by the group extension $\mathbf{Mp}(2,\mathbf{R})$ which is pointwise attached to the one-dimensional center C of G as the group of dynamical symmetries.

The affine wavelet transform includes an attenuation as well as a dephasing factor. The wavelets which are diffracted by the linear gradient switching for spectral localization purposes die out due to the attenuation factor. The gradient reflections or affine symmetries

$$\begin{pmatrix} a & 1 \\ 0 & 1 \end{pmatrix} \rightsquigarrow \begin{pmatrix} -a & 1 \\ 0 & 1 \end{pmatrix}, \quad \begin{pmatrix} a & 0 \\ 1 & 1 \end{pmatrix} \rightsquigarrow \begin{pmatrix} -a & 0 \\ 1 & 1 \end{pmatrix}$$

are able to rewind those phases which are caused by linear gradient switching, hence to eliminate the dispersion spectrum. In view of the inversion formula for transvections [73], the spectral leakage effect due to phase dispersion can be avoided by a repeating the data acquisition experiment with linear magnetic field gradients of opposite polarity. The close analogy to the dephasing effect originating from relaxation, and the technique of spin echo rephasing should be observed. Of course, the linear rewinding procedure has to be in synergy with the successive radiofrequency pulse excitations of the spin isochromats in order to avoid that dispersive wavelets creep into the quantum hologram and then decrease the signal-to-noise ratio.

- Due to the strategy of untwisting by means of reversing the polarity of the linear magnetic field gradient for a time half the length of the $\frac{\pi}{2}$ pulse, or applying a π pulse, the lift out of the tomographic slice $\mathcal{O}_\nu \hookrightarrow \mathbf{P}(\mathbf{R} \times \mathrm{Lie}(G)^\star)$ is brought back and frozen in the rotating coordinate frame of quadrature reference at center frequency $\nu \in \hat{C} - \{0\}$.
- Stepwise incrementation of the linear phase encoding gradient in conjunction with polarity reversal or phase conjugation flip allows for control and recording of the rotational curvature form in the quantum hologram.

In the presence of the frequency gradient of gradient matrix $\begin{pmatrix} -1 & 0 \\ 1 & 1 \end{pmatrix} \in \mathbf{GA}(\mathbf{R})^t$ of polarity -1 which acts via transport by the morphism $\Phi : \mathcal{C}^\infty_{\mathbf{R}} \left(\mathrm{Lie}(G)/\mathrm{Lie}(G)^{[2]}\right) \longrightarrow \mathrm{Z}^1\left(\mathcal{O}_\nu\right)$ on the *connection* differential 1-form

$$\nu(-y \cdot \mathrm{d}x + x \cdot \mathrm{d}y) \in \mathrm{Z}^1\left(\mathcal{O}_\nu\right),$$

the action via Φ of the stepping phase encoding gradient matrices $\begin{pmatrix} a & 1 \\ 0 & 1 \end{pmatrix} \in \mathbf{GA}(\mathbf{R})$ take place. Then the quantum hologram of the Lauterbur subband encoding technique of spectral localization in the trivial line bundle $\mathbf{R} \oplus \mathbf{R}$ on the projectively immersed, affine symplectic plane $\mathcal{O}_\nu \hookrightarrow \mathrm{Lie}(G)^\star\ (\nu \neq 0)$ is generated by $\bigwedge^2 \Phi$ in

$$\bigwedge^2 (\mathcal{O}_\nu) \cong \mathrm{H}^2(\mathbf{R} \oplus \mathbf{R}).$$

It takes the form

$$K^\nu(x,y) \cdot \omega_\nu \qquad (\nu \neq 0)$$

with density $K^\nu \in L^2_{\mathbf{C}}\left(\mathbf{R} \oplus \mathbf{R}\right)$ and non-zero $\nu \in \hat{C} - \{0\}$.

- During the presence of a readout gradient of opposite polarity +1, the quantum hologram $K^{\nu}(x,y)\,\nu\cdot \mathrm{d}x\wedge \mathrm{d}y$ collects in the projectively immersed, affine symplectic plane $\mathcal{O}_{\nu}\,(\nu\neq 0)$ the readout data and stepped phase data of the mode spectra at center frequency $\nu\in\hat{C}-\{0\}$.

It will be established later on that the kernel function K^{ν} admits Hermitian symmetry. Harmonic analysis on the Heisenberg nilpotent group G allows for a detailed analysis of the kernel K^{ν} in terms of the proton density function [69, 70].

The adjoint action Ad_G of G on $\mathrm{Lie}(G)$ represents infinitesimally the action of G onto itself by inner automorphisms. The coadjoint action of G on $\mathrm{Lie}(G)^{\star}$ via the contragredient to Ad_G is denoted by CoAd_G. It is given as

$$\mathrm{CoAd}_G\begin{pmatrix}1 & x & z\\ 0 & 1 & y\\ 0 & 0 & 1\end{pmatrix}=\begin{pmatrix}1 & 0 & -y\\ 0 & 1 & x\\ 0 & 0 & 1\end{pmatrix}.$$

Therefore the action CoAd_G is flat and reads in terms of the coordinates $\{\alpha,\beta,\nu\}$ with respect to the dual basis $\{P^{\star},Q^{\star},I^{\star}\}$ of the dual real vector space $\mathrm{Lie}(G)^{\star}$ as follows:

$$\mathrm{CoAd}_G\begin{pmatrix}1 & x & z\\ 0 & 1 & y\\ 0 & 0 & 1\end{pmatrix}(\alpha P^{\star}+\beta Q^{\star}+\nu I^{\star})=(\alpha-\nu y)P^{\star}+(\beta+\nu x)Q^{\star}+\nu I^{\star}.$$

The linear symplectic affine varieties

$$\mathcal{O}_{\nu}=\mathrm{CoAd}_G\,(G)\,(\nu I^{\star})=\mathbf{R}P^{\star}+\mathbf{R}Q^{\star}+\nu I^{\star}\qquad(\nu\neq 0)$$

are isomorphic to the quotient of $\mathrm{Lie}(G)$ by the radical of the non-zero alternating $\mathbf{R}$-bilinear form

$$\nu\cdot[\cdot,\cdot]$$

The anti-symmetric forms are scaled by the homogeneous line with the origin removed of non-zero alternating bilinear forms on the planar coadjoint orbit $\mathcal{O}_{\nu}\hookrightarrow \mathbf{P}(\mathbf{R}\times\mathrm{Lie}(G)^{\star})\ (\nu\neq 0)$ of G. The driving frequency $\nu\in\hat{C}-\{0\}$ determines the rotating coordinate frame of quadrature reference of the tomographic slice $\mathcal{O}_{\nu}\hookrightarrow\mathrm{Lie}(G)^{\star}$, frequency selected from the canonical foliation, and the associated rotational curvature form.

The homogeneous line with the origin removed of non-zero alternating bilinear forms can be identified with $\hat{C}-\{0\}$, and the frequency selected tomographic slices $\mathcal{O}_{\nu}\,(\nu\neq 0)$ are symplectic affine planes in the sense that they are in the natural way compatibly endowed with both the projectively immersed structure of an affine plane and a symplectic structure. Therefore the projectively immersed, symplectic affine leaves $\mathcal{O}_{\nu}\hookrightarrow\mathbf{P}(\mathbf{R}\times\mathrm{Lie}(G)^{\star})$ through the driving frequencies $\nu\in\hat{C}-\{0\}$ in are predestinate to implement the Kepplerian quadrature detection strategy over the event line $\mathbf{R}$ by a phase-splitting network [68].

- The tomographic slices $\mathcal{O}_{\nu}\,(\nu\neq 0)$ can be frequency addressed by a selective excitation procedure. Adjacent slices are not effected. By using the linear magnetic field gradients in combination, the directional derivatives provide intermediate tomographic slice orientation.

- As projectively immersed, symplectic flats of incidence, the planar coadjoint orbits $\mathcal{O}_\nu \hookrightarrow \mathbf{P}(\mathbf{R} \times \mathrm{Lie}(G)^\star)$ of G through the driving frequency $\nu \in \hat{C} - \{0\}$ carry spin excitation profiles or quantum holograms acting as multichannel reconstructive analysis–synthesis filter banks.

- The Heisenberg group G acts transitively on the planar coadjoint orbits

$$\mathcal{O}_\nu \hookrightarrow \mathbf{P}(\mathbf{R} \times \mathrm{Lie}(G)^\star)$$

through the driving frequency $\nu \neq 0$ via symplectomorphisms on $\mathrm{Z}^1(\mathcal{O}_\nu)$.

- The flatness of the coadjoint orbits implies the triviality of the first cohomology group $\mathrm{H}^1(\mathcal{O}_\nu)$ with coefficients in $\mathbf{R}$.

These high tech implementations emphasize the grandeur of the Kepplerian spatiotemporal quadrature strategy ranging from physical astronomy to very large scale integration (VLSI) microcircuit design of electronic engineering [38, 52].

- In SAR imaging, $\nu \neq 0$ denotes the center frequency of the transmitted pulse train, whereas in clinical MRI the center frequency $\nu \in \hat{C} - \{0\}$ is the frequency of the rotating coordinate frame defined by tomographic slice selection from the canonical foliation in projective space.

The stationary singular plane $\mathcal{O}_\infty \hookrightarrow \mathbf{P}(\mathbf{R} \times \mathrm{Lie}(G)^\star)$ of equation

$$\nu = 0$$

consists of the single point orbits or, in terms of the real projective space $\mathbf{P}(\mathbf{R} \times \mathrm{Lie}(G)^\star)$, the focal points at infinity

$$\left\{\varepsilon_{(\alpha,\beta)} \middle| (\alpha,\beta) \in \mathbf{R} \oplus \mathbf{R}\right\}$$

corresponding to the one-dimensional representations of G. The unifying concepts are the *affine dual* of the frequency selected tomographic slices $\mathcal{O}_\nu \hookrightarrow \mathrm{Lie}(G)^\star\,(\nu \neq 0)$ consisting of all affine $\mathbf{R}$-linear forms on the coadjoint orbit $\mathcal{O}_\nu \hookrightarrow \mathbf{P}(\mathbf{R} \times \mathrm{Lie}(G)^\star)$, and the *projective completion*consisting of the set of homogeneous lines with the origin removed in the dual vector space of the affine dual of each of the affine planes $\mathcal{O}_\nu\,(\nu \neq 0)$.

- The unitary dual $\hat{G}$ of the Heisenberg nilpotent Lie group G can be injected into the projective completion of the dual vector space of the affine dual of each of the tomographic slices $\mathcal{O}_\nu \hookrightarrow \mathrm{Lie}(G)^\star\,(\nu \neq 0)$, frequency selected from the canonical foliation.

- The projective completion of the dual vector space of the affine dual of each of the tomographic slices $\mathcal{O}_\nu \hookrightarrow \mathrm{Lie}(G)^\star\,(\nu \neq 0)$, intrinsically constructed in terms of the single point coadjoint orbits of $\mathcal{O}_\infty$ and the coadjoint orbits $\mathcal{O}_\nu\,(\nu \neq 0)$ of G can be identified with the real projective space $\mathbf{P}(\mathbf{R} \times \mathrm{Lie}(G)^\star)$ of homogeneous event line $\mathbf{R}$.

- The foliated projective space $\mathbf{P}(\mathbf{R} \times \mathrm{Lie}(G)^\star)$ implements the longitudinal dilation controlled transvectional action of the Heisenberg group G.

The complement of the projective plane at infinity $\mathbf{P}(\mathbf{R}\times\mathcal{O}_\infty)$ in the real projective space $\mathbf{P}(\mathbf{R}\times\mathrm{Lie}(G)^\star)$ has the structure of a linear affine variety. Its standard topology inherited from the direction coincides with the relative topology induced by the quotient topology of $\mathbf{P}(\mathbf{R}\times\mathrm{Lie}(G)^\star)$. With respect to this complement of equation $\nu\neq 0$, $\mathbf{R}\times\mathcal{O}_\infty$ defines the plane of direction of the linear projective variety generated by the canonical injection of the symplectic affine leaf $\mathcal{O}_\nu \hookrightarrow \mathbf{P}(\mathbf{R}\times\mathrm{Lie}(G)^\star)$ $(\nu\neq 0)$.

As the observation plane, $\mathcal{O}_\infty \hookrightarrow \mathbf{P}(\mathbf{R}\times\mathrm{Lie}(G)^\star)$ plays a fundamental role in the coherent optical processing of radar data [15, 42, 48, 49], clinico-morphological MRI, clinical magnetic resonance angiography for the clinical management of vascular disease [1, 58, 84], and neurofunctional MRI detecting for the recording of cerebral cortical activities [73].

It follows from this classification of the coadjoint orbits of G in $\mathrm{Lie}(G)^\star$ the highly remarkable fact that there exists no finite dimensional irreducible unitary linear representation of G having dimension > 1. Hence the irreducible unitary linear representations of G which are not unitary characters are infinite-dimensional, and may be realized as unitarily induced group representations. Their coefficient cross-sections for the Hilbert bundle sitting over the event line $\mathbf{R}$ define the holographic transforms.

- Due to the theorem of Stone–von Neumann of quantum physics, the group of invariants of the holographic transform is formed by the metaplectic group $\mathbf{Mp}(2,\mathbf{R})$ which projects onto the underlying special linear group $\mathbf{SL}(2,\mathbf{R})$ with kernel $\mathbf{Z}/2\mathbf{Z}$.
- Due to the covariance identity for the twisting by $\mathbf{SL}(2,\mathbf{R})$, the normalization by the action of $\mathbf{Mp}(2,\mathbf{R})$ of the image group $U^\nu(G)$ under the the irreducible unitary linear representations U^ν of G associated to $\mathcal{O}_\nu$ $(\nu\neq 0)$ in the real projective space $\mathbf{P}(\mathbf{R}\times\mathrm{Lie}(G)^\star)$ provides a planar redistribution of the wavelet energy stored within the quantum hologram by the rotational curvature form for data compression purposes.

Let the set of unipotent upper triangular matrices

$$C=\left\{\left(\begin{array}{ccc}1&0&z\\0&1&0\\0&0&1\end{array}\right)\middle|\, z\in\mathbf{R}\right\}$$

denote the one-dimensional center of G transverse to the projectively immersed, symplectic affine planes of incidence $\mathcal{O}_\nu$ $(\nu\neq 0)$ through the driving frequency $\nu\in\hat{C}-\{0\}$ carrying the spin excitation profiles or quantum holograms. Then

$$C=[G,G]=\exp_G\left(\mathrm{Lie}(G)^{[2]}\right)=\mathbf{R}\exp_G I$$

is spanned by the central transvection $\exp_G I$, hence isomorphic to $\mathbf{R}$, and aligned with the direction of the external static magnetic field along the longitudinal axis of the magnet bore. In coordinate-free terms, G forms the non-split central group extension

$$C\lhd G\longrightarrow G/C$$

where G/C is transverse to the homogeneous line C, and as a complement to the longitudinal line $C\hookrightarrow G$, bicontinuously isomorphic to a linear symplectic affine variety $\mathbf{R}\oplus\mathbf{R}$ which is canonically immersed into the real projective space $\mathbf{P}(\mathbf{R}\times\mathrm{Lie}(G)^\star)$ canonically associated to the dual vector space $\mathrm{Lie}(G)^\star$.

- The group of automorphisms of G which induce the identity on the center $C \hookrightarrow G$ is isomorphic to the semi-direct product of the special linear group $\mathbf{SL}(2,\mathbf{R})$ with the vector group $\mathbf{R}\oplus\mathbf{R}$.

- Provided the central unitary character χ_ν of $\mathcal{O}_\nu \hookrightarrow \mathbf{P}(\mathbf{R}\times \mathrm{Lie}(G)^\star)$ $(\nu \neq 0)$ with center frequency $\nu \in \hat{C}-\{0\}$ defines the identity representation of $K \hookrightarrow \mathbf{SL}(2,\mathbf{R})$, the actions of the holographic transform and the affine wavelet transform associated to the laboratory frame of $G/C\times \mathbf{SL}(2,\mathbf{R})/K$ are synchronized with the rotating coordinate frame of quadrature reference.

An inspection of the spectrum of G described above reveals a continuous open map onto the center $C \hookrightarrow G$ taking a copy of the singular plane $\mathcal{O}_\infty$ onto $\nu = 0$, and a single point onto each non-zero $\nu \in \hat{C}$. In terms of the quantized calculus, the $C^\star$-algebra of G is the algebra of continuous sections vanishing at infinity of a continuous field, or *bundle*, of $C^\star$-algebras $(\mathcal{A}_\nu)_{\nu\in\hat{C}}$, with $\mathcal{A}_\nu$ the quotient corresponding to the closed subset mapping into $\{\nu\}$. Since all points of the projective plane of foci at infinity $\mathbf{P}(\mathbf{R}\times\mathcal{O}_\infty) \hookrightarrow \mathbf{P}(\mathbf{R}\times \mathrm{Lie}(G)^\star)$ which maps into $\{0\}$ are one-dimensional representations of G, it follows

$$\mathcal{A}_0 \cong \mathcal{C}_0(\mathbf{R}\oplus\mathbf{R})$$

For each $\nu \in \hat{C}-\{0\}$, since the spectrum of $\mathcal{A}_\nu$ is a single point, and the irreducible unitary linear representation of G corresponding to the symplectic affine leaf $\mathcal{O}_\nu(\nu \neq 0)$ in the foliated projective space $\mathbf{P}(\mathbf{R}\times \mathrm{Lie}(G)^\star)$ is infinite-dimensional, it follows that $\mathcal{A}_\nu$ is isomorphic to the standard $C^\star$-algebra $\mathcal{LC}\left(L^2_{\mathbf{C}}(\mathbf{R})\right)$ of compact operators acting on the complex Hilbert space $L^2_{\mathbf{C}}(\mathbf{R})$. The simple $C^\star$-algebra

$$\mathcal{A}_\nu \cong \mathcal{LC}\left(L^2_{\mathbf{C}}(\mathbf{R})\right) \qquad (\nu \neq 0)$$

includes the Hilbert–Schmidt operators on the standard modulation space $L^2_{\mathbf{C}}(\mathbf{R})$ as a norm dense ideal.

Let $\hat{C}$ denote the Pontryagin dual of the one-dimensional center $C \hookrightarrow G$. The irreducible unitary linear representations of G associated to the planar coadjoint orbit $\mathcal{O}_\nu(\nu \neq 0)$ of central unitary character $\chi_\nu \in \hat{C}$ may be realized as unitarily induced representations from the maximal abelian, connected subgroups

$$N = \left\{ \left. \begin{pmatrix} 1 & x & z \\ 0 & 1 & 0 \\ 0 & 0 & 1 \end{pmatrix} \right| x,z\in\mathbf{R} \right\}, \quad M = \left\{ \left. \begin{pmatrix} 1 & 0 & z \\ 0 & 1 & y \\ 0 & 0 & 1 \end{pmatrix} \right| y,z\in\mathbf{R} \right\}$$

by arbitrary extensions

$$\tilde{\chi}^N_\nu \in \hat{N}, \quad \tilde{\chi}^M_\nu \in \hat{M}$$

of $\chi_\nu \in \hat{C}$ from C to N and M, respectively.

- The closed normal abelian subgroups $N \hookrightarrow G$ and $M \hookrightarrow G$ represent the local frequency band broadening within the projectively immersed, symplectic affine plane of incidence, frequency selected from the canonical foliation.

These maximal abelian, connected subgroups of G give rise to the associated pair of fibrations

$$(G/N, G/M)$$

of G sitting in quadrature over the pair of semi-direct factors

$$(T, S)$$

which form a pair of homogeneous transverse direction lines, both isomorphic to $\mathbf{R}$. By the usual diagram notation for fiber bundles sitting over their base manifold

$$\begin{array}{ccc} \text{fiber} & \longrightarrow & \text{total space} \\ & & \big\downarrow \\ & & \text{base manifold} \end{array}$$

the situation can be schematically displayed as follows:

$$\begin{array}{ccc} \mathcal{O}_\nu & \longrightarrow & G/N \\ & & \big\downarrow \\ & & T \end{array} \qquad \begin{array}{ccc} \mathcal{O}_\nu & \longrightarrow & G/M \\ & & \big\downarrow \\ & & S \end{array} \qquad (\nu \neq 0)$$

If the generic coadjoint orbit $\mathcal{O}_1 \hookrightarrow \mathbf{P}(\mathbf{R} \times \mathrm{Lie}(G)^\star)$ of G as a projectively immersed, symplectic flat is identified with the realification

$$\mathbf{C}(\mathbf{R} \oplus \mathbf{R})$$

of the field $\mathbf{C}$ of complex numbers by choosing an orthonormal energetic frame of reference of the plane of direction $\mathbf{R} \oplus \mathbf{R}$, the elements $w \in \mathcal{O}_1 \hookrightarrow \mathbf{P}(\mathbf{R} \times \mathrm{Lie}(G)^\star)$ admit a representation by quadrature cell matrices

$$\begin{pmatrix} x & -y \\ y & x \end{pmatrix} = \begin{pmatrix} x & 0 \\ 0 & x \end{pmatrix} + \begin{pmatrix} y & 0 \\ 0 & y \end{pmatrix} \cdot \begin{pmatrix} 0 & -1 \\ 1 & 0 \end{pmatrix}.$$

Thus the realification of $w \in \mathcal{O}_1$ includes the differential phase

$$\begin{pmatrix} x & 0 \\ 0 & x \end{pmatrix},$$

the local frequency

$$\begin{pmatrix} y & 0 \\ 0 & y \end{pmatrix}$$

as real coordinates with respect to the orthonormal energetic frame of reference rotating at the center frequency $\nu = 1$, and the symplectic Weyl quadrature matrix

$$J = \begin{pmatrix} 0 & -1 \\ 1 & 0 \end{pmatrix}$$

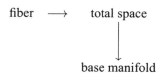

as the imaginary unit $w = i \in \mathcal{O}_+$ which stabilizes $K \cong \mathbf{SO}(2,\mathbf{R})$. The symplectic Weyl quadrature matrix J realized by $i \in \mathcal{O}_+$ give rise to a distinguished element $\neq 0$ on the homogeneous line $\hat{C}$ of *alternating* bilinear forms defined on the copy $\mathbf{R} \oplus \mathbf{R}$ of the generic coadjoint orbit $\mathcal{O}_1$ of G. The distinguished symplectic bilinear form generates cohomologically the closed exterior differential 2-form

$$\omega_1 \in \bigwedge^2 (\mathcal{O}_1).$$

With respect to the orthonormal energetic frame of reference of the plane $\mathbf{R} \oplus \mathbf{R}$, the set of quadrature cell matrices represents the *abelian* subgroup $\mathbf{GO}^+(2,\mathbf{R}) \hookrightarrow \mathbf{GL}(2,\mathbf{R})$ of non-zero direct linear similitudes of the symplectic affine plane $\mathbf{R} \oplus \mathbf{R}$. The group $\mathbf{GO}^+(2,\mathbf{R})$ reflects the stroboscopic and synchronous quadrature format design of the eccentric Kepplerian clockwork dynamics formed by the traces of the tuned in Heisenberg helices[73].

- The group $\mathbf{GO}(2,\mathbf{R})$ of all bijective linear similitudes of the symplectic affine plane $\mathbf{R} \oplus \mathbf{R}$ is the direct product of its normal subgroups consisting of the homothetic transformations of $\mathbf{R} \oplus \mathbf{R}$ of ratio > 0, and the orthogonal group $\mathbf{O}(2,\mathbf{R})$.
- The centralizer of the orthogonal group $\mathbf{O}(2,\mathbf{R})$ in $\mathbf{GL}(2,\mathbf{R})$ is the homothetic group.
- The group $\mathbf{GO}(2,\mathbf{R})$ is the normalizer in $\mathbf{GL}(2,\mathbf{R})$ of its subgroup $\mathbf{O}(2,\mathbf{R}) \hookrightarrow \mathbf{GO}(2,\mathbf{R})$ of orthogonal transformations or linear isometries of $\mathbf{R} \oplus \mathbf{R}$.
- The commutative group $\mathbf{GO}^+(2,\mathbf{R})$ forms a normal subgroup of index two of the non-abelian group $\mathbf{GO}(2,\mathbf{R}) \hookrightarrow \mathbf{GL}(2,\mathbf{R})$.

In $\mathbf{GO}^+(2,\mathbf{R})$, the commutative multiplication law of the quadrature cell matrices reads

$$\begin{pmatrix} x & -y \\ y & x \end{pmatrix} \cdot \begin{pmatrix} x' & -y' \\ y' & x' \end{pmatrix} = \begin{pmatrix} xx' - yy' & -(yx' + xy') \\ yx' + xy' & xx' - yy' \end{pmatrix}.$$

The conjugation identity

$$\begin{pmatrix} 1 & 0 \\ 0 & -1 \end{pmatrix} \begin{pmatrix} x & -y \\ y & x \end{pmatrix} \begin{pmatrix} 1 & 0 \\ 0 & -1 \end{pmatrix}^{-1} = \begin{pmatrix} x & y \\ -y & x \end{pmatrix}$$

yields the area law via the determinant form

$$|w|^2 = \det w,$$

the multiplicator $x^2 + y^2$, and the moment map associated to the rotational *curvature* form

$$(w, w') \rightsquigarrow \Im w \cdot \bar{w'}$$

for $w, w' \in \mathbf{C}$. For the realification of $w \in \mathbf{C} - \{0\}$ in $\mathbf{GO}^+(2,\mathbf{R})$, the inverse of the associated quadrature cell matrix reads in terms of the complex conjugate with reciprocal multiplicator

$$\begin{pmatrix} x & -y \\ y & x \end{pmatrix}^{-1} = \frac{1}{x^2 + y^2} \begin{pmatrix} x & y \\ -y & x \end{pmatrix}.$$

- The bijective similitudes w belonging to the subgroup $\mathbf{GO}^+(2,\mathbf{R}) \hookrightarrow \mathbf{GO}(2,\mathbf{R})$ represent exactly those endomorphisms of the symplectic affine plane $\mathbf{R} \oplus \mathbf{R}$ which commute with the direct linear similitude admitting the symplectic Weyl quadrature matrix J.

- The group $\mathbf{GO}^+(2,\mathbf{R})$ of non-zero direct linear similitudes of the symplectic affine plane $\mathbf{R}\oplus\mathbf{R}$ is the centralizer in $\mathbf{GL}(2,\mathbf{R})$ of any direct linear similitude which is not a homothetic transformation of $\mathbf{R}\oplus\mathbf{R}$.
- The set $\mathbf{GO}^+(2,\mathbf{R})\cup\{0\}$ of direct linear similitudes of the symplectic affine plane $\mathbf{R}\oplus\mathbf{R}$ is a commutative subfield $\mathbf{C}(\mathbf{R}\oplus\mathbf{R})\cong\mathbf{C}$ of the real algebra of endomorphisms of $\mathbf{R}\oplus\mathbf{R}$ with the standard symplectic form $(w,w')\rightsquigarrow\Im w\cdot\bar{w'}$ as rotational curvature form.
- The rotational curvature form is just the second fundamental form of the set of direct similitudes $\mathbf{C}(\mathbf{R}\oplus\mathbf{R})$.

The endomorphisms of the symplectic affine plane $\mathbf{R}\oplus\mathbf{R}$ which commute anti-symmetrically with the direct linear similitude represented by the symplectic Weyl quadrature matrix J, show that the indirect linear similitudes of the plane $\mathbf{R}\oplus\mathbf{R}$ can be represented with respect to an orthogonal energetic frame of reference of $\mathbf{R}\oplus\mathbf{R}$ as self-adjoint endomorphisms of quadrature cell matrices

$$\begin{pmatrix} x & y \\ y & -x \end{pmatrix}$$

with determinant form and multiplicator

$$-|w|^2 = -\det w,$$

and involutory flip matrix

$$\begin{pmatrix} 1 & 0 \\ 0 & -1 \end{pmatrix} \in \mathbf{GO}(2,\mathbf{R}).$$

Inspection of the spectrum shows that each indirect linear similitude of the plane $\mathbf{R}\oplus\mathbf{R}$ forms a reflection or symmetry about the homogeneous line spanned by the vector

$$(y, 1-x).$$

For $x=1, y=1$, the indirect linear similitude

$$\begin{pmatrix} 1 & 1 \\ 1 & -1 \end{pmatrix} \in \mathbf{GO}(2,\mathbf{R})$$

of multiplicator -2 gives rise to the unique continuous involutory automorphism

$$w \rightsquigarrow \bar{w}$$

of the realification $\mathbf{C}(\mathbf{R}\oplus\mathbf{R})$ of the field $\mathbf{C}$.

The multiplicator homomorphism allows for a transition from the direct affine isometries of multiplicator $a=+1$ to the indirect affine isometries of multiplicator $a=-1$. It implies the rephasing or forcing to reconverge process of the spin echo phenomenon by means of Hahn echoes. The spin echo pulse sequence was devised by Erwin Louis Hahn for nuclear magnetic resonance spectroscopy in 1950. It is the most commonly used pulse sequence in clinical MRI. Although faster spin echo techniques are available such as fast spin echo imaging which use the idle time to measure signals from adjacent tomographic slices, the spin echo pulse sequence as applied in two-dimensional Fourier transform MRI reconstructive method is still a workhorse of routine clinical MRI examinations. Most images of MRI anatomy of the body organs and the musculoskeletal system are presented using spin echo sequences which also are extensively used in nuclear magnetic resonance spectroscopy.

- The refocusing procedure of conventional spin echo imaging by phase conjugation flip depends upon the fact that the connected normal subgroup $\mathbf{Is}^+(2,\mathbf{R})$ of direct affine isometries has index two in the non-abelian, disconnected Lie group $\mathbf{Is}(2,\mathbf{R}) \hookrightarrow \mathbf{GA}(2,\mathbf{R})$ of all affine isometries of the symplectic affine plane $\mathbf{R}\oplus\mathbf{R}$.

- The quotient group $\mathbf{Is}(2,\mathbf{R})/\mathbf{Is}^+(2,\mathbf{R})$ is isomorphic to the group $\mathbf{Z}/2\mathbf{Z}$.

In gradient recalled echo imaging, the analogy to the refocusing procedure by spatial linear rewinder gradients should be observed. This procedure actually depends upon the fact that the group $\mathbf{SA}(\mathbf{R})$ of affine transvections has index two in the subgroup of $\mathbf{GA}(\mathbf{R})$ which is generated by the reflections or symmetries of the real line $\mathbf{R}$ about an arbitrary point. To increase the tissue differentiation and enhance the signal-to-noise ratio, a spoiled gradient recalled echo sequence can be used.

In conventional spin echo imaging, the spin echoes between water and fat come back into phase at the center of every echo, even though they differ in local frequency and are spatially misregistered. In gradient recalled echo imaging, however, water and fat protons do not generally come into phase coherence at the center of the echo, since gradient recalled echo imaging lacks the refocusing pulse which accomplishes the rephasing task in conventional spin echo imaging. Therefore, fat and water fall out of phase in gradient recalled echo scans. The characteristic appearance of this type of artifact is a sharply defined black rim around objects such as muscle fascicles on gradient recalled echo images. This artifact arises from boundary pixels that contain both fat and water protons and is manifest by an eerie black halo in all pixels along the entire fat–water interface.

For neurofunctional MRI of cerebral cortical activities it is important to observe that gradient recalled echoes do not refocus the dephasing effects of local inhomogeneities of magnetic flux density associated with the presence of deoxyhemoglobin. If spin echoes are used instead of gradient recalled echoes, then such dephasing effects will be refocused, provided that there is no significant diffusion of water molecules through the linear magnetic field gradients. However, if the water molecules diffuse through local magnetic field gradients during the echo time, then this will result in imperfect refocusing effects, and hence to signal loss in conventional spin echo pulse sequences.

- The direct linear similitude in $\mathbf{GO}^+(2,\mathbf{R})$ admitting the symplectic Weyl quadrature matrix J generates the subgroup $\mathbf{SO}(2,\mathbf{R}) \hookrightarrow \mathbf{O}(2,\mathbf{R})$ of planar rotations. It is isomorphic to the maximal compact, connected component $K \cong \mathbf{T}$ of the Iwasawa decomposition of $\mathbf{SL}(2,\mathbf{R})$.

- The torus group $K \hookrightarrow \mathbf{SL}(2,\mathbf{R})$ is driven by the center frequency $\nu \neq 0$ of the unitary character χ_ν associated to the planar coadjoint orbit $\mathcal{O}_\nu \hookrightarrow \mathbf{P}(\mathbf{R}\times \mathrm{Lie}(G)^\star)$ through the driving frequency $\nu \in \hat{C} - \{0\}$ of the rotating coordinate frame of quadrature reference of the tomographic slice $\mathcal{O}_\nu$, frequency selected from the canonical foliation in projective space.

- At the Lie algebra level, any unitary linear representation of the group of dynamical symmetries $\mathbf{Mp}(2,\mathbf{R})$ is diagonalizable under the action of the generator $J \in \mathbf{GO}^+(2,\mathbf{R})$ of K with eigenvalues in the set $\frac{i}{2}\mathbf{Z}$.

The compact Lie group K of planar rotations forms the stabilizer of the point $w = i$ of the natural action of $\mathbf{SL}(2,\mathbf{R})$ via homographies on the open upper complex half-plane $\mathcal{O}_+$.

In view of the area law, the rotational curvature form of $\mathcal{O}_\nu (\nu \neq 0)$ is exactly the determinant form

$$\nu \cdot \det.$$

The standard symplectic form is generated cohomologically by the moment map of the morphism of $\mathrm{Lie}(G)$ under the Lie bracket operation into the Lie algebra $\mathcal{C}^\infty_{\mathbf{R}}\left(\mathrm{Lie}(G)/\mathrm{Lie}(G)^{[2]}\right)$ under the Poisson manifold structure.

- The rotational curvature form of $\mathcal{O}_\nu \hookrightarrow \mathbf{P}(\mathbf{R} \times \mathrm{Lie}(G)^\star)$ is associated to the moment map of the equivariant Hamiltonian action of G by symplectomorphisms, and dilated by the center frequency $\nu \in \hat{C} - \{0\}$.

The moment map generates cohomologically the distinguished closed exterior differential 2-form $\omega_\nu = \nu \cdot \omega_1$ on $\mathcal{O}_\nu \hookrightarrow \mathbf{P}(\mathbf{R} \times \mathrm{Lie}(G)^\star)$ $(\nu \neq 0)$, and provides the radical of vector fields

$$\mathrm{Z}^1(\mathcal{O}_\nu) = \mathrm{rad}\, \omega_\nu \qquad (\nu \neq 0)$$

Indeed, under the natural pairing between differential forms and vector fields, $\omega_\nu = \nu \cdot \omega_1$ in

$$\bigwedge^2 (\mathcal{O}_\nu) \cong \mathrm{H}^2(\mathbf{R} \oplus \mathbf{R})$$

annihilates the vector fields on the symplectic affine plane $\mathrm{Lie}(G)/\mathrm{Lie}(G)^{[2]}$ and the radical $\mathrm{rad}\, \omega_\nu$ is the only invariant of the exterior differential 2-form ω_ν.

A transfer of the action of the spatial linear magnetic field gradients relative to the laboratory frame to a circle map with respect to the rotating coordinate frame of quadrature reference, and an adaptation of the dynamical system to the diameter of the spherical volume (DSV) of magnetic field homogeneity at the magnet isocenter on the axis of the diametrically bounded magnet bore access allows to shorten the time of imaging and simultaneously to increase the inherent robustness against motion and flow [59,60]. For this transfer to dynamic MRI, it is important to realize that the open upper complex half-plane $\mathcal{O}_+$ is biholomorphically equivalent to the open unit disc

$$D = \{w \in \mathbf{C} \,|\, |w| < 1\}$$

where $w \in \mathbf{C}$ admits the realification by the quadrature cell matrix $\begin{pmatrix} x & -y \\ y & x \end{pmatrix}$ as before, and $|w| = \sqrt{\det w}$. The slope-preserving, biholomorphic Cayley map

$$\Xi : w \rightsquigarrow \frac{w-i}{w+i}$$

which admits the matrix

$$\frac{1}{\sqrt{2}}\begin{pmatrix} 1 & -i \\ 1 & i \end{pmatrix}$$

belongs to the special unitary group $\mathbf{SU}(2,\mathbf{C}) \hookrightarrow \mathbf{SL}(2,\mathbf{C})$. Due to the biholomorphy of the isomorphism

$$\Xi : \mathcal{O}_+ \longrightarrow D,$$

the inverse mapping $\Xi^{-1}: D \longrightarrow \mathcal{O}_+$ is also slope-preserving and admits the matrix

$$\frac{1}{\sqrt{2}}\begin{pmatrix} 1 & 1 \\ i & -i \end{pmatrix} \in \mathbf{SU}(2,\mathbf{C}).$$

It is easy to check that Ξ provides a realization of the Lie group $\mathbf{SL}(2,\mathbf{R})$ of quantized calculus by the conformal subgroup

$$\mathbf{SU}_{\mathbf{C}}(1,1) = \left\{ \begin{pmatrix} u & \bar{v} \\ v & \bar{u} \end{pmatrix} \in \mathbf{SL}(2,\mathbf{C}) \middle| |u|^2 - |v|^2 = 1 \right\}$$

of $\mathbf{SL}(2,\mathbf{C})$. In fact, $\mathbf{SU}_{\mathbf{C}}(1,1)$ is conjugate to $\mathbf{SL}(2,\mathbf{R})$ in $\mathbf{SL}(2,\mathbf{C})$:

$$\mathbf{SU}_{\mathbf{C}}(1,1) = \Xi \circ \mathbf{SL}(2,\mathbf{R}) \circ \Xi^{-1}$$

In the polar coordinate decomposition

$$\mathbf{SU}_{\mathbf{C}}(1,1) = D \times \mathbf{T}$$

of $\mathbf{SU}_{\mathbf{C}}(1,1)$, the center $w = \sqrt{-1} = i \in \mathcal{O}_+$ of the reference unit circle $\mathbf{T} \hookrightarrow \mathbf{C}$ of the eccentric Kepplerian clockwork dynamics is mapped onto the center of $D \hookrightarrow \mathbf{C}$.

- In the polar coordinate decomposition of $\mathbf{SU}_{\mathbf{C}}(1,1)$, the circle group $\partial D = \mathbf{T}$ is phase locked to the eccentric Kepplerian reference clock.
- The open unit disc D is helically parametrized by the local frequency which is driven by the center frequency $\nu \in \hat{C} - \{0\}$ of the rotating coordinate frame of quadrature reference of the tomographic slice $\mathcal{O}_\nu \hookrightarrow \mathbf{P}(\mathbf{R} \times \mathrm{Lie}(G)^\star)$ of driving frequency $\nu \neq 0$.

Whereas two-dimensional Fourier transform MRI reconstructive methods use perpendicular linear magnetic field gradients applied in sequence and with varying duration and slope, radial turbo spin echo imaging techniques employ angular variations of field gradients. Because the homogeneity of the main magnetic flux density has been considerably improved in the new generation hardware, the disadvantages of non-cartesian coordinate parametrizations are only of minor importance. In the radial BURST pulse sequence, for instance, the phase trains of the excitation profiles are equally spaced on the torus $\mathbf{T}$ (Figure 2) with an interpulse delay in the presence of the direction changing projection reconstruction magnetic field gradients [21, 39]. Although the radial BURST technique carries the penalty of a low signal-to-noise ratio, the fact that radial data sets are acquired has a number of advantages over other competing techniques of ultra-fast imaging such as echo-planar imaging (EPI). The pulse sequence of the helical imaging approach is robust and easy to implement. In view of the fact that few gradient switching steps are needed, technical limitations concerning gradient rise times and eddy currents, which make EPI experiments difficult to perform, are not a problem.

Because in MRI heavy emphasis is placed on the phase of the image or processor output, any failure to achieve phase locking with linear magnetic field gradients will inevitably lead to spatial mismapping away from the magnet isocenter, and causes artifacts in MRI [22, 33], including the transition to chaos by iterating circle maps. The mechanism, in the Lauterbur subband encoding technique of spectral localization, leading eventually to chaotic behavior is interactions between the different resonances, caused by the non-linear couplings, and overlap between the resonant regimes of the dynamical system when the couplings exceed a certain

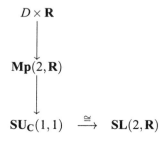

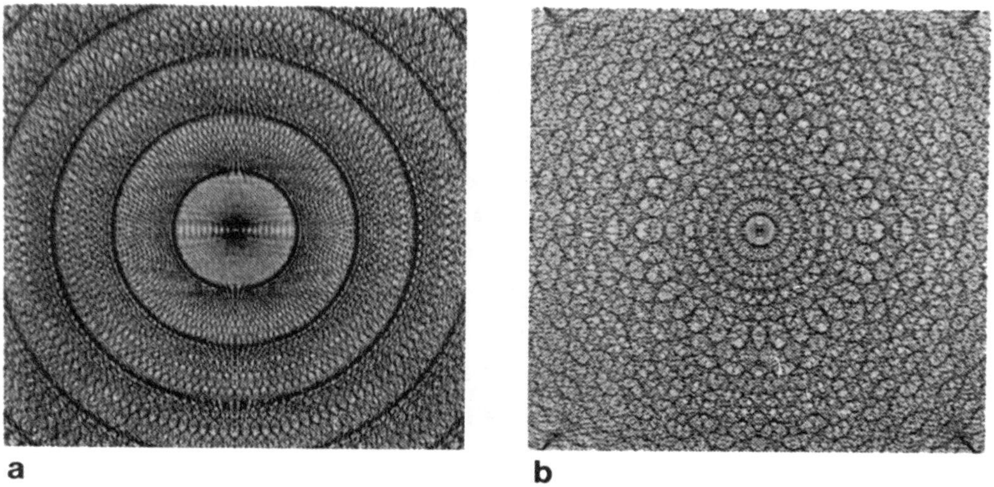

Figure 2. Radial BURST excitation profiles for equally spaced (a) and alternating (b) phase cycles.

critical value. It is easier to identify periodic, quasiperiodic, and chaotic motions by iterating a circle map than by a cumbersome numerical integration of the underlying Bloch–Riccati differential equation. In some sense the spatiotemporal quantization strategy is a renewal of the Kepplerian dynamical system approach, and the analogue, for dissipative systems, of Chirikov's instability of quasiperiodic orbits in Hamiltonian systems. There are, however, several options available to retrospectively correct for the geometric distortions caused by non-linear gradient sequence switching.

The switching on and off of magnetic field gradients during the imaging process induces eddy currents in conductive structures of the magnet. When a linear magnetic field gradient is switched on, the gradient field will not be on instantly, instead it rises exponentially toward its final amplitude. Likewise, when it is turned off, the gradient field will decay exponentially to zero. So even if no gradient is present, a residual magnetic field gradient may persist. A powerful remedy is the shielded gradient. The magnetic flux outside the coil which is the cause of the eddy current but has no function for generating imaging gradients is compensated by a counter-flux density of equal amplitude but opposite direction.

The universal covering group of $\mathbf{SU}_\mathbf{C}(1,1)$ is given by the topological product $D \times \mathbf{R}$. By unwrapping of the cycling of the stroboscopically measured phase, the line $\mathbf{R}$ denotes the time scale of the linear magnetic field gradients and the spatial linear rewinder gradients. The group of dynamical symmetries, the double covering group $\mathbf{Mp}(2,\mathbf{R})$ of $\mathbf{SL}(2,\mathbf{R})$, naturally fits in the following diagram:

$$\begin{array}{ccc}
D \times \mathbf{R} & & \\
\downarrow & & \\
\mathbf{Mp}(2,\mathbf{R}) & & \\
\downarrow & & \\
\mathbf{SU}_\mathbf{C}(1,1) & \xrightarrow{\cong} & \mathbf{SL}(2,\mathbf{R})
\end{array}$$

There is a complex coordinate presentation of G given by the unipotent upper triangular matrices

$$\left\{\left(\begin{array}{ccc}1 & w & iz+\frac{1}{2}|w|^2\\ 0 & 1 & \bar{w}\\ 0 & 0 & 1\end{array}\right)\middle| w\in\mathbf{C}, z\in\mathbf{R}\right\}$$

which admits the center

$$C\cong\mathbf{R}$$

aligned with the static external magnetic field. Its parametrization by the pairs

$$\left(\left(\begin{array}{cc}x & -y\\ y & x\end{array}\right), z\right)$$

gives rise to the symplectic transposition, or alternatively twisting

$$(\cdot)^t = J = \left(\begin{array}{cc}0 & -1\\ 1 & 0\end{array}\right)\in\mathbf{GO}^+(2,\mathbf{R}),$$

which allows for an embedding of G into the symplectic group $\mathbf{Sp}(4,\mathbf{R})$. Moreover, the exterior differential form which includes the driving frequency $\nu\in\hat{C}-\{0\}$ of the rotating coordinate frame of quadrature reference of the tomographic slice $\mathcal{O}_\nu\hookrightarrow\mathbf{P}(\mathbf{R}\times\mathrm{Lie}(G)^\star)$ $(\nu\neq 0)$, frequency selected from the canonical foliation,

$$\omega_\nu = \nu\frac{i}{2}\cdot\mathrm{d}w\wedge\mathrm{d}\bar{w}\qquad(\nu\neq 0)$$

arises.

The bundle-theoretic interpretation of the inducing mechanism gives rise to the pair of isomorphic irreducible unitary linear representations

$$(U^\nu, V^\nu)\qquad(\nu\neq 0)$$

of G acting on the standard modulation space $L^2_{\mathbf{C}}(\mathbf{R})$. They are considered as unitarily induced by the *eccentric* unitary characters

$$(\tilde{\chi}^N_\nu, \tilde{\chi}^M_\nu)$$

of the maximal abelian, connected subgroups

$$(N, M)$$

of G which are embedded in quadrature into G and carry Haar measures adjusted by the Cavalieri principle of volume integration to the Haar measures of T, S, and G. Then

$$U^\nu\cong L^2-\mathrm{ind}_N^G\,\tilde{\chi}^N_\nu,\qquad V^\nu\cong L^2-\mathrm{ind}_M^G\,\tilde{\chi}^M_\nu,$$

and the Weyl commutation relations

$$U^\nu\left(\left(\begin{array}{ccc}1 & x & z\\ 0 & 1 & y\\ 0 & 0 & 1\end{array}\right)\right)\circ V^\nu\left(\left(\begin{array}{ccc}1 & x & z\\ 0 & 1 & y\\ 0 & 0 & 1\end{array}\right)\right)$$
$$= e^{4\pi i\nu xy}V^\nu\left(\left(\begin{array}{ccc}1 & x & z\\ 0 & 1 & y\\ 0 & 0 & 1\end{array}\right)\right)\circ U^\nu\left(\left(\begin{array}{ccc}1 & x & z\\ 0 & 1 & y\\ 0 & 0 & 1\end{array}\right)\right)$$

are satisfied for all triples $(x,y,z)\in\mathbf{R}^3$ and $\nu\neq 0$.

- The centralizers of the image groups $U^\nu(G)$ and $V^\nu(G)$ in the unitary group $\mathbf{U}\left(L^2_\mathbf{C}(\mathbf{R})\right)$ are isomorphic to the subgroup $K \hookrightarrow \mathbf{SL}(2,\mathbf{R})$.
- The normalizers of the image groups $U^\nu(G)$ and $V^\nu(G)$ in the unitary group $\mathbf{U}\left(L^2_\mathbf{C}(\mathbf{R})\right)$ mod $\mathbf{Z}/2\mathbf{Z}$ are isomorphic to the special linear group $\mathbf{SL}(2,\mathbf{R})$. Their maximal compact subgroups are isomorphic to an extension of $K \hookrightarrow \mathbf{SL}(2,\mathbf{R})$ by the dyadic group $\mathbf{Z}/2\mathbf{Z}$.

As a consequence, for non-zero center frequencies $\nu \neq \nu'$ the irreducible unitary linear representations U^ν and $U^{\nu'}$ of G are non-isomorphic, and the same holds for V^ν and $V^{\nu'}$. However, their restrictions to the canonical two-parameter abelian subgroup of generators

$$\{\exp_G P, \exp_G Q\},$$

complementary to the center $C \hookrightarrow G$, are unitary equivalent by the unitary transformation of the standard modulation space $L^2_\mathbf{C}(\mathbf{R})$ arising from a linear homothetic transformation of ratio $a \in \mathbf{R}\,(a \neq 0)$, of the line $\mathbf{R}$.

To get insight to how the metaplectic representation of the double covering group $\mathbf{Mp}(2,\mathbf{R})$ of $\mathbf{SL}(2,\mathbf{R})$ lifts the symplectic Weyl quadrature matrix J to the one-dimensional Fourier transform $\mathfrak{F}_\mathbf{R}$ acting on the standard modulation space $L^2_\mathbf{C}(\mathbf{R})$ and providing signal spectra, let the set of traceless matrices

$$e_+ = \begin{pmatrix} 0 & 1 \\ 0 & 0 \end{pmatrix}, \quad e_- = \begin{pmatrix} 0 & 0 \\ 1 & 0 \end{pmatrix}, \quad h = \begin{pmatrix} 1 & 0 \\ 0 & -1 \end{pmatrix}$$

denote the canonical basis of the smallest nonabelian simple Lie algebra

$$\mathrm{Lie}\,(\mathbf{SL}(2,\mathbf{R})) = \left\{ \begin{pmatrix} a & b \\ c & -a \end{pmatrix} \middle|\, a,b,c \in \mathbf{R} \right\}.$$

Then the elements $\{h, e_+, e_-\}$ of $\mathrm{Lie}\,(\mathbf{SL}(2,\mathbf{R}))$ satisfy the commutation relations

$$[h,e_+] = 2e_+, \quad [h,e_-] = -2e_-, \quad [e_+,e_-] = h.$$

These equations characterize $\mathrm{Lie}\,(\mathbf{SL}(2,\mathbf{R}))$.

- The element h generates the closed subgroup $A_0 = \{\exp_{\mathbf{SL}(2,\mathbf{R})}((\log a)h) \mid a > 0\} \cong \mathbf{R}$ of the solvable component $A_0 \cdot N_0$ of the Iwasawa decomposition of $\mathbf{SL}(2,\mathbf{R})$.

It follows that the conformal group $\mathbf{SU}_\mathbf{C}(1,1) \hookrightarrow \mathbf{SL}(2,\mathbf{C})$ which is characterized by the invariance of the Hermitian form on the complex plane $\mathbf{C}^2$

$$(w,w') \rightsquigarrow \det\begin{pmatrix} w & w' \\ \bar{w}' & \bar{w} \end{pmatrix} = |w|^2 - |w'|^2$$

satisfies the commutation relation

$$\begin{pmatrix} \bar{u} & \bar{v} \\ v & u \end{pmatrix} \cdot h = h \cdot \begin{pmatrix} \bar{u} & -\bar{v} \\ -v & u \end{pmatrix} \qquad (u \in \mathbf{C}, v \in \mathbf{C}).$$

Conversely, the preceding commutation relation implies the invariance under the action of the conformal group $\mathbf{SU}_\mathbf{C}(1,1) \hookrightarrow \mathbf{SL}(2,\mathbf{C})$ of the Hermitian form on the complex plane

$\mathbf{C}^2$. It follows that Lie $(\mathbf{SL}(2,\mathbf{R}))$ transports onto the complex Lie algebra of traceless matrices with purely imaginary entries on their main diagonals:

$$\operatorname{Lie}(\mathbf{SU_C}(1,1)) = \left\{ \begin{pmatrix} i\xi & \eta \\ \bar{\eta} & -i\xi \end{pmatrix} \middle| \xi \in \mathbf{R}, \eta \in \mathbf{C} \right\}$$

The quotient $\mathbf{SU_C}(1,1)/(\pm\mathrm{id})$ together with its image under the complex conjugation flip $w \rightsquigarrow \bar{w}$ provides the Lie group of all isometries of the Riemannian manifold D.

- The element e_+ generates the closed subgroup $N_0 = \{\exp_{\mathbf{SL}(2,\mathbf{R})}(te_+) \mid t \in \mathbf{R}\} \cong \mathbf{R}$ of the solvable component $A_0 \cdot N_0 \hookrightarrow \mathbf{SL}(2,\mathbf{R})$.

Moreover, the elements $\{e_+, e_-, h\}$ are related to the basis of Lie $(\mathbf{SU}(2,\mathbf{C}))$ formed by the Pauli spin matrices

$$\varepsilon_1 = \begin{pmatrix} 0 & 1 \\ 1 & 0 \end{pmatrix}, \quad \varepsilon_2 = \begin{pmatrix} 0 & -i \\ i & 0 \end{pmatrix}, \quad \varepsilon_3 = \begin{pmatrix} 1 & 0 \\ 0 & -1 \end{pmatrix}$$

via the complex linear combinations

$$e_+ = \frac{1}{2}(\varepsilon_1 + i\varepsilon_2), \quad e_- = \frac{1}{2}(\varepsilon_1 - i\varepsilon_2), \quad h = \varepsilon_3.$$

Then the Fourier transform $\mathcal{F}_\mathbf{R}$ acting as a unitary operator on the standard modulation space $L^2_\mathbf{C}(\mathbf{R})$ can be written in terms of these bases as

$$\mathcal{F}_\mathbf{R} = e^{-\frac{\pi}{4}i} J = e^{-\frac{\pi}{4}i} \exp_{\mathbf{SL}(2,\mathbf{R})}\left(\frac{\pi}{2}(e_+ - e_-)\right) = e^{-\frac{\pi}{4}i} \exp_{\mathbf{SU}(2,\mathbf{C})}\left(\frac{\pi}{2} i\varepsilon_2\right),$$

where the phase factor is given via the Maslov index by the cocycle of the group extension

$$\begin{array}{ccccccc} \{1\} & \longrightarrow & \mathbf{Z}/2\mathbf{Z} & \longrightarrow & \mathbf{Mp}(2,\mathbf{R}) & & \\ & & & & \downarrow & & \\ & & & & \mathbf{SL}(2,\mathbf{R}) & \longrightarrow & \{1\} \end{array}$$

as the Bernoulli expression

$$e^{-\frac{\pi}{4}i} = \frac{1}{\sqrt{i}} = \frac{\sqrt{2}}{1+i}.$$

Notice that the preceding identity is in accordance to Harish-Chandra's restriction theorem which asserts that the smallest positive eigenvalue of

$$(e_+ - e_-) = i\varepsilon_2 \in \operatorname{Lie}(\mathbf{SL}(2,\mathbf{R}))$$

is given as

$$m = \frac{1}{2}.$$

It represents another form of the Heisenberg uncertainty principle which governs the quadrature format design of the Kepplerian spatiotemporal strategy.

- At the Lie algebra level, any unitary linear representation of the group of dynamical symmetries $\mathbf{Mp}(2,\mathbf{R})$ is diagonalizable under the action of the generator $\varepsilon_2 = i(e_- - e_+)$ of K with eigenvalues $m \in \frac{1}{2}\mathbf{Z}$ of half-integral or integral value.

In the generic case, associated to the planar coadjoint orbit $\mathcal{O}_1 \hookrightarrow \mathbf{P}(\mathbf{R} \times \mathrm{Lie}(G)^\star)$ of G, the intertwining identity

$$\mathcal{F}_{\mathbf{R}} \circ U^1 = V^1 \circ \mathcal{F}_{\mathbf{R}}$$

holds. By an affine homothetic transformation of C to the center frequency $\nu \neq 0$ as in the transition $\omega_1 \rightsquigarrow \omega_\nu$ from the generic coadjoint orbit $\mathcal{O}_1$ to the tomographic slice $\mathcal{O}_\nu (\nu \neq 0)$, frequency selected from the canonical foliation in the real projective space $\mathbf{P}(\mathbf{R} \times \mathrm{Lie}(G)^\star)$, the Fourier transform $\mathcal{F}_{\mathbf{R}}$ gives rise to a lifted intertwining operator $\mathcal{F}^\nu_{\mathbf{R}}$ of the isomorphic irreducible unitary linear representations U^ν and V^ν of G acting on the standard complex Hilbert space $L^2_{\mathbf{C}}(\mathbf{R})$ as modulation space:

$$\mathcal{F}^\nu_{\mathbf{R}} \circ U^\nu = V^\nu \circ \mathcal{F}^\nu_{\mathbf{R}}$$

In accordance to the Stone-von Neumann theorem of quantum physics, both representations admit the same central unitary character

$$\chi_\nu = U^\nu \mid C = V^\nu \mid C \qquad (\nu \neq 0)$$

which has the form

$$\chi_\nu = \tilde{\chi}^N_\nu \mid C = \tilde{\chi}^M_\nu \mid C : z \rightsquigarrow e^{2\pi i \nu z}$$

with center frequency $\nu \in \hat{C} - \{0\}$. Adjacent tomographic slices are not effected. An infinitesimal version of the unitary representation U^ν is given by its differentiated form. The differentiated form of U^ν provides by the evaluation

$$U^\nu(P) = \frac{\mathrm{d}}{\mathrm{d}t}$$

at $P = \begin{pmatrix} 0 & 1 & 0 \\ 0 & 0 & 0 \\ 0 & 0 & 0 \end{pmatrix} \in \mathrm{Lie}(G)$ the temporal derivative on the event line,

$$U^\nu(Q) = 2\pi i \nu t \times$$

provides by evaluation at $Q = \begin{pmatrix} 0 & 0 & 0 \\ 0 & 0 & 1 \\ 0 & 0 & 0 \end{pmatrix} \in \mathrm{Lie}(G)$ the multiplication with the imaginary time scale, and finally

$$U^\nu(I) = 2\pi i \nu \times$$

provides by evaluation at $I = \begin{pmatrix} 0 & 0 & 1 \\ 0 & 0 & 0 \\ 0 & 0 & 0 \end{pmatrix} \in \mathrm{Lie}(G)$ the multiplication with the imaginary angular frequency, with the usual maximal domains as skew-adjoint Hilbert space operators. Similarly, an application of the symplectic Weyl quadrature matrix

$$J = -i\varepsilon_2$$

yields for the differentiated form of the unitary representation V^ν of G

$$V^\nu(P) = 2\pi i \nu t \times, \quad V^\nu(Q) = -\frac{\mathrm{d}}{\mathrm{d}t}, \quad V^\nu(I) = 2\pi i \nu \times$$

when evaluated at the canonical basis $\{P, Q, I\}$ of the Heisenberg Lie algebra Lie(G). The induced Hilbert bundles sitting in quadrature over the event line $\mathbf{R}$, admit for any Fourier transformed pair of excitation profiles

$$(\psi, \varphi)$$

in the modulation space $L^2_{\mathbf{C}}(\mathbf{R})$, and element $z \in C$ the contiguous cross-sections of a phase-splitting network of uncorrelated multichannels in quadrature format

$$\left(x_0, e^{2\pi i \nu(z-(x-x_0)y)} \cdot \psi(-x)\right), \quad \left(y_0, e^{2\pi i \nu(z+x(y-y_0))} \cdot \varphi(y)\right) \qquad ((x_0, y_0) \in T \oplus S)$$

where $x_0 \in T$ denotes the phase reference of the stroboscopic phase cycling at which system state change. Moreover, $y_0 \in S$ denotes the intermediate frequency reference of the synchronous period cycling clockwork of transitions which is determined by the computer's programming, and

$$\varphi = \mathcal{F}_{\mathbf{R}} \psi.$$

In terms of the $C^\star$-algebra of the Heisenberg group G, the Kepplerian quadrature conchoid trajectory construction in the projectively immersed, symplectic affine plane may be naturally viewed as the crossed product of $\mathcal{C}_0(\mathbf{R} \oplus \mathbf{R})$ by the action of the central factor $C \hookrightarrow G$ which in each line $\{\nu\} \times \mathbf{R}$ of the bundle of lines parallel to the second coordinate axis S of the projectively immersed, symplectic affine plane $\mathbf{R} \oplus \mathbf{R}$ consists of translations, but scaled by the first coordinate ν of this line, so that each point of the second coordinate axis S itself is left fixed under the scaling operation.

Quadrature detection has two main advantages over detection using a single phase-sensitive detector. First, noise is not folded about the quadrature reference frequency, and as a result there is an improvement in signal-to-noise ratio by a factor of $\sqrt{2}$. This corresponds to a saving in accumulation time of a factor of two, which can be extremely valuable. Secondly, the quadrature reference frequency can be placed as intermediate frequency y_0 in the middle of the frequency range. This considerably reduces bandwidth problems that may arise from the effects of finite pulse width.

- In the helical imaging approach to dynamic MRI, the helical multichannel network reflects the invariance properties of the slope-preserving biholomorphic Cayley map $\Xi : \mathcal{O}_+ \longrightarrow D$ of the Lauterbur subband encoding technique of spectral localization by directional derivatives, or linear magnetic field gradients.

An increase of flexibility of the eccentric Kepplerian clockwork dynamics can be achieved by employing wavelet packets from a library of bases to the excitation profiles. The term library in this context refers to a collection of bases linked together by some common feature. Beyond the Haar–Hadamard wavelet packet library of piecewise constant functions, libraries of smooth wavelet bases can be considered for the purpose of phase encoding [32,87]. For fast MRI study protocols, multiwavelets can be used.

The symplectic affine plane, internal direct sum

$$T \oplus S$$

of the homogeneous transverse direction lines, may be identified with the complex plane

$$\mathbf{C}(\mathbf{R} \oplus \mathbf{R}) \cong (\mathcal{O}_1, \omega_1)$$

by complexification via identification of the symplectic Weyl quadrature matrix $J = i \cdot (-\varepsilon_2)$ with $i \in \mathbf{C}$.

- The phase reference x_0 and the intermediate frequency reference y_0 are derived directly from the stable master oscillator governing the system-wide timing of the MRI scanner architecture.
- Fast cycling schemes in the projectively immersed, symplectic affine plane of incidence as realized by the MRI scanner system are implemented by means of area-efficient first-in/first-out queue buffers.

The unitary forms associated to the cross-sections represent the phase coherent wavelets transmitted in parallel synchronously by the contiguous local frequency encoding subband multichannels.

- The contiguous local frequency encoding subband multichannels are driven by the relaxing nuclear spins selectively excited inside planar spin isochromats via a broadband low-noise preamplifier covering the range of the Larmor frequencies y of the sample.

Broadband low-noise preamps are operated by the amplification mode of junction field-effect transistors in an integrated circuit module. The gates of the transistors form semiconductor junctions with the underlying channels. Thermal stability is assured by the mechanism of negative feedback. A transformer balun (balancing unit) coupling to the main receiving coil ensures by the conjugation symmetry of the circuitry that the same interfering voltage is generated on both sides of the receiving coil. In view of the fact that the involutory flip matrix

$$\varepsilon_3 = \begin{pmatrix} 1 & 0 \\ 0 & -1 \end{pmatrix} \in \mathrm{Lie}\,(\mathbf{SU}(2,\mathbf{C}))$$

has determinant -1 and therefore transforms the direct linear similitudes of $\mathbf{GO}^+(2,\mathbf{R})$ into indirect similitudes in $\mathbf{GO}(2,\mathbf{R})$, the aforementioned conjugation identity

$$\begin{pmatrix} 1 & 0 \\ 0 & -1 \end{pmatrix} \begin{pmatrix} x & -y \\ y & x \end{pmatrix} \begin{pmatrix} 1 & 0 \\ 0 & -1 \end{pmatrix}^{-1} = \begin{pmatrix} x & y \\ -y & x \end{pmatrix}$$

by the involutory flip matrix in $\mathbf{GO}(2,\mathbf{R})$ is at the basis of the common-mode rejection technique of balanced coupling to antennae. A ground loop effects the matching condition so that no interference current flows in the main receiving coil, and no interference is gathered by the receiver circuitry. Clearly, any lack of dynamical symmetry degrades the effectiveness of the balanced circuitry leading eventually to chaotic behavior. An additional shield round the coupling coil helps to prevent its receiving interference directly.

The Hilbert bundles are G-homogeneous in the sense that the Heisenberg group G moves their fibers around by linear transformations. The G-homogeneity allows for adjustment of x_0 and y_0 by phase and frequency shifts, respectively.

- By reducing the intermediate frequency reference y_0, the demands on the analog-to-digital converter are significantly reduced.

The contiguous local frequency encoded subband multichannels are locked-in to integrated electronic circuitry hardware realizing the symplectic Weyl quadrature matrix J by a voltage controlled local oscillator chip and frequency range extending baluns at the interface of analog and digital techniques [38]. In this way, the resonant response wavelets are processed. An implication of the weakness of the detected signals is the non-invasiveness of the MRI modality.

- Linear phase detection is performed by a broadband ring modulator. Its output is used to direct the frequency of the on-chip voltage controlled local oscillator of a phase locked loop which pulls in to resonance by the lock-in technique.

The local oscillator frequency can be above or below the Larmor precession frequency y by an amount of the intermediate frequency, though operation above by a single-sideband modulator is advantageous.

- The single-sideband technique requires an input organization in the symplectic format design. The wideband generation of quadrature components is based on phase sequence networks. The quadrature phase shift of buffered data, or alternatively data swapping, is performed by the data routing process.

The electronic control is performed by a special purpose computer, the pulse programmer, which interprets the instructions received from the host computer, controls nuclear spin choreography, directs the phase-sensitive detectors, phase-locked loops, and frequency synthesizers, as well as overseeing analog-to-digital and digital-to-analog conversions of data.

- The sampling theorem, or equivalently, the Poisson summation formula, are compatible with the symplectic affine structure of the frequency selected tomographic slice $(\mathcal{O}_\nu, \omega_\nu)$ rotating with driving frequency $\nu \neq 0$.

Data transfer is via a bus which is an extension of one which is used inside the host computer, appropriately buffered. Synchronization is performed by pulses on additional strobing bus lines. The frequency synthesizer derives all the different frequencies of its output from the single master oscillator.

Because an MRI scanner forms a synchronous system which requires great clock accuracy, and the system timing is distributed to many circuits, the clock generation is external to the chip. The period of the stable master oscillator is typically controlled by a crystal mounted in an oven with temperature control.

The linear representation U^ν of G and its copy V^ν swapped by the symplectic Weyl quadrature matrix J, are globally square integrable modulo C. Indeed, it is well known that a coadjoint orbit is a linear symplectic affine variety if and only if one (and hence all) of the corresponding irreducible unitary linear representations is globally square integrable modulo its kernel. This forces the dimension of G to be *odd*.

- The flatness of the coadjoint orbits $\mathcal{O}_\nu \hookrightarrow \mathbf{P}(\mathbf{R} \times \mathrm{Lie}(G)^\star)$ $(\nu \neq 0)$ of G implies the discrete series trace formula for the holographic transforms on the transverse plane G/C.

- Due to the discrete series trace formula for the holographic transforms on G/C, the contiguous local frequency encoding subband multichannels are uncorrelated and therefore each subband channel can be encoded independently for storage or wavelet transmission.

Because the choice of the L^2 norm as well as the flatness of the coadjoint orbits $\mathcal{O}_\nu \hookrightarrow \mathbf{P}(\mathbf{R} \times \mathrm{Lie}(G)^\star)$ $(\nu \neq 0)$ have quantum physical impact, it is reasonable to regard global square integrability as an essential part of the Stone–von Neumann theorem of quantum physics. Due to the fact that a representation of a nilpotent Lie group is determined by its central unitary character χ_ν if and only if it is globally square integrable modulo center, $\chi_\nu : z \leadsto e^{2\pi i \nu z}$ allows for frequency selection of the tomographic slice $(\mathcal{O}_\nu, \omega_\nu)$ $(\nu \neq 0)$ rotating with center frequency $\nu \in \hat{C} - \{0\}$, and the coadjoint orbit $(\mathcal{O}_\nu, \omega_\nu)$ of G allows for mathematically modelling the conceptual trick of the rotating coordinate frame of quadrature reference. The corresponding equivalence classes of irreducible, unitarily induced, linear representations U^ν of G acting on the complex Hilbert space of globally square integrable cross-sections for the Hilbert bundle sitting over the event line $\mathbf{R}$ are infinite-dimensional.

According to the Stone–von Neumann theorem of quantum physics, the unitary representation U^ν of G can be realized as a Hilbert–Schmidt integral operator in $\mathcal{LC}\left(L^2_{\mathbf{C}}(\mathbf{R})\right)$ with attached kernel $K^\nu \in L^2_{\mathbf{C}}(\mathbf{R} \oplus \mathbf{R})$. See the references [67, 86]. The kernel function admits the Hermitian symmetry

$$K^\nu(x,y) = \bar{K}^\nu(y,x) \qquad (x,y) \in \mathbf{R} \oplus \mathbf{R}$$

so that the associated Hilbert–Schmidt integral operator is self-adjoint, or alternatively, a Hermitian operator. It is this kernel symmetry which reflects the symmetry inherent to the geometric quantization approach.

- The Hermitian kernel function $K^\nu \in L^2_{\mathbf{C}}(\mathbf{R} \oplus \mathbf{R})$ attached to the irreducible unitary linear representation $U^\nu (\nu \neq 0)$ of G acting with central unitary character $\chi_\nu = U^\nu \mid C$ in the standard modulation space $L^2_{\mathbf{C}}(\mathbf{R})$ implements in the quadrature format design of a phase-splitting network a multichannel coherent wavelet reconstructive analysis–synthesis filter bank of matched filter type in the projectively immersed, symplectic affine plane of incidence $(\mathcal{O}_\nu, \omega_\nu)$.

- The phase histories in contiguous local frequency encoding subband multichannels are transmultiplexed and finally recorded by the quantum hologram K^ν. The unitary reconstruction processing is performed by the symplectically reformatted two-dimensional Fourier transform of period 2.

- The symplectic Fourier transform defines a phase-sensitive average over the focal points of the observation plane at infinity $\mathbf{P}\left(\mathbf{R} \times \mathcal{O}_\infty\right)$ in the projective completion $\mathbf{P}(\mathbf{R} \times \mathrm{Lie}(G)^\star)$ of the dual vector space $\mathrm{Lie}(G)^\star$.

- The Hermitian symmetry inherent to the kernel function allows for an application of the one-half Fourier, or alternatively, $\frac{1}{2}$-NEX reconstructive method.

The center of the product group

$$\mathbf{S}_3 \times \mathbf{S}_3$$

is given by the set

$$\{1, -1\} \times \{1, -1\}.$$

Due to the antipody identification of $\mathbf{S}_3 \hookrightarrow \mathbf{R}^4$, the center of $\mathbf{S}_3 \times \mathbf{S}_3$ gives rise to the symplectic spinor

$$\star(1_\nu \otimes 1_\nu)$$

It forms the *reproducing kernel* associated to the symplectic affine leaf $(\mathcal{O}_\nu, \omega_\nu)$. The action of the symplectic convolution operator has to be symplectically adjusted to the inhomogeneous transverse direction line $\mathbf{R}$ of $\mathcal{O}_\nu \hookrightarrow \mathbf{P}(\mathbf{R} \times \mathrm{Lie}(G)^\star)$. See the reference [73]. The symplectic Fourier transform reconstructive method is another crucial topic which justifies the non-commutative geometric analysis approach to clinical MRI.

The reproducing kernel in the complex vector space of symplectic spinors $\mathcal{S}'_{\mathbf{C}}(\mathbf{R} \oplus \mathbf{R})$ corresponds to the symplectic direct linear similitude

$$\begin{pmatrix} 1 & -1 \\ 1 & 1 \end{pmatrix} \in \mathbf{GO}^+(2, \mathbf{R})$$

of the copy $\mathbf{R} \oplus \mathbf{R}$ of $\mathcal{O}_\nu\,(\nu \neq 0)$ with multiplicator 2, and via reflection to the indirect linear similitude

$$\begin{pmatrix} 1 & 1 \\ 1 & -1 \end{pmatrix} \in \mathbf{GO}(2, \mathbf{R})$$

with multiplicator -2. Generated by the involutory flip matrix in $\mathbf{GO}(2, \mathbf{R})$, it forms the reflection or symmetry

$$w \rightsquigarrow \bar{w}$$

about the real axis $\Im w = 0$ which changes the sign of the rotational curvature form. The $\frac{1}{2}$-NEX reconstruction reduces the data acquisition time by 50 % by retaining the spatial resolution. However, the signal-to-noise ratio is reduced by a factor of $\frac{1}{\sqrt{2}}$. Practical experience shows that fast imaging methods such as the radial BURST method are superior to the $\frac{1}{2}$-NEX reconstruction technique.

The compact selfadjoint integral operator defined by the Hermitian kernel

$$K^\nu \in L^2_{\mathbf{C}}(\mathbf{R} \oplus \mathbf{R})$$

has a singular value decomposition associated to its discrete spectrum as a least square fit. The Karhunen–Loève basis is known to form the minimizer of the number of non-negligible amplitudes in the computational realization of the quantum holograms associated to U^ν. Whereas ultra-fast imaging techniques such as radial turbo spin echo and EPI drastically reduce the imaging time, the Karhunen–Loève transform (KLT) can be applied in order to reparametrize the spatial coordinates of the quantum hologram via the normalizing action of the metaplectic group [86]

$$\begin{array}{c} \mathbf{Mp}(2, \mathbf{R}) \\ \Big\downarrow \\ \mathbf{SL}(2, \mathbf{R}) \end{array}$$

of dynamical symmetries. The KLT both decorrelates the input and optimizes the redistribution of the wavelet energy in the L^2-sense within the projectively immersed, symplectic affine plane of incidence $\mathcal{O}_\nu \hookrightarrow \mathbf{P}(\mathbf{R} \times \mathrm{Lie}(G)^\star)$ $(\nu \neq 0)$. As an adaptive image transform coding algorithm [87] beyond the still picture image compression standard of the Joint Photographic Experts Group (JPEG), it allows to extract the prominent features of the final image with the fewest number of measurements. Such a block compression data design performed by the best zonal sampler is of particular importance for use in teleradiology as part of a distributed hospital picture and archiving system (PACS).

Since typically commutativity, as opposed to non-commutativity, is considered as contributing to simplicity, it is a remarkable fact that the embedding of the two-dimensional Fourier transform as a non-local operator into non-commutative affine geometry is the basic strategy for setting the mood for the symbol calculus associated to the spin-warp technique of standard clinical MRI. It is the full symbol calculus in the theory of pseudodifferential operators which establishes the final proton density reconstruction formula [69, 70]. Due to the symplectic Fourier slice or projection theorem for the Radon transform, the reconstruction in radial turbo spin echo imaging techniques is performed by filtered back projection under the polar angle of the radial data set [60]. Computer correction can be applied to the data set during the fast Fourier transform (FFT) process. However, this tactic is of little avail for correcting problems involving tomographic slice selection where accurate refocusing is needed.

In 1952 Otto E. Neugebauer discovered the remarkable fact that the Babylonian astronomers used already a primitive kind of Fourier series for the prediction of celestial events. The Fourier transform, however, grew from the desire to understand black body radiation in the context of the cooling characteristics of military cannons. The application of the symplectically reformatted two-dimensional Fourier transform underlying the Kepplerian quadrature detection strategy, and the operational calculus of Fourier integral operators to the visualization of MRI scans is of considerably higher benefit to humankind.

The Heisenberg nilpotent Lie group approach leads to the non-locality phenomenon of quantum physics as approved by the double-slit interference experiment of photonics [68], and to major application areas of pulsed signal recovery methods, the corner turn algorithm in the digital processing of high resolution SAR data [85], the spin-warp procedure in standard clinical MRI, and finally to the variants of the ultra-high-speed EPI technique of neurofunctional MRI [14, 43, 73, 82]. Combined with multi-slice imaging via interleaving of data acquisition, it is the spin-warp version of the two-dimensional Fourier transform MRI reconstruction technique which is used almost exclusively in current routine clinical examinations and now forms a general basis for the majority of MRI studies [26].

Long data acquisition time is a characteristic of MRI limiting its clinical use in certain diagnostic areas. This problem is particularly enhanced in the field of cardiology where electrocardiographic (ECG) gating is typically required. As the scan length in cardiac MRI is mainly determined by the number of gated radiofrequency excitations required to collect the samples of the entire quantum holograms (Figure 3), reducing this number is the key to reducing data acquisition time.

The most effective ultra-fast imaging approach is EPI which samples the quantum holograms by using a single excitation. Apart of cardiac MRI, neurofunctional MRI requires drastically reduced data acquisition time. The EPI modality is an exceptionally powerful tool for neurofunctional MRI because combined with the BOLD technique 20 or more contiguous tomographic brain slices covering the whole head can be acquired every 3 s for a total duration of several minutes [47]. However, this approach requires substantial hardware modifications in order to achieve high magnetic field gradients, and short rise time. EPI also suffers from the inherent limitation that the high slew rates can lead to nerve stimulations. A clinical alternative to EPI in neurofunctional MRI is the PRESTO technique [54] which allows for a

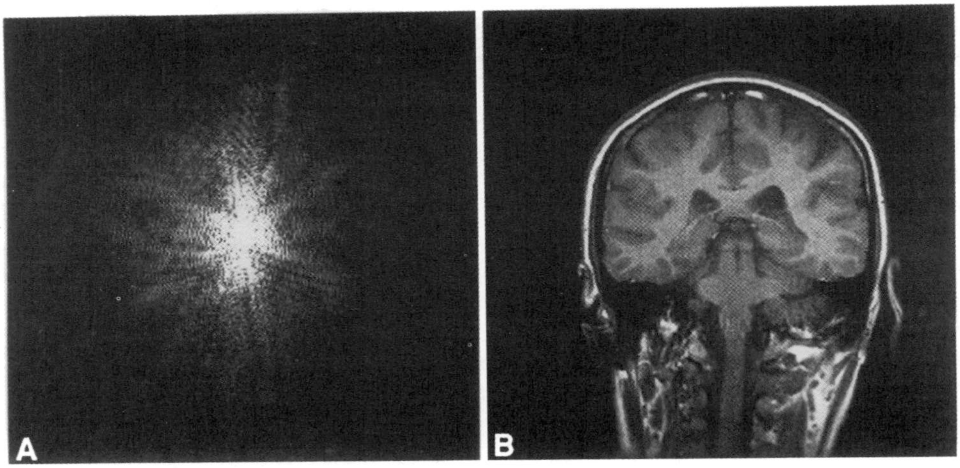

Figure 3. Quantum holograms (A) and their two-dimensional Fourier transform MRI reconstructions (B).

rapid three-dimensional approach for neurofunctional MRI of the human brain, and the high external magnetic flux density approach to cognitive function [80].

Although Lauterbur's original back projection technique for image reconstruction is restricted to fast imaging methods such as the radial BURST technique, and not currently used for routine examinations on clinical MRI scanners, the employment of linear magnetic field gradients for the purpose of spectral localization, the distinctive feature of Lauterbur's solvable affine encoding approach, has remained widely used. It is at the basis of the data acquisition by standard MRI study protocols.

The MRI scan acquired often reflects a compromise between quality and cost factors. Postprocessing with wavelet-based multiscale edge detectors in an offline mode on stored scans for the purpose of enhancing diagnostically useful features and reducing the interference caused by noise allows for improvement of the raw image quality. This technique offers a great deal of flexibility with respect to the MRI parameters.

For many physicists, the 20th century begins in 1895, with Wilhelm Conrad Röntgen's discovery of X-ray imaging. It needed almost 80 years until the first X-ray CT scanner was installed by Geoffrey N. Hounsfield at Hammersmith College in London 1973. Although the physics as well as the method of data manipulation of MRI are far more subtle than the physical and data acquirement principles underlying X-ray CT, the speed with which clinical MRI spread throughout the world as a diagnostic imaging tool was phenomenal. In the early 1980s when the first commercial MRI scanner, a permanent magnet scanner, was placed in a diagnostic imaging center in Cleveland, Ohio, the clinical MRI modality burst onto the scene with even more intensity than X-ray CT in the 1970s with its intrinsically poor soft tissue contrast capability. Whereas at the end of 1981 there were only three working MRI scanner systems available in the United States, presently there are more than 4.000 imagers performing in a non-invasive manner more than 8.5 million examinations per year. Today many radiologists are convinced that if history was rewritten, and X-ray CT invented after

MRI, nobody would bother to pursue the CT modality with its intrinsically poor soft tissue contrast performance.

The speed of growth is a testimony of the clinical significance of the MRI technique. Today the modality is firmly established as a core diagnostic tool in the fields of neuroradiology and musculoskeletal imaging [7, 22, 24, 35], , routinely used in all medical centers in Western Europe, the United States, and Japan. It is rare to find there a neurosurgeon or an orthopedic surgeon who do not order or review MRI scans on a daily basis. Frequently, MRI is the definitive examination procedure, providing invaluable information to help the surgeon not only to understand the underlying pathology, but also to make the critical decision regarding surgical intervention.

For the clinicians, high quality MRI atlases of the human cross-sectional anatomy are helpful with the interpretation of MRI scans [2, 6, 8–11, 13, 16, 20, 23], so that radiologists, not only anatomists, can acquire a depth of understanding of clinico-morphologic structure. Because 70 % of the MRI examinations are concerned with the central nervous system (CNS), and advances in MRI has changed the practice of medicine nowhere more than in the care of patients with CNS malignancies, neuroradiological competence is of utmost importance [27, 88].

There have been dramatic advances in the methods used to display MRI scans, which are able now to display finer details and more subtle lesions. Only with the advent of MRI have radiologists become familiar with uncommon pathology such as soft tissue tumors. Advanced MRI guarantees the most accurate diagnosis of neurogenic, fibrous, and vascular tumors. Even more important is that MRI accurately detects various stages of hemorrhage, multiple sclerosis (MS) plaques, intracanalicular acoustic neuromas, subtle brainstem abnormalities, and spinal cord cavities. Lesions adjacent to dense bones are easily identified. MRI has had a major influence on the evaluation of patients with the classical white matter disorder MS [2–4, 64, 66, 82, 83]. The non-invasive detection of MS plaques provided one of the early success stories of clinical MRI. The presence of contrast enhancement in an MS plaque is currently taken as a sign of disease activity, and therefore its detection is important in assessing acute disease burden [29]. Vascular abnormalities such as basilar artery occlusion, venous thrombosis, and arteriovenous malformations can be displayed. The normal MRI scan excludes cerebral and spinal cord abnormalities with a much higher degree of confidence than does the X-ray CT modality [29, 30].

One of the most recent improvements is the use of an array of receiving coils in phased array MRI [62]. Each coil of the phased array is linked to a separate receiver channel including low-noise preamplifier, demodulator, and data acquisition system. Phased array MRI allows direct visualization of the long spinal cord and nerve roots as opposed to viewing the secondary effects of a lesion on a spinal column of contrast.

- In long spine scanning, phased array MRI reconstitutes the partite image consisting of the cervical, cervicothoracic, thoracolumbar and upper lumbar spine into a single spine scan with improved spatial resolution compared to standard surface coil technique.

Direct visualization of spinal lesions on X-ray CT scans is not possible without intrathecal contrast. This is one of the various reasons for the strong trend to replace in today's fast changing medical environment the invasive X-ray CT modality by the non-invasive MRI modality [23] in order to study disc herniations, spinal trauma, vertebral tumors, paraspinal masses, infections of the spine, congenital malformations of the spinal cord, as well as joint abnormalities.

The Kepplerian quadrature detection strategy is not only used in SAR imaging and clinical MRI, but also in sonographic imaging to improve the signal-to-noise ratio. In the case of diagnostic sonography, the holographic recording in quadrature format provides striking results, too. Contrary to popular belief, the bioeffects and safety issues of sonographic examinations are not negligible.

Whereas today sonography is the most important imaging modality of mammography [37], it has not proved sensitive enough in the detection of small and early malignancies. In contrast to the sonographic mammography and the invasive X-ray mammography modality [37], the sensitivity of magnetic resonance mammography is greater than 95 % for the detection of carcinoma of the mammae, and the multifocality of breast cancer can be adequately recognized *only* by the MRI modality [18, 36, 41]. Further research using dedicated coils, and clinical tests under standardized examination conditions of a higher number of breast cancer patients, however, will be required to increase the specificity of magnetic resonance mammography in order to establish its superiority in the discrimination of benign and malignant lesions over the other mammographic imaging modalities presently available. The new generation of microprocessors will support this advances. The role of MRI in mammography and gynecology has been limited in the evaluation of breast and gynecologic malignancies by the unfamiliarity of referring physicians with the study, and by the relative inexperience of most radiologists in the community with detailed breast and pelvic MRI.

Since the pioneering work of Paul Broca (1824–1880) and Carl Wernicke (1848–1905), and up to the 1970's the understanding of the implementation of cognitive functions has relied on studies of patients bearing cerebral lesions. The recent development of neurofunctional MRI has demonstrated that in addition to providing clinico-morphological scans of exquisite detail, the MRI modality can be used to obtain neurofunctional maps in the human brain. The primary motor, sensory, visual, and language regions of the cerebral cortex can be identified using neurofunctional MRI. Accurate spatially localization of cerebral cortical activities that correlates with the temporal format of the study protocol is important for surgical planning and preoperative assessment in the treatment of such conditions as intractable seizure disorders in epilepsy, vascular malformations, and neoplasms [44, 82]. Dissecting the substrates of the human symptomatic epilepsies has become a reality with the advances in MRI [46, 75]. The neurofunctional MRI techniques rely on changes in the blood supply to the brain that accompany sensory stimulation or changes in cognitive state. Among the method that has received the greatest attention in neuroscience research and that has produced the most impressive MRI-based neurofunctional cerebral cortical maps is BOLD contrast imaging. BOLD has its origin in the magnetic properties of hemoglobin and the fact that the hemodynamic and metabolic response of the brain to increased neuronal activity is expected to lead to a decrease in the deoxyhemoglobin content in the microvasculature of the activated region. Indeed, neuronal activation is accompanied by an increase in regional cerebral blood flow, but oxygen consumption does not increase commensurately [14, 44]. It becomes apparent that there is considerable overlap between MRI and metabolic studies. As the technology matures, this overlap will even increase.

The role of neurofunctional MRI in the evaluation of acute stroke is best understood when placed in the context of hemodynamics and ischemia. The key finding is that there is a level of cerebral blood flow at which neurons stop functioning but have not undergone cell death, and therefore the damage from ischemia may be reversible. One of the goals of neurofunctional MRI is to visualize the ischemic penumbra, and ideally identify the difference between salvageable, non-salvageable, and undamaged cerebral parenchyma [74]. Taking into account that stroke is diagnosed 400.000 times per year in the United States, and contributes to approximately 150.000 deaths per year, the importance of neurofunctional MRI as a non-invasive MRI technique, sensitive to local changes of regional cerebral blood flow, volume, and oxygenation which accompanies neuronal activation, becomes evident.

In biochemical and chemical applications of the nuclear magnetic resonance phenomenon, the quest for ever-increasing external magnetic flux densities has been and continues to be pursued. This particular aspect, however, does not apply to the field of clinical MRI. As early as 1979 it was predicted that clinical MRI would not possible at carrier frequencies > 10 MHz because of limitations imposed by radiofrequency penetration. This dire prediction was fortunately proven to be erroneous, and MRI scanner systems operating at carrier frequency of 63.8 MHz, or external magnetic flux density of 1.5 T by the Larmor equation, became the accepted standard at the high end of the clinical imaging market. Although 1.5 T and even 2.0 T MRI scanner systems matured into the preferred instruments for demanding applications, and there is no conclusive evidence for irreversible or hazardous bioeffects related to exposure, higher external magnetic flux densities were regarded by clinicians with skepticism. The expectations for higher external magnetic flux densities were minimal based on diminishing contrast, dielectric and penetration effects with radiofrequency, and increasing susceptibility effects leading to potentially undesirable artifacts, and loss of peak signal-to-noise ratio. Early results have in fact confirmed these negative expectations to some extent. Recent results obtained at 4.0 T, however, demonstrate that these problems are surmountable, and properties that were deemed to be detrimental to human imaging studies at high external magnetic flux densities can, in fact, be used to the advantage of neurofunctional MRI.

The configuration of conventional clinical MRI scanner systems excludes direct contact with the patient under examination. Vertically open configuration magnets, however, allow full access to the exposed anatomy of the patient. The physician while located between the "double doughnuts" of the 0.5 Tesla superconducting magnet system can perform various MRI guided interventional procedures. At an external magnetic flux density of 0.5 T, the vertically open configuration magnet system has three important engineering features. First, the system does not require cryogens. No liquid He is used. The wires within the magnet are made from a special alloy which experiences superconductivity at a higher temperature than those used in conventional clinical MRI scanner systems. A closed cycle system provides sufficient cooling to maintain the superconducting state. The second notable feature of the vertically open configuration magnet system is the lack of gradient coils within the open part of the system. The coils are hidden in the doughnuts where they can switch the spatial linear gradient sequences of the spin-warp imaging technique without precluding direct access. In conventional clinical MRI scanner systems the patient is not only surrounded by the gradient coils but either by the head or the body coil. The open configuration magnet system does not need a a body or head coil. The third unique feature is the lack of a fixed transmitting radiofrequency coil. Instead a series of transmit–receive coils are specifically designed for the imaging particular body parts. These coils are flexible and therefore adapt perfectly to the shape of the anatomic region under investigation. These flexible coils are integrated into the surgical drape, can be sterilized and allow full access to the image volume [40].

Target definition for biopsy, and minimally invasive interventions require image guidance. MRI guided nonferromagnetic fine needle aspiration is an example of a minimally invasive procedure that is used to obtain cytologic specimens of suspicious lesions in the breast. Because contrast-enhanced MRI of the breast is able to reveal suspicious lesions that are not palpable and are not depicted with mammography or ultrasonic imaging, they must be localized under MRI guidance and then either aspirated, biopsied, or excised. Presently MRI guided nonferromagnetic needle localization is going to assume a role as the initial procedure in the evaluation and management of breast disease.

Operations done under MRI guidance have a decisive advantage over endoscopy, namely more accurate spatial localization. Recently, the first MRI guided biopsy of benign thyroid lesions without craniotomy in a vertically open MRI scanner system has been performed at the University Hospital in Zürich, Switzerland. To avoid projectile effects and artifacts, mechanical instruments must be made of nonferromagnetic materials, typically titanium, platinum, stainless steel, special plastics, or superelastic nitinol. Compared to awake craniotomy, the time needed for minimally invasive intracranial operations inside a vertically open MRI scanner has been shortened up to 80 %. In addition, the stereotactic resection of cavernous malformations using a MRI guided frameless stereotactic system has been reported.

It will be highly interesting to see how the emerging field of tomographic microtherapy will develop, as well as MRI guided stereotactic techniques for neurosurgical procedures, including craniotomy for primary and metastatic brain tumors, MRI guided frameless stereotactic resection of lesions, and telesurgery [5,40]. Nevertheless, it will be only an intermediate step toward a more clinical goal of interventional radiology.

Summarizing the significant breakthrough which MRI represents in conjunction with the recent hardware and software developments, the future of clinical MRI as a non-invasive diagnostic imaging modality seems to be bright. With its many advantages, including unrestricted multiplanar imaging capability, high spatial resolution imaging, exquisite contrast imaging of soft tissues, in addition to great versatility offering the ability to image blood flow, motion during the cardiac cycle, temperature effects, and chemical shifts, clinico-morphological MRI is a well-recognized tool in the evaluation of anatomic, pathologic, and functional processes. Specifically, clinical MRI allows for greater depiction of tumor extension and staging [2,22,63,64,66,77,79]. In light of the several dozens of scans that need to be analyzed and semantically interpreted in order to acquire comprehensive information from morphological studies which give consistent help in terms of earlier diagnosis, lesion characterization, and definition of the extent of disease, it is worth looking for some laborious routine tasks which could be automated and done by computers. As the applications of functional MRI in clinical radiology become more evident, automation is an even more important requirement for neurofunctional MRI studies which are based on the evaluation of hundreds of scans to detect signal changes well below the visual detection threshold under exclusion of changes that originate in head motion which correlate with the motor or visual stimuli, and simulate activiation of the human brain.

Although MRI has not reached the end of its development, this diagnostic imaging modality has already undoubtedly saved many lives, and patients the world over enjoy a higher quality of life, thanks to MRI. The previously impenetrable black holes of lung air spaces are finally yielding their secrets to MRI. Utilizing inhaled ^{3}He or ^{129}Xe gases that are hyperpolarized by laser light, MRI scans can be acquired in a breath-hold that promise to reveal new insights into pulmonary anatomy and function. Because the exhaled gases can be recycled, MRI will play a role also in the earlier detection of chest diseases and bronchiectasis, and surgical planning of lung transplantation.

The dramatic advances made in clinical MRI within the last few years, the resulting enhancement of the ability to evaluate morphologic and pathologic changes, and the non-invasive window on human brain activation offered by neurofunctional MRI to the preoperative assessment, demonstrate the unity of mathematics, science, and engineering in an impressive manner. In conclusion, it can only be assumed that the inexorable progress of quantum holography [50] and MRI will continue, and that there are many more improvements and discoveries of new clinical applications around the corner. The reader should try to accept these extensions of knowledge as part of interesting mathematics for the benefit of humankind.

ACKNOWLEDGMENT

The author gratefully acknowledges the hospitality extended to him as a visiting radiology fellow by his mentors at the Departments of MRI of Stanford University School of Medicine at Stanford, California, University of California School of Medicine at San Francisco, California, Massachusetts General Hospital at Charlestown, Massachusetts, and Harvard Medical School at Boston, Massachusetts, and the Russell H. Morgan Department of Radiology and Radiological Science, The Johns Hopkins Medical Institutions at Baltimore, Maryland. He deeply appreciates the bedside knowledge he learned from the radiologic diagnosticians and clinicians of these institutions in *theoria cum praxi*.

Moreover, the author is grateful to Professors George L. Farre (Georgetown University, Washington DC) and Erwin Kreyszig (Carleton University, Ottawa) for their generous advice and continuing support of this work.

REFERENCES

1. C. M. Anderson, R. R. Edelman, and P. A. Turski, Clinical Magnetic Resonance Angiography. Raven Press, New York 1993.
2. S. W. Atlas, editor, Magnetic Resonance Imaging of the Brain and Spine. Second edition, Lippincott–Raven Publishers, Philadelphia, New York 1996.
3. A. J. Barkovich, Pediatric Neuroimaging, Second edition, Raven Press, New York 1995.
4. A. J. Barkovich, C. L. Truwit, Practical MRI Atlas of Neonatal Brain Development. Raven Press, New York 1990.
5. G. H. Barnett, C. P. Steiner, and J. Weisenberger, Intracranial meningioma resection using frameless stereotaxy. J. Image Guided Surgery 1, 46–52 (1955).
6. R. Bauer, E. van de Flierdt, K. Mörike, and C. Wagner-Manslau, MR Tomography of the Central Nervous System. Gustav Fischer Verlag, Stuttgart, Jena, New York 1993.
7. J. Beltran, editor, Current Review of MRI. First edition, Current Medicine, Philadelphia 1995.
8. J. H. Bisese, A.-M. Wang, Pediatric Cranial MRI: An Atlas of Normal Development. Springer-Verlag, New York, Berlin, Heidelberg 1994.
9. S. Braitinger, J. Pahnke, Hrsg., editors, MR-Atlas der HNO-Anatomie, MR Atlas of ENT Anatomy. Bilingual Eurobook, F. K. Schattauer, Stuttgart, New York 1995.
10. J. J. Brown, F. J. Wippold II, Practical MRI: A Teaching File. Lippincott–Raven Publishers, Philadelphia, New York 1996.
11. D. R. Cahill, M. J. Orland, and G. M. Miller, Atlas of Human Cross-Sectional Anatomy, with CT and MR Images. Third edition, Wiley–Liss, New York, Chichester, Brisbane 1995.
12. W. G. Carrara, R. S. Goodman, and R. M. Majewski, Spotlight Synthetic Aperture Radar: Signal Processing Algorithms. Artech House, Boston, London 1995.
13. M. Castillo, S. K. Mukherji, Imaging of the Pediatric Head, Neck, and Spine. Lippincott–Raven Publishers, Philadelphia, New York 1996.
14. M. S. Cohen, Rapid MRI and functional applications. In: Brain Mappping — The Methods, A. W. Toga, J. C. Mazziotta, editors, pp. 223–255, Academic Press, San Diego, New York, Boston 1996.
15. L. J. Cutrona, E. M. Leith, L. J. Porcello, and W. E. Vivian, On the application of coherent optical processing techniques to synthetic-aperture radar. Proc. IEEE 54, 1026–1032 (1966).
16. H. Damasio, Human Brain Anatomy in Computerized Images. Oxford Univiversity Press, Oxford, New York 1995.
17. E. R. Davies, Electronics, Noise and Signal Recovery. Academic Press, London, San Diego, New York 1993.
18. P. L. Davis, editor, Breast Imaging. MRI Clinics of North America, Vol. 2, No. 4, November 1994, pp. 505–740, W. B. Saunders Company, Philadelphia, London, Toronto 1994.
19. G. Deleuze, F. Guattari, Q'est — ce que la philosophie? Les Éditions de Minuit, Paris 1991.

20. P. De Potter, C. L. Shields, and J. A. Shields, MRI of the Eye and Orbit. Lippincott–Raven Publishers, Philadelphia, New York 1995.
21. S. J. Doran, P. Jakob, and M. Décorps, Rapid repetition of the "burst" sequence: The role of diffusion and consequences for imaging. Magn. Reson. Med. 35, 547–553 (1996).
22. R. R. Edelman, J. R. Hesselink, and M. B. Zlatkin, Clinical Magnetic Resonance Imaging. Two volumes, second edition, W. B. Saunders Company, Philadelphia, London, Toronto 1996.
23. G. Y. El-Khoury, R. A. Bergman, and W. J. Montgomery, Sectional Anatomy by MRI. Second edition, Churchill Livingstone, New York, Edinburgh, London 1995.
24. J. Fleckenstein, J. V. Crues III, and C. D. Reimers, Muscle Imgaging in Health and Disease. Springer-Verlag, Berlin, Heidelberg, New York 1996.
25. E. Fukushima, editor, NMR in Biomedicine: The Physical Basis: Key Papers in Physics, Number 2, American Institute of Physics, New York 1989.
26. D. G. Gadian, NMR and its Applications to Living Systems. Second edition, Oxford University Press, Oxford, New York, Tokyo 1996.
27. A. E. George, Neurodegenerative diseases: Alzheimer's disease and related disorders. Neuroimaging Clinics of North America, Vol. 5, No. 1, February 1995, pp. 1–159, W. B. Saunders Company, Philadelphia, London, Toronto 1995.
28. O. Gingerich, Kepler's place in astronomy. In Kepler: Four Hundred Years. Proceedings of Conferences held in Honour of Johannes Kepler, A. Beer, and P. Beer, editors, Vistas in Astronomy, Vol. 18, pp. 261–278, Pergamon Press, Oxford, New York, Toronto 1975.
29. C. B. Grossman, Magnetic Resonance Imaging and Computed Tomography of the Head and Spine. Second edition, Williams & Wilkins, Baltimore, Philadelphia, London 1996.
30. R. I. Grossman, D. M. Yousem, Neuroradiology. Mosby-Year Book, St. Louis, Baltimore, Berlin 1994.
31. B. L. Hart, E. C. Benzel, and C. C. Ford, Fundamentals of Neuroimaging. W. B. Saunders Company, Philadelphia, London, Toronto 1997.
32. D. M. Healy, Jr., J. Lu, and J. B. Weaver, Two applications of wavelets and related techniques in medical imaging. Ann. Biomed. Eng. 23, 637–665 (1995).
33. R. M. Henkelman, M. J. Bronskill, Artifacts in magnetic resonance imaging. Rev. Magn. Reson. Med. 2, 1–126 (1987).
34. A. Heuck, G. Luttke, and J. W. Rohen, MR-Atlas der Extremitäten. F. K. Schattauer, Stuttgart, New York 1994.
35. L. Heuser, M. Oudkerk, editors, Advances in MRI. Blackwell Science, Oxford, London, Edinburgh 1996.
36. S. H. Heywang-Köbrunner, R. Beck, Contrast-Enhanced MRI of the Breast. Second edition, Springer-Verlag, Berlin, Heidelberg, New York 1996.
37. S. H. Heywang-Köbrunner, I. Schreer, Bildgebende Mammadiagnostik: Untersuchungstechnik, Befundmuster und Differentialdiagnostik in Mammographie, Sonographie und Kernspintomographie. Georg Thieme Verlag, Stuttgart, New York 1996.
38. P. Horowitz, W. Hill, The Art of Electronics. Second edition, Cambridge University Press, Cambridge, New York, Port Chester 1990.
39. P. M. Jakob, F. Kober, and A. Haase, Radial BURST Imaging. Magn. Reson. Med. 36, 557–561 (1996).
40. F. A. Jolesz, MRI-guided interventions. In: Progressi in RM, Note di tecnica, a cura di M. Cammisa, T. Scarabino, pp. 199–220, Guido Gnocchi, Editore, Napoli 1995.
41. W. A. Kaiser, MR Mammography (MRM). Springer-Verlag, Berlin, Heidelberg, New York 1993.
42. M. King, Fourier optics and radar signal processing. In: Applications of Optical Fourier Transforms. H. Stark, editor, pp. 209–251, Academic Press, Orlando, San Diego, San Francisco 1982.
43. H.-J. Kretschmann, W. Weinrich, Dreidimensionale Computergraphik neurofunktioneller Systeme: Grundlagen für die neurologisch-topische Diagnostik und die kranielle Bilddiagnostik (Magnetresonanztomographie und Computertomographie). Georg Thieme Verlag, Stuttgart, New York 1996.
44. J. Kucharczyk, M. E. Moseley, T. Roberts, and W. W. Orrison, Jr., editors, Functional neuroimaging. Neuroimaging Clinics of North America, Vol. 5, No. 2, May 1995, pp. 161–308, W. B. Saunders Company, Philadelphia, London, Toronto 1995.
45. A. Kumar, D. Welti, and R. R. Ernst, NMR Fourier zeugmatography. J. Magn. Reson. 18, 69–83 (1975).
46. R. I. Kuzniecky, G. D. Jackson, Magnetic Resonance in Epilepsy. Raven Press, New York 1995.
47. K. Kwong, Functional magnetic resonance imaging with echo planar imaging. Magn. Reson. Quart. 11, 1–20 (1995).
48. E. N. Leith, Synthetic aperture radar. In: Optical Data Processing, D. Casasent, editor, pp. 89–117, Topics in Applied Physics, Vol. 23, Springer-Verlag, Berlin, Heidelberg, New York 1978.
49. E. N. Leith, Optical processing of synthetic aperture radar data. In: Photonic Aspects of Modern Radar, H. Zmuda, E. N. Toughlian, editors, pp. 381–401, Artech House, Boston, London 1994.

50. P. J. Marcer, W. Schempp, A mathematically specified template for DNA and the genetic code in terms of the physically realisable processes of quantum holography. In: Proc. Symp. Living Computers: The Nature of Turing and Non-Turing Reproducible Order in Living Organisms, A. M. Fedorec, P. J. Marcer, editors, pp. 45–62, The British Computer Society, Greenwich University Press, London 1996.
51. J. Mattson, M. Simon, The Pioneers of NMR and Magnetic Resonance in Medicine: The Story of MRI. Bar-Ilan University Press, Ramat Gan 1996.
52. C. Mead, L. Conway, Introduction to VLSI Systems. Addison–Wesley Publishing Company, Reading, Menlo Park, London 1980.
53. T. B. Möller, E. Reif, MRI Atlas of the Musculoskeletal System. Blackwell Scientific Publications, Boston, Oxford, London 1993.
54. C. T. W. Moonen, P. van Gelderen, N. Ramsey, G. Liu, J. H. Duyn, J. Frank, and D. R. Weinberger, PRESTO, a rapid 3D approach for functional MRI of human brain. In: Syllabus Functional MRI, P. Pavone and P. Rossi, editors, pp. 105–110, Springer-Verlag, Berlin, Heidelberg, New York 1996.
55. P. L. Munk, C. A. Helms, MRI of the Knee. Second edition, Lippincott–Raven Publishers, Philadelphia, New York 1996.
56. M. Nägele, G. Adam, Moderne Kniegelenkdiagnostik: Bildgebende Verfahren und klinische Aspekte. Springer-Verlag, Berlin, Heidelberg, New York 1995.
57. W. Noack, editor, X-SAR Picture Book. Springer-Verlag, Berlin, Heidelberg, New York 1997.
58. E. J. Potchen, E. M. Haacke, J. E. Siebert, and A. Gottschalk, Magnetic Resonance Angiography: Concepts and Applications. Mosby-Year Book, St. Louis, Baltimore, Boston 1993.
59. V. Rasche, R. W. de Boer, D. Holz, and R. Proksa, Continuous radial data acquisition for dynamic MRI. Magn. Reson. Med. 34, 754–761 (1995).
60. V. Rasche, D. Holz, and W. Schepper, Radial turbo spin echo imaging. Magn. Reson. Med. 32, 629–638 (1994).
61. A. W. Rihaczek, Principles of High-Resolution Radar. Artech House, Boston, London 1996.
62. P. B. Roemer, W. A. Edelstein, C. E. Hayes, S. P. Souza, and O. M. Mueller, The NMR phased array. Magn. Reson. Med. 16, 192–252 (1990).
63. V. M. Runge, editor, Magnetic Resonance Imaging: Clinical Principles. J. B. Lippincott Company, Philadelphia, New York, London 1992.
64. V. M. Runge, Magnetic Resonance Imaging of the Brain. J. B. Lippincott Company, Philadelphia 1994.
65. J. A. Sanders, Functional magnetic resonance imaging. In: Functional Brain Imaging, W. W. Orrison, Jr., J. D. Lewine, J. A. Sanders, and M. F. Hartshorne, editors, pp. 239–326, Mosby-Year Book, St. Louis, Baltimore, Berlin 1995.
66. K. Sartor, MR Imaging of the Skull and Brain. Springer-Verlag, Berlin, Heidelberg, New York 1995.
67. W. Schempp, Harmonic Analysis on the Heisenberg Nilpotent Lie Group, with Applications to Signal Theory. Pitman Research Notes in Mathematics Series, Vol. 147, Longman Scientific and Technical, London 1986.
68. W. Schempp, Geometric analysis: The double-slit interference experiment and magnetic resonance imaging. Cybernetics and Systems '96, Vol. 1, pp. 179–183, Austrian Society for Cybernetic Studies, Vienna 1996.
69. W. Schempp, Geometric analysis and symbol calculus: Fourier transform magnetic resonance imaging and wavelets. In: Synergie, Syntropie, Nichtlineare Systeme, Wiener-Symposium, Heft 4, W. Eisenberg, U. Renner, S. Trimper, M. Kunz und K. Vogelsang, Hrsg., pp. 133–186, Verlag im Wissenschaftszentrum Leipzig, Leipzig 1996.
70. W. Schempp, Non-commutative affine geometry and symbolic calculus: Fourier transform magnetic resonance imaging and wavelets. In: Signal and Image Representation in Combined Spaces, J. Zeevi and R. R. Coifman, editors, pp. 1–47, Academic Press, London, San Diego, New York 1997.
71. W. Schempp, Wavelets in high-resolution radar imaging and clinical resonance tomography. Cybernetics and Systems: An International Journal 28, 1–23 (1997).
72. W. Schempp, Wavelets in high resolution radar imaging and clinical magnetic resonance imaging. Proc. IWISP '96: Third International Workshop on Image and Signal Processing on the Theme of Advance in Computational Intelligence, Manchester, United Kingdom, B. G. Mertzios, P. Liatsis, editors, pp. 73–80, Elsevier, Amsterdam, Lausanne, New York 1996.
73. W. Schempp, Magnetic Resonance Imaging: Mathematical Foundations and Applications. John Wiley & Sons, New York, Chichester, Brisbane (in print).
74. A. G. Sorensen, MR imaging in hyperacute stroke. In: Syllabus Functional MRI, P. Pavone and P. Rossi, editors, pp. 99–102, Springer-Verlag, Berlin, Heidelberg, New York 1996.
75. H. Stefan, Epilepsien: Diagnose und Behandlung. Chapman & Hall, London, Glasgow, Weinheim 1995.
76. B. Stephenson, Kepler's Physical Astronomy. Princeton University Press, Princeton, NJ 1994.
77. P. Stoeter, P. Gutjahr, und K. Brühl, Tumoren bei Kindern: Moderne Bildgebung mit MRT und CT, Band 1: ZNS. Georg Thieme Verlag, Stuttgart, New York 1996.
78. D. W. Stoller, editor, Magnetic Resonance Imaging in Orthopaedics & Sports Medicine. Second edition, Lippincott–Raven Publishers, Philadelphia, New York 1997.

79. H. Strunk, P. Gutjahr, Tumoren bei Kindern: Moderne Bildgebung mit MRT und CT, Band 2: Körperstamm und Extremitäten. Georg Thieme Verlag, Stuttgart, New York 1996.
80. K. R. Thulborn, J. Voyvodic, B. McCurtain, J. Gillen, S. Chang, M. Just, P. Carpenter, and J. A. Sweeney, High field functional MRI in humans: Applications to cognitive functions. In: Syllabus Functional MRI, P. Pavone and P. Rossi, editors, pp. 91–96, Springer-Verlag, Berlin, Heidelberg, New York 1996.
81. C. L. Truwit, T. E. Lempert, High Resolution Atlas of Cranial Neuroanatomy. Williams & Wilkins, Baltimore, Philadelphia, Hong Kong 1994.
82. D. Uhlenbrock, MRT und MRA des Kopfes: Indikationsstellung, Wahl der Untersuchungsparameter, Befund-interpretation. Georg Thieme Verlag, Stuttgart, New York 1996.
83. M. S. van der Knaap, J. Valk, Magnetic Resonance of Myelin, Myelination, and Myelin Disorders. Second edition, Springer-Verlag, Berlin, Heidelberg, New York 1995.
84. T. J. Vogl, MR-Angiographie und MR-Tomographie des Gefäßsystems: Klinische Diagnostik. Springer-Verlag, Berlin, Heidelberg, New York 1995.
85. D. R. Wehner, High Resolution Radar. Artech House, Norwood, MA 1987.
86. A. Weil, Sur certains groupes d'opérateurs unitaires. Acta Math. 111, 143–211 (1964). In: Œuvres Scientifiques, Collected Papers, Vol. III (1964–1978), pp. 1–69, Springer-Verlag, New York, Heidelberg, Berlin 1980.
87. M. V. Wickerhauser, Costum wavelet packet image compression design. Proc. IWISP '96: Third International Workshop on Image and Signal Processing on the Theme of Advance in Computational Intelligence, Manchester, United Kingdom, B. G. Mertzios, P. Liatsis, editors, pp. 47–52, Elsevier, Amsterdam, Lausanne, New York 1996.
88. D. H. Yock, Jr., Magnetic Resonance Imaging of CNS Disease: A Teaching File. Mosby-Year Book, St. Louis, Baltimore, Berlin 1995.

RAY TRANSFORM OF SYMMETRIC TENSOR FIELDS FOR A SPHERICALLY SYMMETRIC METRIC

V. A. Sharafutdinov*

Institute of Mathematics
Russian Academy of Sciences
Novosibirsk, 630090, Russia

ABSTRACT

The ray transform I on a Riemannian manifold (M,g) with boundary is the linear operator on the space of symmetric tensor fields of degree m that sends a tensor field into the set of its integrals over all maximal geodesics. The principal question on the ray transform is formulated as follows: for what Riemannian manifolds and values of m does the kernel of I coincide with the space of potential fields? A tensor m-field f is called potential if it is the symmetric part of the covariant derivative of another tensor field of degree $m-1$. The conjecture is proved in the case when M is the ball in Euclidean space and the metric g is spherically symmetric.

1. INTRODUCTION

In [1, 2] G. Herglotz, E. Wiechert and K. Zoeppritz considered the following inverse kinematic problem of seismics: one has to recover a function $n(\rho)$ $(0 \le \rho \le \rho_1)$ from the known distances in the metric

$$ds^2 = n^2(\rho)(d\rho^2 + \rho^2 d\theta^2) \tag{1.1}$$

between points belonging to the boundary circle $\{\rho = \rho_1\}$. They solved the problem under the assumption

$$\frac{d}{d\rho}(\rho n(\rho)) > 0. \tag{1.2}$$

*Partly supported by RFBR (Grant 96–01–01558) and by RFBR — DFG (Grant 96–01–00094)

The solution is based on the following well-known fact: in the case of the surface of revolution the equation for geodesics possesses the first integral (Clairaut's integral).

V. G. Romanov in [3,4] investigated the integral geometry problem (linearized inverse kinematic problem of seismics) of determining a function f in the ring

$$D = \{(\rho\cos\theta, \rho\sin\theta) \mid 0 < \rho_0 \leq \rho \leq \rho_1\} \tag{1.3}$$

from the known its integrals over geodesics of metric (1.1), joining points of the circle $\rho = \rho_1$. Using Clairaut's integral he derived some second integral Volterra equation for every Fourier coefficient of the function $f(\rho\cos\theta, \rho\sin\theta)$. The equation implies uniqueness of a solution to the problem under assumption (1.2).

It is shown in Section 3.7 of the book [4] that the linearization of the inverse kinematic problem for anisotropic media leads to the integral geometry problem for a symmetric second degree tensor field. A solution to the latter problem is not unique. Theorem 3.6 of [4] allows us to find only some part of components of the sought tensor fields under the assumption that other components are known.

The integral geometry problem for symmetric higher degree tensor fields is of some interest too. For instance, as is shown in Ch. 7 of [5], the problem of determining the elasticity tensor of a quasi-isotropic medium from measurement of compression waves is equivalent to the integral geometry problem for a symmetric tensor field of degree 4.

The present article is devoted to integral geometry of symmetric tensor fields over geodesics of a spherically symmetric Riemannian metric. We define the ray transform I on such fields and find the kernel of I in the case of metric (1.1). The main result is that Ker$I$ coincides with the space of potential fields. A symmetric tensor field f of degree m is called potential if there exists a symmetric tensor field v of degree $m-1$ vanishing on the circle $\rho = \rho_1$, and such that f is the symmetric part of the covariant derivative of v.

A similar statement is true in the case of the metric

$$ds^2 = n^2(x_1)\sum_{i=1}^{n} x_i^2$$

in the half-space $\mathbf{R}^n_+ = \{(x_1, \ldots, x_n) \mid x_1 \geq 0\}$. The arguments are the same as in the present article, but one has to use the Fourier transform instead of Fourier series. This version of the result was used in [6] for investigating some geotomography problems for slightly anisotropic elastic media.

As mentioned in [4], for scalar functions, the integral geometry problem in the ring has logarithmic stability. In the present article we do not discuss the stability problem. Here we note only that in the case of tensor fields, the setting of the stability problem is not evident because of nontriviality of Ker$I$. Considering the corresponding problem for compact dissipative Riemannian manifolds (see Ch. 4 of [5]), we got over this difficulty by introducing the notion of the solenoidal part of a tensor field. In the present case, such approach is impossible because the potential v does not vanish on the inner boundary $\rho = \rho_0$ of ring (1.3).

Our method is similar to that of Section 3.4 of [4]. Instead of metric (1.1) we will use the metric

$$ds^2 = \omega^2(r)dr^2 + r^2 d\theta^2. \tag{1.4}$$

The equations for geodesics are simpler for metric (1.4) than for metric (1.3). On the other hand, using (1.4) we do not lose in generality because, under assumption (1.2), these two metrics are transformed to one other by the change of coordinates $r = \rho n(\rho)$, $\omega(r) = n(\rho)/(\rho n(\rho))'$.

We present detailed formulations for all definitions and statements. As for proofs, we give only short sketches here. The detailed proofs will be published later in the Siberian Math. J.

2. POSING THE PROBLEM AND FORMULATING THE RESULT

We use terminology and notations concerning tensor analysis that are presented in Ch. 3 of [5]. In particular, for a Riemannian manifold (M,g), by $S^m\tau'_M$ we denote the bundle of symmetric tensors of degree m. The inner derivative

$$d : C^l(S^m\tau'_M) \to C^{l-1}(S^{m+1}\tau'_M)$$

is defined by the equality $d = \sigma\nabla$, where ∇ is the covariant derivative and σ is the symmetrization. There is the inner product in fibers of $S^m\tau'_M$ which is expressed in local coordinates as follows:

$$\langle u, v\rangle = u^{i_1\dots i_m}\bar{v}_{i_1\dots i_m}. \tag{2.1}$$

In particular, for $u \in C^l(S^m\tau'_M)$, a point $x \in M$, and a tangent vector $\xi \in T_xM$

$$\langle u(x), \xi^m\rangle = u_{i_1\dots i_m}(x)\xi^{i_1}\dots\xi^{i_m}.$$

Given a tensor field $v \in C^l(S^{m-1}\tau'_M)$ $(l \geq 1)$ and a geodesic $\gamma : [a,b] \to M$ the equality

$$\frac{d}{dt}\langle v(\gamma(t)), \dot\gamma^{m-1}(t)\rangle = \langle (dv)(\gamma(t)), \dot\gamma^m(t)\rangle,$$

holds which implies

$$\langle v(\gamma(b)), \dot\gamma^{m-1}(b)\rangle - \langle v(\gamma(a)), \dot\gamma^{m-1}(a)\rangle = \int_a^b \langle (dv)(\gamma(t)), \dot\gamma^m(t)\rangle\, dt. \tag{2.2}$$

We fix a domain G in the boundary ∂M of M and denote by Γ_G the manifold of all geodesics $\gamma : [a,b] \to M$ whose endpoints belong to G. The ray transform

$$I_G : C(S^m\tau'_M) \to C(\Gamma_G) \tag{2.3}$$

is the linear operator defined by the equality

$$(I_G f)(\gamma) = \int_a^b \langle f(\gamma(t)), \dot\gamma^m\rangle\, dt. \tag{2.4}$$

Observe that the ray transform I introduced in Ch. 4 of [5] is the special case of operator (2.3) corresponding to $G = \partial M$.

A tensor field $f \in C^l(S^m\tau'_M)$ $(l \geq 0)$ is called potential if there exists a field $v \in C^{l+1}(S^{m-1}\tau'_M)$ vanishing on G and such that $dv = f$. As follows from (2.2), potential fields constitute the subspace of the kernel $\mathrm{Ker} I_G$. The principal question of the ray transform is formulated as follows: for what Riemannian manifolds (M,g), domains $G \subset \partial M$ and values of m does the kernel KerI_G coincide with the space of potential fields? Of course, the answer can be positive only in the case when G is large enough such that at least one geodesic of Γ_G passes through every point of M.

Remind that an oriented hypersurface in M is called strictly convex if its second quadratic form is positively definite.

Our main result is formulated as follows.

Theorem 2.1. *Let a Riemannian metric g in the domain*

$$D = \{x \in \mathbf{R}^n \mid \rho_0 \le |x| \le \rho_1\} \qquad (0 < \rho_0 < \rho_1, \quad (n \ge 2) \tag{2.5}$$

be such that (1) g is invariant with respect to all orthogonal transforms of $\mathbf{R}^n$, *and (2) the sphere* $S_\rho = \{x \mid |x| = \rho\}$ *is strictly convex for every* $\rho \in [\rho_0, \rho_1]$. *Let* $G = S_{\rho_1}$. *If a symmetric tensor field* $f \in C^l(S^m\tau'_D)$ $(l \ge 1, m \ge 0)$ *belongs to the kernel of the ray transform* I_G, *then there exists a tensor field* $v \in C^l(S^{m-1}\tau'_D)$ *satisfying the boundary condition* $v|_G = 0$ *and such that*

$$dv = f. \tag{2.6}$$

Note that the theorem claim does not perfectly correspond to the above posed question because of the following two circumstances. First, the theorem claims nothing in the case $l = 0$. Second, in the case $l \ge 1$ it claims only that v belongs to C^l, but does not claim that v belongs to C^{l+1}. The following two remarks are valid on these circumstances.

The theorem remains valid in the case $l = 0$ if equality (2.6) is understood in the sense of distribution theory.

If $f \in C^l(S^m\tau'_D)$ and $l \ge m$, then every solution to equation (2.6) belongs to C^{l+1}. This claim follows from the fact: being differentiated $m-1$ times equation (2.6) can be solved with respect to $\nabla^m v$. This fact is proved in Theorem 2.2 of [5] for Euclidean metric. The same proof is valid for arbitrary Riemannian metric, since the covariant derivatives $\nabla^m v$ in any two metrics differ in terms of degree $m-1$.

Given a metric meeting the assumption of Theorem 2.1, every geodesic is in a two-dimensional plane through the origin. On the base of this fact the theorem can be easily reduced to its two-dimensional case. In the latter case our metric looks in polar coordinates as follows

$$ds^2 = a^2(\rho)\,d\rho^2 + b^2(\rho)\,d\theta^2.$$

Strict convexity of circles $\rho = \text{const}$ is equivalent to the inequality $b'(\rho) > 0$. After the change $r = b(\rho)$, $\omega(r) = a(\rho)/b'(\rho)$, we arrive at metric (1.4). In coordinates (r, θ) the ring D is defined by the equality

$$D = \{(r\cos\theta, r\sin\theta) \mid R_0 \le r \le R_1\}. \tag{2.7}$$

In what follows the numbers $0 < R_0 < R_1$ and positive function $\omega \in C^\infty([R_0, R_1])$ are fixed. For $M = D$ and $G = \{R_1\cos\theta, R_1\sin\theta\}$, henceforth we denote the ray transform (2.3) by I.

3. VOLTERRA EQUATION FOR THE FOURIER COEFFICIENTS

For metric (1.4), every geodesic γ in the ring (2.7) with endpoints on the circle $r = R_1$ has a unique point (ρ, α) nearest to the origin. The latter is called the top of γ. Such geodesics can be parameterized by their tops: $\gamma = \gamma_{\rho,\alpha}$. The top (ρ, α) divides the geodesic $\gamma = \gamma_{\rho,\alpha}$ into two symmetric branches that are given in polar coordinates (r, θ) by the equation

$$\theta(r) = \alpha \pm \psi(\rho, r), \quad \psi(\rho, r) = \int_{\rho}^{r} \frac{\omega(r')\, dr'}{r'\sqrt{r'^2 - \rho^2}}. \tag{3.1}$$

Being measured from the top, the arc length t of $\gamma_{\rho,\alpha}$ is expressed by the formula

$$t(r) = \pm \int_{\rho}^{r} \frac{r'\omega(r')\, dr'}{\sqrt{r'^2 - \rho^2}}. \tag{3.2}$$

On a two-dimensional manifold a symmetric tensor field of degree m has only $m+1$ different components. So it is reasonable to use the following notation, for tensor components, which have only one index: for $f \in C(S^m \tau'_D)$ we put

$$f_j = f_{\underbrace{r\ldots r}_{j}\underbrace{\theta\ldots\theta}_{m-j}} \quad (0 \le j \le m). \tag{3.3}$$

It is also convenient to assume that $f_j = 0$ for $j < 0$ and $j > m$.

For a geodesic $\gamma(t) = (r(t), \theta(t))$ $(a \le t \le b)$, definition (2.4) for the ray transform is written in the new notation as follows:

$$If(\gamma) = \int_{a}^{b} \sum_{j=0}^{m} \binom{m}{j} f_j(r(t), \theta(t)) \dot{r}^j(t) \dot{\theta}^{m-j}(t)\, dt.$$

With the help of (3.2) and (3.3) the last formula is transformed to the form

$$If(\rho, \alpha) \equiv If(\gamma_{\rho,\alpha}) =$$

$$= \sum_{j=0}^{[m/2]} \binom{m}{2j} \int_{\rho}^{R_1} \frac{\rho^{m-2j}(r^2 - \rho^2)^{(2j-1)/2}}{r^{2m-2j-1}\omega^{2j-1}(r)} [f_{2j}(r, \alpha + \psi(\rho, r)) + f_{2j}(r, \alpha - \psi(\rho, r))]\, dr +$$

$$+ \sum_{j=0}^{[m/2]-1} \binom{m}{2j+1} \int_{\rho}^{R_1} \frac{\rho^{m-2j-1}(r^2 - \rho^2)^j}{r^{2m-2j-2}\omega^{2j}(r)} [f_{2j+1}(r, \alpha + \psi(\rho, r)) - f_{2j+1}(r, \alpha - \psi(\rho, r))]\, dr. \tag{3.4}$$

The Fourier coefficients of the ray transform

$$If(\rho, \alpha) = \sum_{k=-\infty}^{\infty} (If)_k(\rho) e^{ik\alpha} \tag{3.5}$$

are related to the Fourier coefficients of the field $f \in C(S^m \tau'_D)$

$$f_j(r, \theta) = \binom{m}{j}^{-1} r^{2m-j-1} \omega^{j-1}(r) \sum_{k=-\infty}^{\infty} f_{j|k}(r) e^{ik\theta}. \tag{3.6}$$

by the equations

$$\int_\rho^{R_1}\left[\sum_{j=0}^{[m/2]}\rho^{m-2j}(r^2-\rho^2)^{(2j-1)/2}\cos k\psi(\rho,r)f_{2j|k}(r)+\right.$$

$$\left.+i\sum_{j=0}^{[m/2]-1}\rho^{m-2j-1}(r^2-\rho^2)^j\sin k\psi(\rho,r)f_{2j+1|k}(r)\right]dr=\frac{1}{2}(If)_k(\rho). \tag{3.7}$$

that is obtained from (3.4) by a routine calculation.

Equation (3.7) gives us the following important statement: the ray transform commutes with expansion of a tensor field into Fourier series. More exactly: if, given $f\in C(S^m\tau'_D)$ and an integer k, we define $\overset{k}{f}\in C(S^m\tau'_D)$ by putting

$$(\overset{k}{f})_j(r,\theta)=\binom{m}{j}^{-1}r^{2m-j-1}\omega^{j-1}(r)f_{j|k}(r)e^{ik\theta}\quad(0\le j\le m) \tag{3.8}$$

where $f_{j|k}(r)$ are the Fourier coefficients of (3.6), then

$$(I\overset{k}{f})(\rho,\alpha)=(If)_k(\rho)e^{ik\alpha},$$

where $(If)_k(\rho)$ are the coefficients of (3.5). In particular, if $If=0$, then $I\overset{k}{f}=0$ for every k.

Due to the singularity in the first term of the integral, (3.7) can be transformed to the second kind Volterra integral equation

$$\int_s^{R_1}\sum_{j=0}^{m}R_{j|k}(s,r)f_{j|k}(r)\,dr-f_{0|k}(s)=\frac{1}{\pi}\frac{d}{ds}\int_s^{R_1}\frac{(If)_k(\rho)\,d\rho}{\rho^{m-1}\sqrt{\rho^2-s^2}} \tag{3.9}$$

with the kernels

$$R_{2j|k}(s,r)=\frac{2}{\pi}\frac{\partial}{\partial s}\int_s^r\frac{(r^2-\rho^2)^{(2j-1)/2}\cos k\psi(\rho,r)}{\rho^{2j-1}\sqrt{\rho^2-s^2}}\,d\rho,$$

$$R_{2j+1|k}(s,r)=\frac{2i}{\pi}\frac{\partial}{\partial s}\int_s^r\frac{(r^2-\rho^2)^j\sin k\psi(\rho,r)}{\rho^{2j}\sqrt{\rho^2-s^2}}\,d\rho. \tag{3.10}$$

4. THE FORMAL SOLUTION OF THE EQUATION $DV=F$

It turns out that the kernels (3.10) are connected by some differential equations. The equations can not be easily derived from definition (3.10). However there is another way of deriving the equations. Indeed, we know that, given a tensor field $v\in C^1(S^{m-1}\tau'_D)$ meeting the boundary condition $v|_{r=R_1}=0$, the identity $I(dv)\equiv 0$ holds. Consequently, the Fourier coefficients $f_{j|k}(r)$ of the field $f=dv$ satisfy the homogeneous equation

$$\int_s^{R_1}\sum_{j=0}^{m}R_{j|k}(s,r)f_{j|k}(r)\,dr=f_{0|k}(s). \tag{4.1}$$

In such a way we arrive at some identity including m arbitrary functions, the components of the field v. This arbitrariness leads to the desired equations on the kernels. Let us realize our plan.

For a tensor field $v \in C^1(S^{m-1}\tau'_D)$, the inner derivative with respect to metric (1.4) is given in notation (3.3) by the formula

$$(dv)_j = \frac{1}{m}\left[j\frac{\partial v_{j-1}}{\partial r} + (m-j)\frac{\partial v_j}{\partial \theta} - j\left((j-1)\frac{\omega'}{\omega} + 2\frac{m-j}{r}\right)v_{j-1} + \right.$$

$$\left. + (m-j-1)(m-j)\frac{r}{\omega^2}v_{j+1}\right]. \tag{4.2}$$

For brevity, arguments are not designated here, but it is meant that $\omega = \omega(r)$ and $v_j = v_j(r,\theta)$.

If the fields v and $f = dv$ are expanded into Fourier series

$$v_j(r,\theta) = \sum_{k=-\infty}^{\infty} v_{j|k}(r)e^{ik\theta} \quad (0 \le j \le m-1), \tag{4.3}$$

$$f_j(r,\theta) = (dv)_j(r,\theta) = \sum_{k=-\infty}^{\infty} (dv)_{j|k}(r)e^{ik\theta} \quad (0 \le j \le m), \tag{4.4}$$

then the series (3.6) and (4.4) coincide. Therefore (4.2) implies the relations

$$f_{j|k} = \frac{1}{m}\binom{m}{j} r^{j-2m+1}\omega^{1-j}(dv)_{j|k} = \frac{1}{m}\binom{m}{j} r^{j-2m+1}\omega^{1-j} \times$$

$$\times \left[jv'_{j-1|k} - j\left((j-1)\frac{\omega'}{\omega} + 2\frac{m-j}{r}\right)v_{j-1|k} + \right.$$

$$\left. + ik(m-j)v_{j|k} + (m-j-1)(m-j)\frac{r}{\omega^2}v_{j+1|k}\right] \quad (0 \le j \le m). \tag{4.5}$$

Formula (4.5) allows us to make the following remark: the inner derivative d commutes with expansion of a tensor field into Fourier series. More exactly: if, given $v \in C^1(S^{m-1}\tau'_D)$ and an integer k, we define $\overset{k}{v} \in C^1(S^{m-1}\tau'_D)$ by putting

$$(\overset{k}{v})_j(r,\theta) = v_{j|k}(r)e^{ik\theta} \quad (0 \le j \le m-1), \tag{4.6}$$

where $v_{j|k}(r)$ are the coefficients of (4.3), then

$$(d\overset{k}{v})_j(r,\theta) = (dv)_{j|k}(r)e^{ik\theta},$$

where $(dv)_{j|k}(r)$ are the coefficients of (4.4).

Given a tensor field $v \in C^1(S^{m-1}\tau'_D)$ satisfying the boundary condition

$$v_{j|k}(R_1) = 0, \tag{4.7}$$

the field $f = dv$ meets equation (4.1). Substituting values (4.5) for $f_{j|k}$ into (4.1), after simple transformations we arrive at the identity

$$\frac{1}{m}\sum_{j=0}^{m-1}\binom{m}{j}(m-j)\int\limits_{s}^{R_1}\Big[-r\frac{\partial R_{j+1|k}(s,r)}{\partial r}+jR_{j+1|k}(s,r)+$$

$$+ik\omega(r)R_{j|k}(s,r)+jR_{j-1|k}(s,r)\Big]\frac{r^{j-2m+1}}{\omega^j(r)}v_{j|k}(r)\,dr=$$

$$=\frac{1}{s^{2m-1}}\big(ik\omega(s)+sR_{1|k}(s,s)\big)\,v_{0|k}(s)+\frac{m-1}{s^{2m-1}\omega(s)}\big(1+sR_{2|k}(s,s)\big)\,v_{1|k}(s)+$$

$$+\frac{1}{ms^{2m-2}}\sum_{j=2}^{m-1}\binom{m}{j}(m-j)\frac{s^j}{\omega^j(s)}R_{j+1|k}(s,s)v_{j|k}(s).$$

This equality holds for arbitrary functions $v_{j|k}\in C^1([R_0,R_1])$ meeting (4.7), and for every $s\in[R_0,R_1]$. It implies the desired differential equation

$$r\frac{\partial R_{j+1|k}(s,r)}{\partial r}-jR_{j+1|k}(s,r)-ik\omega(r)R_{j|k}(s,r)-jR_{j-1|k}(s,r)=0\quad(0\le j\le m-1)$$

connecting the kernels of integral equation (4.1) as well as the relations

$$R_{1|k}(s,s)=-ik\frac{\omega(s)}{s},\qquad R_{2|k}(s,s)=-\frac{1}{s},\qquad R_{j|k}(s,s)=0\quad(3\le j\le m).$$

Inverting the argument of the current section, we prove the following

Lemma 4.1. *Let a tensor field $f\in C(S^m\tau'_D)$ be in the kernel of the ray transform, i.e., $If\equiv 0$. Expand every component of f into Fourier series (3.6) and define the tensor field $\overset{k}{f}\in C(S^m\tau'_D)$ by equality (3.8) for every integer k. Then the field $\overset{k}{f}$ is potential for every k, i.e., there exists a tensor field $\overset{k}{v}\in C^1(S^{m-1}\tau'_D)$ such that*

$$\overset{k}{v}|_{r=R_1}=0 \tag{4.8}$$

and

$$d\overset{k}{v}=\overset{k}{f}. \tag{4.9}$$

Relations (3.6) and (4.9) imply that the components of the field $\overset{k}{v}$ can be represented in form (4.6). The rest of the paper is devoted to proving convergence of Fourier series (4.3) whose coefficients are expressed through the tensor field $\overset{k}{v}$ by formula (4.6). In what follows we use only properties (4.8) and (4.9) of the fields $\overset{k}{v}$.

5. COERCIVENESS OF THE OPERATOR D IN THE C^L-NORM

Given tensor fields $u, v \in C^l(S^m \tau'_D)$, the inner product (2.1) is expressed in notations (3.3) by the formula

$$\langle u(r,\theta), v(r,\theta)\rangle = \sum_{j=0}^{m} \binom{m}{j} r^{2m-2j} \omega^{2j}(r) u_j(r,\theta)\overline{v_j(r,\theta)}, \quad |u(r,\theta)|^2 = \langle u(r,\theta), u(r,\theta)\rangle.$$

For a domain $U \subset D$ we denote

$$(u,v)_{L_2(U)} = \iint_U r\omega(r)\langle u(r,\theta), v(r,\theta)\rangle \, dr\, d\theta, \quad \|u\|_{C^l(U)} = \sum_{j=0}^{m} \|u_j\|_{C^l(U)}.$$

The following statement is a version of Poincaré's inequality and can be proved in a full analogy with the proof of Lemma 4.5.2 of [5].

Lemma 5.1. *Let $D_{r_0} = \{(r,\theta) \mid r_0 \le r \le R_1\}$ be the subring of the ring D. If a tensor field $v \in C^1(S^m \tau'_D)$ meets the boundary condition $v|_{r=R_1} = 0$, then the estimate*

$$\|v\|^2_{L_2(D_{r_0})} \le C(R_1 - r_0)\|dv\|^2_{L_2(D_{r_0})} \quad (R_0 \le r_0 \le R_1) \tag{5.1}$$

holds with some constant C independent of v and r_0.

If a tensor field $f \in C(S^m \tau'_D)$ is expanded in Fourier series (3.6) and the fields $\overset{k}{f} \in C(S^m \tau'_D)$ are defined by (3.8), then the series

$$f = \sum_{k=-\infty}^{\infty} \overset{k}{f} \tag{5.2}$$

converges to f in $L_2(S^m \tau'_D)$ and by the Parseval equality

$$\frac{1}{2\pi}\|f\|^2_{L_2(D)} = \sum_{k=-\infty}^{\infty} \|\overset{k}{f}\|^2_{L_2(D)}. \tag{5.3}$$

Let a tensor field $f \in C(S^m \tau'_D)$ be in the kernel of the ray transform and let $\overset{k}{v} \in C^1(S^{m-1}\tau'_D)$ be the fields existing by Lemma 4.1. Applying Lemma 5.1 to $\overset{k}{v}$ and using (5.3), we see that the series

$$v = \sum_{k=-\infty}^{\infty} \overset{k}{v} \tag{5.4}$$

converges in $L_2(S^{m-1}\tau'_D)$ and the estimate

$$\|v\|^2_{L_2(D_{r_0})} \le C(R_1 - r_0)\|f\|^2_{L_2(D)}$$

holds with a constant C independent of v and r_0. Convergence of series (5.4) in the space $L_2(S^{m-1}\tau'_D)$ implies its convergence in the sense of distribution theory. Since every series can be differentiated in the sense of distribution theory, (5.2) and (5.4) imply

$$dv = \sum_{k=-\infty}^{\infty} d\overset{k}{v} = \sum_{k=-\infty}^{\infty} \overset{k}{f} = f.$$

We have thus proved

Lemma 5.2. *If a tensor field $f \in C(S^m \tau'_D)$ is in the kernel of the ray transform, then there exists a tensor field $v \in L_2(S^{m-1}\tau'_D)$, such that the equality*

$$dv = f \tag{5.5}$$

holds in the sense of distribution theory, and

$$\lim_{r \to R_1} \|v\|_{L_2([r,R_1]\times[0,2\pi])} = 0. \tag{5.6}$$

We assume now, additionally to conditions of Lemma 5.2, that $f \in C^1(S^m \tau'_D)$. Applying the divergence operator δ to equation (5.5), we obtain

$$\delta dv = \delta f. \tag{5.7}$$

The operator δd is elliptic as is shown in [5, p. 93]. The right-hand side of equation (5.7) is continuous in D. Since an elliptic operator is hypoelliptic, we derive that $v \in H^2_{\mathrm{loc}}(S^{m-1}\tau'_{\overset{\circ}{D}})$, where

$$\overset{\circ}{D} = \{re^{i\theta} \mid R_0 < r < R_1\}$$

is the interior of D. Applying the imbedding theorem $H^2_{\mathrm{loc}}(\overset{\circ}{D}) \subset C(\overset{\circ}{D})$, we arrive at

Lemma 5.3. *If a tensor field $f \in C^1(S^m \tau'_D)$ is in the kernel of the ray transform, then there exists a tensor field $v \in L_2(S^{m-1}\tau'_D) \cap C(S^{m-1}\tau'_{\overset{\circ}{D}})$, satisfying (5.5) and (5.6).*

Using the machinery of averaging functions, one can easily generalize formula (2.2) to the case of continuous tensor fields so as to obtain

Lemma 5.4. *Let the tensor fields $v \in C(S^{m-1}\tau'_D)$ and $f \in C(S^m \tau'_D)$ satisfy the equation $dv = f$ in the sense of distribution theory. Then for every geodesic $\gamma\colon [a,b] \to D$*

$$\langle v(\gamma(b)), \dot\gamma^{m-1}(b)\rangle - \langle v(\gamma(a)), \dot\gamma^{m-1}(a)\rangle = \int_a^b \langle f(\gamma(t)), \dot\gamma^m(t)\rangle\, dt. \tag{5.8}$$

To prove Theorem 2.1 we need the following main property of the operator d.

Lemma 5.5. *Choose numbers R'_0 and R'_0 such that $R_0 < R'_0 < R'_1 < R_1$, and denote $D' = \{re^{i\theta} \mid R'_0 \le r \le R'_1\}$ the corresponding subring of D. If $v \in C(S^m \tau'_D)$ and $dv \in C^l(S^{m+1}\tau'_D)$ $(l \ge 0)$, then $v \in C^l(S^m \tau'_D)$, and the estimate*

$$\|v\|_{C^l(D)} \le C_1 \|dv\|_{C^l(D)} + C_2 \|v\|_{C(D')} \tag{5.9}$$

holds with some constants C_1 and C_2 depending only on m, R_0, R_1, R'_0, R'_1, and the function $\omega(r)$.

We will not present the formal proof of the lemma which is rather cumbersome. Here we explain only the idea of the proof.

Given a domain $U \subset D$, assume that there exist points $y_0, y_1, \ldots, y_m$ in D' such that every point $x \in U$ can be joint with y_n $(0 \le n \le m)$ by some geodesic $\gamma_n(t)$ $(0 \le t \le 1)$ depending smoothly on x. By (5.8)

$$\langle v(x), \dot\gamma_n^m(1)\rangle = \langle v(y_n), \dot\gamma_n^m(0)\rangle + \int_{\gamma_n} \langle dv, \dot\gamma_n^{m+1}\rangle\, dt \quad (0 \le n \le m). \tag{5.10}$$

We consider (5.10) as a system of linear algebraic equations in the functions $v_j(x)$ $(0 \le j \le m)$. Coefficients of the system depend smoothly on x, and its right-hand sides belong to C^l. If the determinant of the system is nonzero, then the solution belongs to C^l and satisfies the estimate

$$\|v\|_{C^l(U)} \le C_1 \|dv\|_{C^l(U)} + C_2 \max_n |v(y_n)|.$$

It remains to convince ourselves that the ring D can be covered by a finite number of domains U with the above-mentioned properties.

Applying Lemma 5.5 to subrings of the ring D, we derive

Corollary 5.6. *Let v be a continuous in $\overset{\circ}{D}$ symmetric tensor field of degree m. If $dv \in C^l(S^{m+1}\tau'_{\overset{\circ}{D}})$ $(l \ge 1)$ and the norm $\|dv\|_{C^l(\overset{\circ}{D})}$ is finite, then v can be extended to the closed ring D in such a way that the extension belongs to $C^{l-1}(S^m\tau')$.*

Proof of Theorem 2.1: Let a tensor field $f \in C^l(S^m\tau'_D)$ $(l \ge 1)$ belongs to the kernel of the ray transform. By Lemma 5.3, there exists a tensor field $v \in L_2(S^{m-1}\tau'_D) \cap C(S^{m-1}\tau'_{\overset{\circ}{D}})$ satisfying (5.5) and (5.6). Applying Corollary 5.6, we extend v to a continuous tensor field in the closed ring D. Then, with the help of Lemma 5.5, we see that $v \in C^l(S^{m-1}\tau'_D)$. Finally, (5.6) implies the boundary condition $v|_{r=R_1} = 0$.

REFERENCES

1. Herglotz G. Uber die Elastität der Erde bei Berücksichtigung ihrer variablen Dichte, Zeitschr. füf Math. und Phys., 52, No 3 (1905), 275–299.
2. Wiechert E. und Zoeppritz K. Über Erdbebenwellen, Nachr. Königl. Geselschaft Wiss, Göttingen, 4 (1907), 415–549.
3. Romanov V. G. On determing a function from its integrals over the curves of a given family. Siberian Math. J., V. 8, No 5, 1967, 1206–1208. (in Russian)
4. Romanov V. G. *Inverse Problems of Mathematical Physics.* NVU: Science Press, Utrecht, the Netherlands, 1979.
5. Sharafutdinov V. A. *Integral Geometry of Tensor Fields.* NVU: Science Press, Utrecht, the Netherlands, 1994.
6. Sharafutdinov V. A. Linearized inverse problems of determining parameters of transversally isotropic elastic media from measurements of refracted waves. J. Inverse Ill-posed Problems. 1996, V. 4, No 2, 211–230.

12

REDUCING NOISE IN IMAGES BY FORCING MONOTONIC CHANGE BETWEEN EXTREMA

John B. Weaver*

Department of Radiology
Dartmouth-Hitchcock Medical Center
Lebanon, NH

ABSTRACT

A novel method of reducing noise in images is presented. The significant extrema (maxima and minima) in the image are selected using a simple low pass Fourier filter. The method forces the pixel values in the image to vary monotonically between the selected extrema. For example, the pixel values in the filtered image should decrease monotonically in all directions from an isolated maximum. Because the algorithm that performs the monotonic fits is one dimensional, we approximate monotonic change in all directions by doing monotonic fits along line segments throughout the image. The filtering operation on each line segment replaces the pixel values on that segment with a monotonic sequence that fits the original pixel values best in a least squares sense. Monotonic change is enforced along line segments in as many directions as desired. The method is simple, reasonably fast and quite stable. Good results can be obtained for images with SNR's as low as 0.5.

1. BACKGROUND

There are many methods of removing noise from images. The basic idea is almost always to represent the signal and noise in a basis that separates the true signal from the noise as completely as possible. In Fourier filters, the noise is assumed to be dominant in the high frequencies and the signal dominant in the low frequencies so removing high frequencies removes mostly noise. However, removing or damping the high frequencies produces band-limited blurring. Wavelet denoising [1–6] adds another twist by allowing the bandwidth passed to be different at different positions in the image. The high frequencies are allowed to

*Supported by a grant from the National Cancer Institute, CA23108 and by a grant from the Department of Defense, DAMD17-96-1-6119. The author takes pleasure in acknowledging his introduction to monotonic fits by Jian Lu and Dennis M. Healy, Jr. The help and ideas of Peter J. Kostelec is also gratefully acknowledged.

Inverse Problems, Tomography, and Image Processing, edited by Ramm,
Plenum Press, New York, 1998

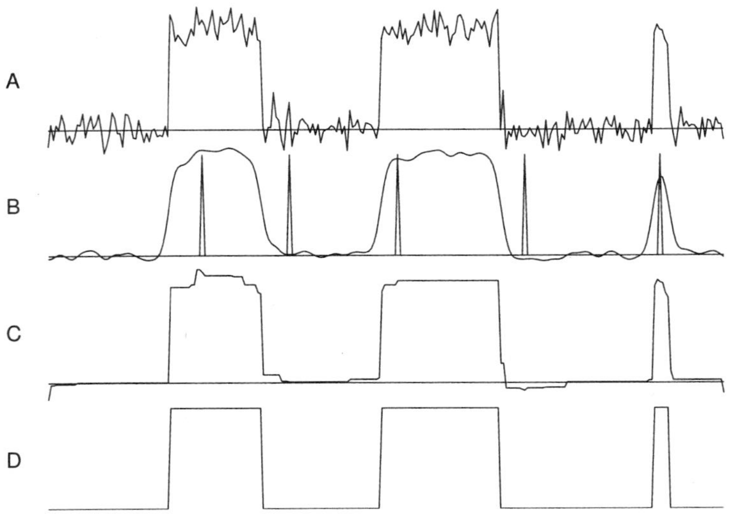

Figure 1. An example of suppressing noise on a line segment with a simulated signal and normally distributed random noise. The signal is three boxcars. The height of the boxcars is 1. The boxcars, from left to right, are 35, 45 and 6 pixels wide. The signal with added noise is shown in A. The standard deviation of the normally distributed random noise is 0.1. The Gaussian smoothed signal with the extrema selected are shown in B. Standard deviation of the Gaussian is 4 percent of the total bandwidth and the extrema were required to change by 20 percent of the maximum signal. The result of forcing monotonic change between the extrema is shown in C. The original signal before noise was added is shown in D for comparison.

pass where edges have been identified or are likely and the high frequencies are more strongly suppressed where edges are not likely. Edges produce extrema in the wavelet transform domain so a wider bandwidth is passed around large values of the wavelet transform. One of the keys in wavelet denoising is deciding when an edge is present and when the large wavelet response is from noise. An alternative method of preferentially suppressing noise is presented here. Instead of identifying extrema of the derivative as in wavelet denoising, the extrema of the signal itself (peaks) are found; the signal is then forced to change monotonically between the extrema. The method should be more robust than wavelet denoising because averages are more stable than differences. However, identifying the correct extrema is again the key to the performance of the method. The filter is made possible by an elegant algorithm due to Demetriou and Powell that finds the monotonic series that fits data points best in a least squares sense [7]. It basically averages large enough groups of adjacent points in the series to achieve a monotonic progression. Monotonically decreasing series can be found by reversing the order of the data. It is a robust and relatively fast method. Our noise reduction method for images has two parts: selecting the important extrema and forcing monotonic change between those extrema. Extrema selection is best done in two dimensions because extra stability is gained by smoothing in both dimensions rather than only one. The process of forcing monotonic change in all directions is accomplished by forcing monotonic change along many line segments. We will first look at the relevant properties of the algorithm that forces monotonic change along a single line segment. Then we will describe the two dimensional algorithm in detail, show some results, give some applications, and propose future improvements.

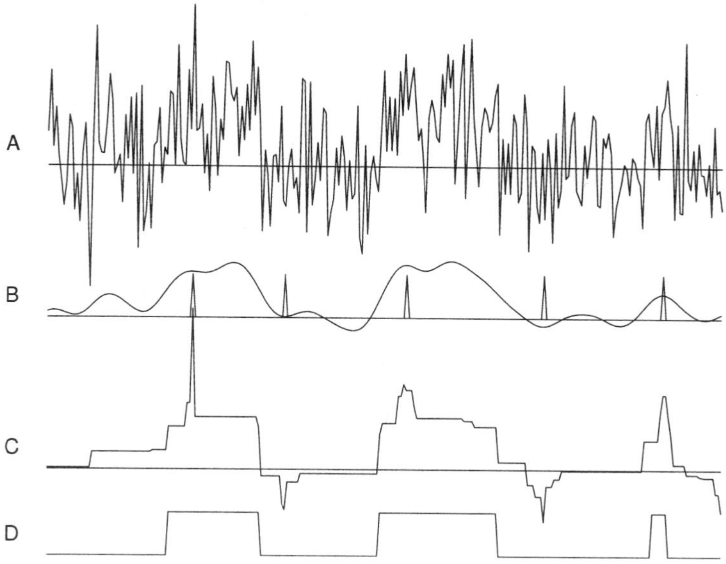

Figure 2. The result when the noise is much larger. The same signal as in Figure 1 was corrupted with noise with a standard deviation of 1 instead of 0.1. The format is the same as in Figure 1.

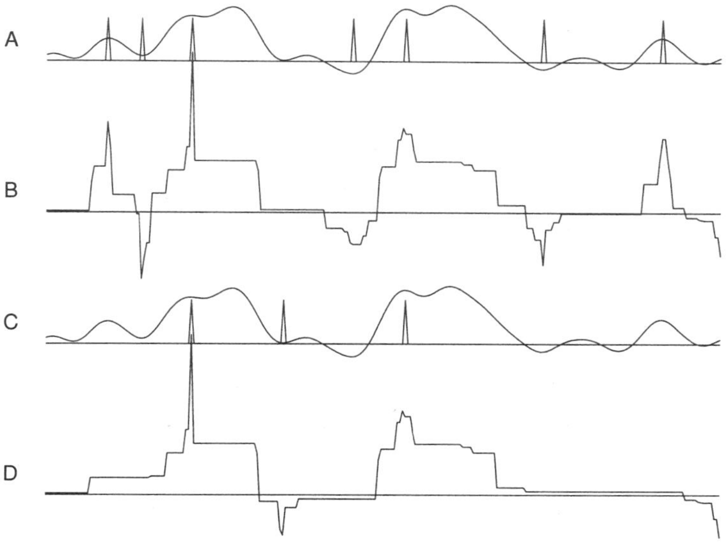

Figure 3. The result of suboptimal selection of extrema. Figure 2 was reconstructed with extrema that were larger than 15 percent of the maximum. Figures A and B show the result of selecting extrema larger than 10 percent of the maximum. Figures A and C correspond to B in Figure 2 and Figures B and D correspond to C in Figure 2. The lower threshold result in two new extrema seen to the far left of the segment. That extra extrema produces a rather large peak in the final result. Figures C and D show the result of selecting the extrema larger than 20 percent of the maximum. The extrema over the 6 pixel wide spike in the signal is lost and does not appear in the final result.

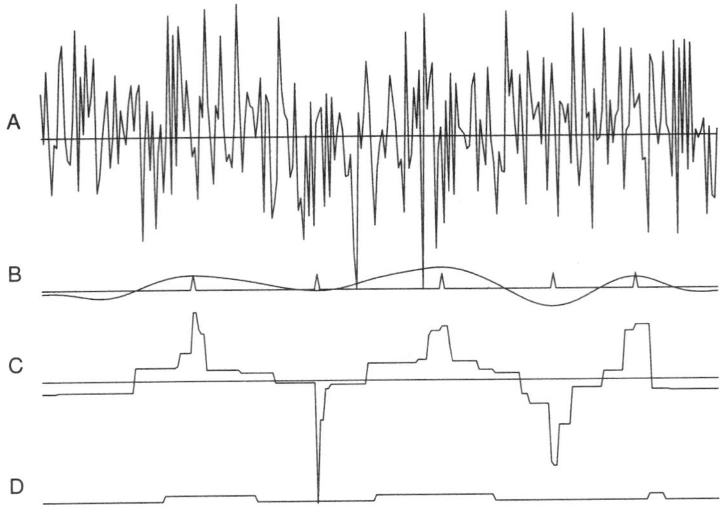

Figure 4. The result with extremely large noise. The same signal as in Figure 1 was corrupted with noise with a standard deviation of 10. The format is the same as in Figure 1. Figures A-D are scaled the same.

2. ONE DIMENSIONAL EXAMPLES

The values of a function at points between two adjacent extrema must vary monotonically essentially by definition. Therefore, a function of one variable in additive noise can be retrieved by identifying the positions of the extrema and fitting the points bounded by each pair of adjacent extrema to a monotonic function. For any segment bounded by a pair of adjacent extrema, the monotonic series that fits the points best in a least squares sense can be found using the Demetriou and Powell algorithm [7]. This algorithm has several very interesting properties. The result is not just a fit to a limited set of basis functions. Any monotonic series can be recovered. The result is not band-limited; edges are not blurred. The algorithm takes the first element of the series as the starting value and advances through the series element by element. If an element in the series is smaller than the previous element, the algorithm averages past points in the series to bring the past values down and the present element up enough to maintain monotonic increase. The algorithm is fast, works in place so memory requirements are minimal and is relatively robust. Figures 1 to 4 demonstrates the important properties. Figure 1 shows a simulated signal made up of three boxcars with moderate added noise. The local SNR over the boxcars is approximately ten. The ratio of the total signal energy to the total noise energy is six. This is generally a relatively poor SNR for medical imaging; a good, crisp MR image generally has a SNR of at least 80. The blurred signal and the extrema selected are shown as well as the final noise suppressed signal. Two features of the noise suppressed signal should be noted: the edges are not blurred at all and there are spurious peaks at the boundaries between monotonic segments. Demetriou and Powell's algorithm is very happy with sharp edges; they are not blurred at all. This is obviously very important because edges are among the most important features we use to interpret images. Blurring is also the most limiting property of many noise reduction techniques especially the Fourier based methods. Wavelet based noise suppression methods have been promising largely because they promise to leave edges unblurred. The spurious peaks at the boundaries between monotonic segments are the only deformation of the signal resulting from the noise suppression. It is caused by the lack of averaging at the ends of the segments. A large value caused by noise in the center of the segment will be balanced by random small values on both sides of it while a large value caused by noise at the end of the segment satisfies the monotonic criteria and is not changed. Another way to see the effect is to run the algorithm over a series of random values. Some part of the noise energy is monotonic and it is primarily at the ends of the segment as shown in Figure 5. That monotonic part of the random noise can not be distinguished from real monotonically increasing signal. Figure 2 shows the results at very low SNR's. The noise has a standard deviation of one and the signal peaks have a height of one. The SNR over the peaks is one and the ratio of the total signal energy to the total noise energy is 0.6. The peaks are recovered and the edges are sharp. The leakage of noise at the boundaries between the segments is much more pronounced than at higher SNR, as might be expected. Figure 3 demonstrates the importance of extrema selection. All three peaks were recovered when the thresholds were properly selected. However, if the threshold for extrema selection was too low, too many extrema were selected and extraneous peaks were introduced as in Figure 3B. If the threshold for extrema selection was too high, too few extrema were selected and features with small energy were lost as the 6 pixel wide peak was lost in Figure 3D. As the SNR was reduced to extremely low levels, approximately 0.1, the noise leakage at the boundaries between monotonic segments dominates the result as shown in Figure 4. Features that have a large enough area were still found and the sharp edges were recovered effectively. However, the noise leakage at the boundaries between monotonic segments overwhelms the recovered signal. The noise leakage at the boundaries can be reduced by averaging the monotonic fits obtained with several (5 to 11) boundary points near the maximum. If the average is weighted by the error between the data and the fit, sharp peaks can still be recovered. However, computation times increase enough to discourage use of this technique on images.

3. METHODS

The first method of processing images to try is to simply process the rows of the image, then rotate the result and process the rows again. Then iterate by rotating the result and processing the rows until nothing is changing and quit. This simple method works pretty well but it needs to be modified a bit because of two directional effects.

3.1. Directional Effects

The first is that there are many kinds of extrema in two dimensions. It is a directional property in two dimensions; i.e., a point can be an extrema in one direction but not in another. For example, a saddle point is an extrema in all directions but two. Therefore, the extrema must be determined independently for each direction processed in an image. The second directional effect is somewhat more subtle. When an image is processed in multiple directions, most of the noise is suppressed in the first direction processed. The leakage of noise at the boundary between monotonic segments is greatest perpendicular to the first direction processed and much less in other directions. The results of making the columns monotonic first and then the rows is different from those obtained by making the rows monotonic first and then the columns. If this effect were limited to the edges of the image it would be tolerable but it occurs at each and every boundary between segments throughout the image. The leakage of noise at

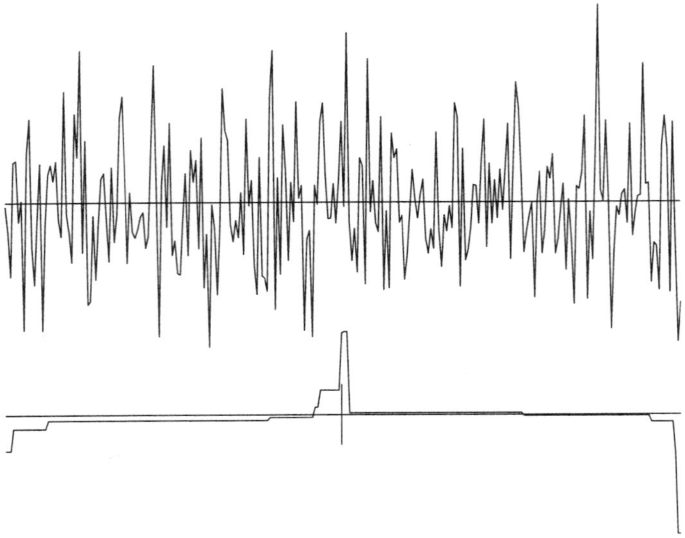

Figure 5. The result of forcing monotonic change on normally distributed random noise shows the leakage of noise at the boundaries between monotonic segments. The random series was monotonically fit to two segments: the first increasing and the second decreasing. There is always a false peak at the boundaries between monotonic segments because the monotonic fit allows negative noise to pass at the beginning of the segment and positive noise to pass at the end of an increasing segment. In the middle of the segment, values to either side are enough to average out the positive and negative noise.

boundaries leads to the widening of a peak perpendicular to the first direction made monotonic. The effect is demonstrated in Figure 6. Just noise was processed to show how it is blurred. If the rows are made monotonic first, the rows stay essentially monotonic after the columns are made monotonic. Therefore, each direction needs to be made monotonic only once.

3.2. Algorithm

Our method of processing images attempts to handle these directional effects. An intermediate image was found for each angle used. To obtain the an intermediate image, the original image was rotated to the appropriate angle. The rotated images were obtained by interpolating to a rotated grid using cubic B-splines [8, 9]. The rotated version of the image was blurred using a simple Gaussian filter in the Fourier domain. The extrema along the rows and along the columns of the blurred image were identified. The two sets of extrema were examined and those that differed from adjacent extrema by less than the threshold were eliminated. Each row of the image was made monotonic between extrema. Then the columns of the row processed image were made monotonic between extrema. The row-column processed image was averaged with the column-row processed image to obtain the intermediate image. Making the image monotonic in two directions is sufficient to suppress most of the noise and keep most of the features. Processing the image at more angles to get the intermediate image takes too much processing time. Each intermediate image had the noise leakage primarily perpendicular to the first direction made monotonic. To remove the noise leakage, intermediate images at several angles were averaged together. Actually the intermediate images were least squares fit to the original image to obtain the final processed image. A simple average can also

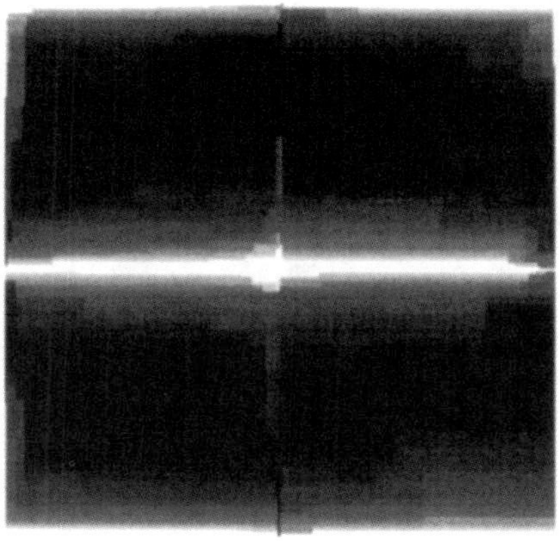

Figure 6. A field of random numbers with standard deviation 1024 was made monotonic along the columns first and then along the rows. The center row were the maxima when the columns were processed and the central column were the maxima when the rows were processed. The result shows the directional blurring of noise perpendicular to the direction first processed.

be used instead of a least squares fit. The final processed image is almost monotonic between extrema in all directions and contains no preferred directional effects.

4. RESULTS

The preliminary results are very promising. Noise can be suppressed significantly. Good quality images can be extracted from noise that would otherwise make the images of very limited usefulness. The first example is an MRI of a phantom shown in Figure 7. The imaging technique selected produced very noisy images. The 'true' image was obtained from averaging 64 of the images to suppress noise through averaging. Four angles were used in the noise suppression. The edges and most of the small features are recovered well. The first two rows of small pins in the black field on the upper left section of the phantom are retained. The edges remain sharp. However, the fan shaped resolution pattern is less well seen. Smaller parts of the fan pattern could probably be visualized if more angles were used. Most of the noise remaining in the noise suppressed image is leakage at the boundaries between segments. The second example is of a functional MRI (fMRI) image. Functional MRI is a procedure that identifies areas of the brain that are used to perform mental tasks such as the motor strip or the areas used for different kinds of memory. Surgeons need such information to avoid critical areas of the brain when operating. It is also important to understand damage and reorganization of the brain following injury such as stroke or trauma. In fMRI many sequential images of the brain are obtained during a mental task and during rest from that task. The area of the brain that is active during the task has very small signal intensity changes that correlate with the task being on and off. These signal changes are caused by increased blood flow during activation and are only around two percent of the signal. Noise or patient movement can render the study inconclusive. The image shown in Figure 8 is a single image from an fMRI study. The monotonic noise suppression produces excellent results. Eight angles were used in the noise suppression. The noise suppressed image has almost all the features present in the original but the noise is reduced significantly. The gray and white matter can also be more

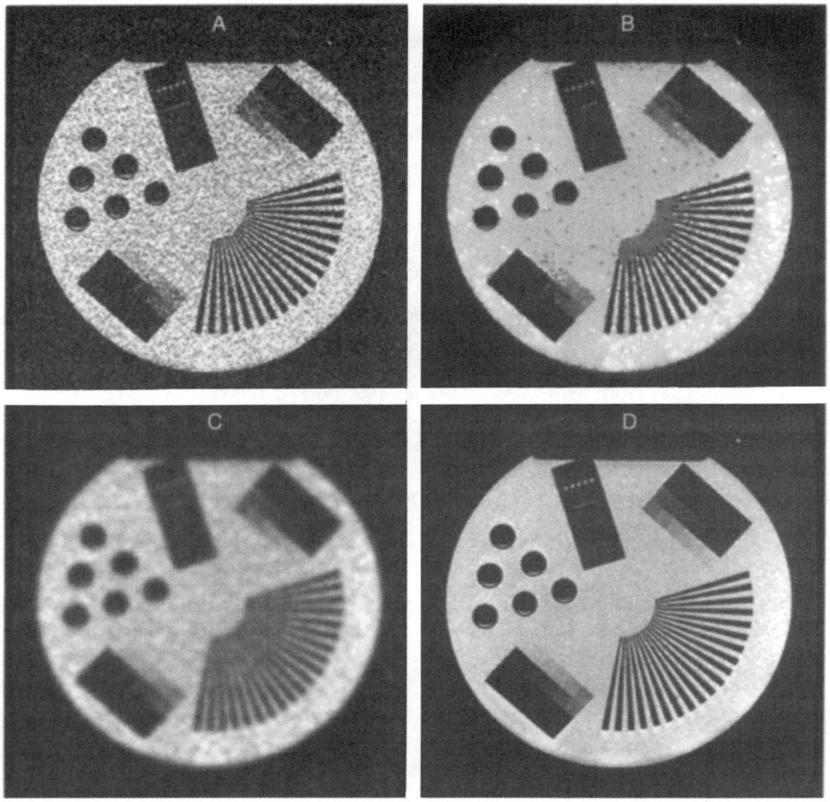

Figure 7. Figure A shows an MRI image of a phantom. The imaging technique used produced a very poor SNR image, shown in Figure A. Figure B shows the results of noise reduction using monotonic fits between extrema. Figure C shows a Fourier filtered image with the same SNR as in Figure B; the blurring limits the usefulness of the image. Figure D shows the average of 64 acquisitions averaged together to reduce noise. The SNR in Figure D is 8 times that in Figure A.

easily segmented in the noise suppressed image. The regions of similar signal intensity are grouped very well. The third example is an T1 weighted MR image of a brain study. One of the important features of T1 weighted images is to differentiate gray and white matter. The gray matter is the less bright shell of tissue forming the cortical surface. The brighter white matter is inside the gray and the dark cerebrospinal fluid that cushions the brain is between the gray matter and the skull. Eight angles were used in the noise suppression. Noise was added to the image to reduce the SNR from 80 to 16 and more noise was added to decrease the SNR farther to 4. The monotonic noise suppression increased the SNR from 16 to 85 and from 4 to 30. The gray-white matter separation is recovered well.

4.1. Applications

There are many potential applications of monotonic noise suppression but two applications are the most promising. Segmentation is the most natural. Areas that have similar signal intensities are grouped into contiguous regions very effectively. Recovery of images in very

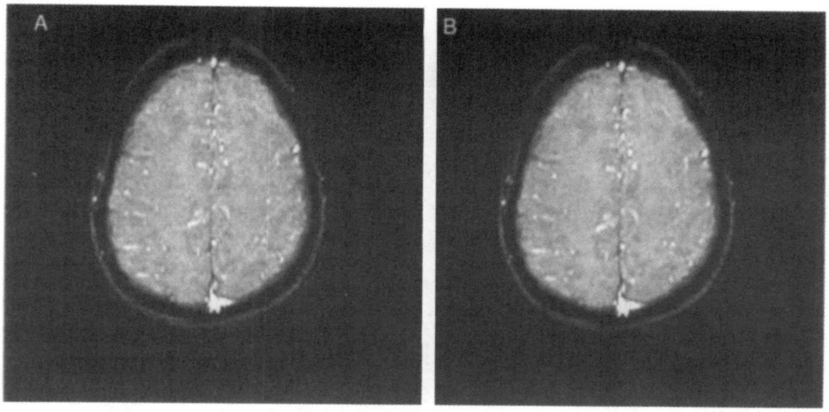

Figure 8. Figure A shows the original axial MR image and Figure B shows the results of forced monotonic noise suppression. The parameters were set to produce uniform areas that could be useful in segmentation. The SNR is improved significantly by forced monotonic noise suppression.

high noise is the other natural application because this technique works well at high SNR's and at very low SNR's. Most noise reduction methods do not perform well at low SNR's. For example, in mammography we are using monotonic noise suppression as a preprocessing step for a watershed algorithm that is used to segment the digitized mammograms. Monotonic noise suppression can be adjusted to remove the small features that tend to make the watershed algorithm oversegment.

4.2. Future Improvements

This technique is still being actively developed and there are many improvements to be made. Many of the improvements necessary require better theoretical understanding. For example, how many angles need to be used to suppress noise adequately? The answer will depend on the area of the regions between extrema; more angles will be needed for larger areas. How fast can extrema change with angle? Most extrema are found if only four angles are used. Can the leakage at the boundaries be suppressed without eliminating smaller features? The most important improvement to make is to make the selection of extrema more robust and automatic. The same tricks that are used to find maximum gradient points in wavelet denoising can be applied here as well. For example, tracking extrema across multiple scales and using continuity would probably help. Also estimating the cutoffs that determine the extrema automatically from the estimated SNR would help. Now the selected extrema are shown on the screen to select the correct cutoff parameters.

5. CONCLUSIONS

Forcing monotonic change between extrema is a very promising noise suppression technique. Edges are not blurred and it works well over a wide range of SNR's. As the SNR drops, features that have less energy than the noise spikes are lost. The key to recovering the image accurately is to identify the correct extrema.

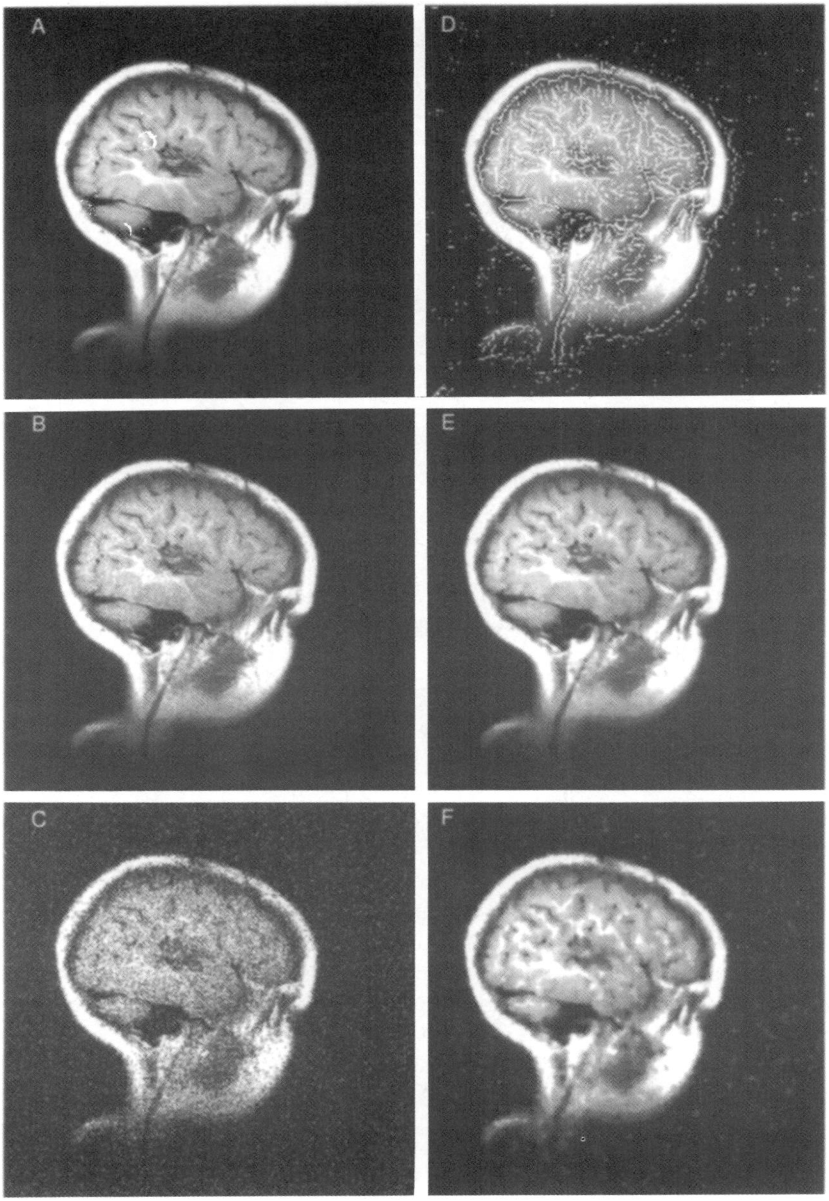

Figure 9. Figure A shows the original T1 weighted sagital MR image that has a relatively high SNR, SNR = 80 within the brain. Figures B and C show the original image with added normally distributed random noise, SNR = 16 and SNR = 4 within the brain for Figures B and C respectively. Figure D shows the Gaussian filtered image with the selected extrema superimposed. Figure E shows the result of forced monotonic noise suppression on Figure B. The SNR increased from 16 to 85. Figure F shows the result of monotonic noise suppression on Figure C. The SNR is increased to from 4 to 30.

REFERENCES

1. S.G. Mallat, A theory of multiresolution signal decomposition: the wavelet representation, *IEEE Trans. Patt. Anal. Machine Intell., Vol. PAMI-11, No. 7, pp. 674–693, 1989.*
2. J.B. Weaver, Yansun Xu, D.M. Healy, Jr., L.D. Cromwell, Filtering Noise From Images With Wavelet Transforms., *Magnetic Resonance in Medicine, 21:288-295, 1991.*
3. S. Mallat, Characterization of Signals from Multiscale Edges, *IEEE Trans on PAMI, Vol. 14, 1992, pp. 710–732.*
4. Jian Lu, J.B. Weaver, D.M. Healy, Jr., Yansun Xu, Noise Reduction with Multiscale Edge Representation and Perceptual Criteria., *Proceeding of the IEEE-SP International Symposium on Time-Frequency and Time-Scale Analysis, Victoria, B.C., October 1992..*
5. Yansun Xu, J.B. Weaver, D.M. Healy, Jr., Jian Lu, Wavelet Transform Domain Filters: A Spatially Selective Noise Filtration Technique., *IEEE Trans. on Image Processing, 3(6) 747-758 Nov 1994.*
6. D.L. Donoho, De-noising by soft-thresholding., *IEEE Trans on Info Theory, Vol. 41, 1995, pp. 613–627.*
7. I.C. Demetriou and M.J.D. Powell, Least Squares Smoothing of Univariate Data to Achieve Piecewise Monotonicity, *IMA Journal of Numerical Analysis, Vol. 11, No. 2, 1991, pp. 411–432.*
8. M. Unser, A. Aldroubi, M. Eden, Fast B-Spline Transforms for Continuous Image Representation and Interpolation, *IEEE Trans. Patt. Anal. Machine Intell., Vol. 13, No. 3, pp. 277–285, Mar. 1991.*
9. M. Unser, A. Aldroubi, M. Eden, The L_2 Polynomial Spline Pyramid, *IEEE Trans. Patt. Anal. Machine Intell., Vol. 15, No. 4, pp. 364–379, April 1993.*

13

APPLIED NONLINEAR ILL-POSED PROBLEMS AND THE VARIATIONAL APPROACH FOR CONSTRUCTING OF REGULARIZING ALGORITHMS

I. V. Kochikov[1], G. M. Kuramshina,[2] and A. G. Yagola[1]

[1]Department of Mathematics
Faculty of Physics
Moscow State University
Moscow 119899, Russia
[2]Department of Physical Chemistry
Faculty of Chemistry
Moscow State University
Moscow 119899, Russia

1. INTRODUCTION

At present, the theory of ill-posed problems is widely used to solve inverse problems in optics, spectroscopy, astrophysics, geophysics, plasma diagnostics, electronic microscopy, and other applied sciences. In the paper we discuss some questions connected with constructing and application of regularizing algorithms to nonlinear ill-posed problems in physics. As examples of successful implementation we consider certain inverse problems in vibrational spectroscopy.

Many problems of science, technology and engineering are posed in the form of operator equation of the first kind with operator and right part approximately known. Often such problems turn out to be ill-posed. It means that they may have no solutions, or may have non-unique solution, or/and these solutions may be unstable. Usually, non-existence and non-uniqueness can be overcome by searching some "generalized" solutions, the last is left to be unstable. So for solving such problems is necessary to use the special methods — regularizing algorithms. The theory of solving linear ill-posed problems is advanced greatly today [1]. It is not so in the case of nonlinear ill-posed problems, since the direct transfer of linear theory to the nonlinear case is not possible in general. A general scheme for constructing regularizing algorithms on the base of Tikhonov variational approach has been considered [2, 3], and iterative methods for linear and nonlinear ill-posed problems were advanced [4]. Here we

Inverse Problems, Tomography, and Image Processing, edited by Ramm,
Plenum Press, New York, 1998

have no enough place to describe these results in details, we shall discuss only some general questions and results of implementation of regularized algorithms in applied sciences.

It is very well known that ill-posed problems have unpleasant properties even in the cases when there exist stable methods (regularizing algorithms) of their solution. So at first it is recommended to study all *a priori* information, to find all physical constraints, which may make it possible to construct a well-posed mathematical model of the physical phenomena. For some inverse problems of astrophysics we proposed to use natural physical assumptions on monotonicity of unknown brightness and absorption distribution on discs for constructing stable numerical methods and obtaining physical results [5]. Of course, it is necessary to understand that all these results are in frame of chosen mathematical model only. Computational programs for linear ill-posed problems with *a priori* information (monotonicity, convexity, known number of extremes, etc.) are available [1], and could be generalized for nonlinear problems also. If the constraints are not sufficient to make a problem well-posed, then it is necessary to use all these constraints but we must also know errorlevel of experimental data. Bakushinsky firstly showed impossibility of constructing of regularized algorithms for ill-posed problems without knowledge of errorlevel in the right-hand side of an ill-posed operator equation [6]. For systems of linear algebraic equations this fact has been emphasized by Tikhonov in his last publications [7]. Simple generalization of these results has been proposed [8]. As an example of successful application of variational regularizing algorithms with *a posteriori* choice of regularization parameter to practical problems we consider below an inverse problem of vibrational spectroscopy [9].

Vibrational spectra are among the most important sources of our knowledge about molecular structure. From the viewpoint of analyzing experimental data (obtained by means of infrared and Raman spectroscopy) a number of inverse problems arise. One of the most important is so-called inverse vibrational problem of determining parameters of the molecular force field from given experimental data (vibrational frequencies, isotope frequency shifts, Coriolis constants, centrifugal distortion constants, etc.). The accumulation of data on molecular constants helps us to predict spectra and other properties of compounds not yet investigated and assists in development of physical models in a theory of molecular structure. In this paper we describe stable methods (regularizing algorithms) for the solution of inverse problems in vibrational spectroscopy, which we can consider as nonlinear ill-posed problems in finite-dimensional spaces.

2. TIKHONOV'S VARIATIONAL APPROACH FOR CONSTRUCTING REGULARIZING ALGORITHMS

We consider nonlinear ill-posed problems in finite-dimensional (for simplicity) case and describe Tikhonov's approach for constructing regularizing algorithms (stable methods), proposed at first by A. N. Tikhonov and developed later in publications by A. V. Goncharsky, A. S. Leonov and A. G. Yagola. Full list of references and detailed description of the theory and numerical methods can be found elsewhere [2, 3, 10]. In this section the main problem for us is an operator equation

$$Az = u, \quad z \in D \subseteq Z, \quad u \in U \tag{2.1}$$

where D is a nonempty set of constraints, Z and U are finite-dimensional normed spaces, A is a class of operators from D into U. Let us give a general formulation of Tikhonov's scheme of constructing a regularizing algorithm for solving the main problem: for the operator Eq. (2.1) on D find an element z^* for which

$$\rho(Az^*,u) = \inf\{\rho(Az,u) : z \in D\} \equiv \mu \tag{2.2}$$

(ρ is the distance in the normed space U). We call this problem as the quasisolution problem for Eq. (2.1). In the case $D = Z$ problem (2.2) gives pseudosolution of (2.1). If the measure of incompatibility is equal to zero, then the solutions of (2.2) are the solutions of Eq. (2.1) on D. The quasisolution problem (2.2) may be ill-posed. Namely, problem (2.2) is not solvable for some equations of the form (2.1). The solution of (2.2) may be not unique and unstable in the metrics of Z with respect to perturbations of the data (A,u).

We assume that to some element $u = \bar{u}$ there corresponds the nonempty set $Z^* \in D$ of quasisolutions and that Z may consist of more than one element. Furthermore, we suppose that a functional $\Omega(z)$ is defined on D and bounded below:

$$\Omega(z) \geq \Omega^* \equiv \inf\{\Omega(z) : z \in D\} \geq 0.$$

The Ω-optimal quasisolution problem for Eq. (2.1) is formulated as follows:
find a $\bar{z} \in Z^*$ such that

$$\Omega(\bar{z}) = \inf\{\Omega(z) : z \in Z^*\} \equiv \bar{\Omega} \tag{2.3}$$

We denote the set of Ω-optimal quasisolutions of Eq. (2.1) by $\bar{Z}$. If $D = Z$, then $\bar{Z}$ is the set of the Ω-optimal pseudosolutions of Eq. (2.1). For simplicity we use only the name "pseudosolution" below.

We suppose that, instead of the unknown exact data (A,u), we are given approximate data which satisfy the following conditions:

$$u_\delta \in U, \quad \rho(\bar{u},u_\delta) \leq \delta; \quad A_h \in A, \rho(Az,A_hz) \leq \psi(h,\Omega(z)) \forall z \in D.$$

Here the function ψ represents the known measure of approximation of the precise operator A by the approximate operator A_h. We are given also numerical characterizations $h,\delta \geq 0$ of the "closeness" of (A_h,u_δ) to $(A,\bar{u})$. The main problem is to construct from the approximate data $(A_h,u_\delta,\psi,h,\delta)$ in Eq. (2.1) an element $z_\eta = z_\eta(A_h,u_\delta,\psi,h,\delta) \in D$ which converges to the set $\bar{Z}$ of Ω-optimal solutions as $\eta = (h,\delta) \to 0$.

Let us formulate our basic assumptions [3]:

1. The class A consists of the operators A continuous from D to U.

2. The functional $\Omega(z)$ is lower semicontinuous (for example continuous) on D:

$$\forall z_0 \in D, \quad \forall \{z_n\} \in D : z_n \to z_0 \Rightarrow \lim_{h\to\infty} \inf \Omega(z_n) \geq \Omega(z_0).$$

3. If K is an arbitrary number such that $K \geq \Omega^*$, then the set $\Omega_k = \{z \in D : \Omega(z) \leq K\}$ is compact in Z.

4. The measure of approximation $\psi(h,\Omega)$ is assumed to be defined for $h \geq 0$, $\Omega \geq \Omega^*$, to depend continuously on all its arguments, to be monotonically increasing with respect to Ω for any $h > 0$, and to satisfy the equality $\psi(0,\Omega) = 0$, $\forall \Omega \geq \Omega^*$. Conditions 1)–3)

guarantee that $\bar{Z} \neq \emptyset$. Tikhonov's scheme for constructing of a regularizing algorithm is based on using the smoothing functional [2, 3]

$$M^\alpha[z] = f[\rho(A_h z, u_\delta)] + \alpha\Omega(z), \quad z \in D, \quad \alpha > 0 \tag{2.4}$$

in the conditional extreme problem: for fixed $\alpha > 0$, find an element $z^\alpha \in D$ such that

$$M^\alpha[z^\alpha] = \inf\{M^\alpha[z] : z \in D\}. \tag{2.5}$$

Here $f[x]$ is an auxiliary function. A common choice is $f[x] = x^m$, $m \geq 2$. We denote the set of extremals of (2.5) which correspond to a given $\alpha > 0$ by Z^α. Conditions 1)–3) imply that $Z^\alpha \neq \emptyset$. The scheme of construction of an approximation to the set $\bar{Z}$ includes:

(i) the choice of the regularization parameter $\alpha_\eta(A_h, u_\delta, h, \delta)$;

(ii)the fixation of the Z^{α_η} corresponding to α_η, and a special selection of an element Z^{α_η} in this set.

We take the element z^{α_η} chosen in this way as a solution of the main problem. Procedures (i), (ii) must be accomplished so as to guarantee the convergence $z^{\alpha_\eta} \to \bar{Z}$ as $\eta \to 0$. Thus, the Tikhonov's regularizing algorithm differ from each other by the method of choosing α_η and by the method of selecting z^{α_η}.

It is in this way that the generalized analogs of a posteriori parameter choice strategies are used. They were introduced by A. S. Leonov, their descriptions it is possible to find also in [2]. We define for their formulations some auxiliary functions and functionals:

$$\begin{aligned} &\gamma(\alpha) = \Omega(z^\alpha), \quad \beta(\alpha) = f[\rho(A_h z^\alpha, \quad u_\delta)] \equiv \mathrm{I}(z^\alpha), \\ &\pi(\alpha) = f[\psi(h, \gamma(\alpha)) + \delta + \mu_\eta] \equiv \Pi(z^\alpha), \\ &\rho(\alpha) = \beta(\alpha) - \pi(\alpha) \equiv \mathrm{P}(z^\alpha), \quad \forall z^\alpha \in \mathrm{Z}^\alpha; \alpha > 0. \end{aligned} \tag{2.6}$$

Here $\mu_\eta = \inf\{\rho(A_h z, u_\delta) + \psi(h, \Omega(z)) + \delta : z \in D\}$ is a generalized measure of incompatibility for nonlinear problems having the properties: $\mu_\eta > \mu$, $\mu_\eta \to \mu$ as $\eta \to 0$ [2]. All the functions (2.6) are generally many-valued. They have the following properties.

Lemma 2.1 (see [3]). *The functions γ, β, π, ρ are single-valued and continuous everywhere for $\alpha > 0$ except perhaps not more a countable set of their common points of discontinuity of the first kind, which are points of multiple-valuedness, then there exists at least two elements z_+^α) and z_-^α in the set Z^α such that $\gamma(\alpha \pm 0) = \Omega(z_\pm^\alpha)$, $\rho(\alpha \pm 0) = P(z_\pm^\alpha)$. The functions β, ρ are monotonically nondecreasing and γ, π are nonincreasing.*

The generalized discrepancy principle (GDP) for nonlinear problems consists of the following steps.

(i) The choice of the regularization parameter as a generalized solution $\alpha > 0$ of the equation

$$\rho(\alpha) = 0. \tag{2.7}$$

Here and in the sequel we say that α is the generalized solution of Eq. (2.7) for a monotone function ρ if α is an ordinary solution or if is a "jump"-point of this function over 0.

(ii) The method of selecting an approximate solution z^{α_η} from the set Z^{α_η} by means of the following selection rule. Let $q > 1$ and $C > 1$ be fixed constants, $\alpha_1 = \alpha_\eta / q$ and $\alpha_2 = \alpha_\eta \cdot q$

are auxiliary regularization parameters, and let z^{α_1} and z^{α_2} be extremals of (3.2) for $\alpha = \alpha_{1,2}$. If the inequality

$$I(z^{\alpha_2}) \geq C\Pi(z^{\alpha_1}) - (C-1)f(\mu_\eta) \tag{2.8}$$

holds for z^{α_1} and z^{α_2}, then any elements $z^{\alpha_\eta} \in Z^{\alpha_\eta}$ subject to the condition $P(z^{\alpha_\eta}) \leq 0$ can be taken as the approximate solution. For instance we can take $z^{\alpha_\eta} = z_-^{\alpha_\eta}$. But if

$$I(z^{\alpha_2}) < C\Pi(z^{\alpha_1}) - (C-1)f(\mu_\eta) \tag{2.9}$$

then we choose z^{α_η} so as to have $P(z^{\alpha_\eta}) \geq 0$, for example, $z^{\alpha_\eta} = z_+^{\alpha_\eta}$.

Note that we do not need any selection rule if α_η is an ordinary solution of Eq. (2.7). In this case the equality $P(z^{\alpha_\eta}) = \rho(\alpha_\eta) = 0$ holds, and an arbitrary element $z^{\alpha_\eta} \in Z^{\alpha_\eta}$can be taken as an approximate solution.

Theorem 2.2 (see [3,11]). *Suppose that for any quasisolution $z^* \in D$ of Eq. (2.1) the inequality $\Omega(z^*) > \Omega^* = \inf\{\Omega(z) : z \in D\}$ holds. Then (a) Eq. (2.7) has positive generalized solution; (b) for any sequence $\eta_n = (h_n, \delta_n)$ such that $\eta_n \to 0$ as $n \to \infty$, the corresponding sequence $\{z_n\}$ of approximate solutions, which is found by GDP has the following properties:*

$$z_n \to \bar{z}, \quad \Omega(z_n) \to \Omega, \quad as \quad n \to \infty.$$

In many practical cases it is very convenient to take $\Omega(z) = \|z\|^r$ (r is a constant, $r > 1$). If it is known in addition that when Eq. (2.7) has a solution on D, then the value μ_η can be omitted. GDP in linear and nonlinear cases has some optimal properties [2].

3. INVERSE VIBRATIONAL PROBLEM

Among the variety of ill-posed problems in natural sciences bounded to an analyzing experimental data there are very important inverse problems connected with processing experimental data in vibrational spectroscopy. Two of the most important ones are so-called inverse vibrational problem (finding parameters of the molecular force field from given spectral data) and inverse electrooptical problem (defining of electrooptical parameters determined the intensity distribution in IR and Raman spectra). These problems are examples of nonlinear ill-posed problems. The main purpose of solving the inverse problems in vibrational spectroscopy is to determine parameters of the molecular force field using experimental data. The idea of the force field arises from the attempt to consider a molecule as a mechanical system of nuclei while all the interactions due to the electrons are included in an effective potential function $U(q_1, ..., q_n)$, where $q_1, ..., q_n$ denote the $n = 3N - 6$ generalized coordinates of the N atomic nuclei of the molecule. The force field of a molecule determines many of it's important physical properties. The force field minimum (with respect to nucleus coordinates) assigns the equilibrium geometry of the molecule and the second derivatives of the potential with respect to nucleus coordinates in the point of equilibrium

$$f_{ij} = \frac{\partial^2 U}{\partial q_i \partial q_j} \Big|_{eq} \; (i,j = 1, ..., n)$$

constitute a positive definite matrix F determining all the molecular characteristic connected with small vibrations. Describe briefly what kind of experimental information can be used for finding parameters of molecular force field. The vibrational frequencies (obtained from IR and Raman spectra) are the main type of experimental information on molecular vibrations. They are connected with the matrix of the force constants F by the eigenvalue equation (main equation of a normal coordinate analysis)

$$GFL = L\Lambda \tag{3.1}$$

where Λ is a diagonal matrix consisting of the squares of the molecular normal vibration frequencies $\omega_1, ..., \omega_n$, $\Lambda = diag\{\omega_1^2, ..., \omega_n^2\}$, and G is the kinetic energy matrix in the momentum representation. L is a matrix of normalized relative amplitudes (so-called forms of vibrations).

While Eq. (3.1) is the main source of data determining the force constants, it is evident that (except for diatomic molecules) the $n(n+1)/2$ parameters of F cannot be found from n experimental frequencies $\omega_1, ..., \omega_n$. If we have only the experimental frequencies of one isotopomer of the molecule, inverse vibrational problem of finding force constant matrix F reduces to the inverse eigenvalue problem (Eq. (3.1)); hence, when G is not singular it follows that as a solution of Eq. (3.1) we have any matrix F such that

$$F = G^{-1/2}C^*\Lambda CG^{-1/2} \tag{3.2}$$

where C is an arbitrary orthogonal matrix (the asterisk symbol denotes the transposed matrix). This formula describes all the variety of possible solutions of inverse vibrational problem. To choose the definite solution it is necessary to use additional information or to take into account some model assumption narrowing a class of possible solutions.

The additional information can be extracted from vibrational spectra of isotopic species (isotopomeres) of the molecule because within the approximation considered, the force field of the molecule is independent on the nuclear masses, and hence for the spectra of m isotopic molecular species we have, instead of Eq. (3.1), the system

$$(G_iF)L_i = L_i\Lambda_i, \; i = 1, ..., m. \tag{3.3}$$

Usually, the introduction of isotopomeres frequencies leads to a limited number of independent equations in (3.3), thus leaving the inverse problem undetermined. Important additional information of the molecular force field is provided by the Coriolis constants, which characterize the vibrational-rotational interaction in a molecule, mean square amplitudes, of vibrations (obtained from gas-phase electron diffraction), constants of the centrifugal distortion, connected with splitting of the degenerate vibrational levels etc. [9]. The dependencies of these experimentally measured values on the elements of the matrix F can be written in terms of the eigenvalues Λ and eigenvectors L of Eq. (3.1).

We consider the set of Eqs. (3.1) and (3.3) and additional similar equations (or only some of them, depending on the experimental information available) to be summarized in a single operator equation

$$AF = \Lambda. \tag{3.4}$$

where nonlinear operator A corresponds the real symmetrical matrix F with the set Λ of vibrational frequencies of the molecule (and its isotopomeres, if available), the Coriolis constants, the mean square amplitudes, etc.. This set of data may be presented as a vector in finite-dimensional space R^m, where m is a number of known experimental data. Also consider matrix F as a vector of finite-dimensional space Z, consisting either of the elements of the matrix F or of the quantities by means of which this matrix can be parametrized.

In our opinion the main problem is to find the normal pseudosolution of Eq. (3.1) [9,12]: It is required to obtain

$$\bar{F}_n = \arg\min \|F - F^0\|, \quad F \in \{F : F \in D, \quad \|AF - \Lambda\| = \mu\}$$

where $\mu = \inf \|AF - \Lambda\|$, $F \in D$.

The element $F^0 \in D$ should be specified from *a priori* consideration on the solution, using both approximate quantum mechanical calculations [13] and other ideas (for example, the transferability of the force constants to similar fragments of molecules). The choice of the set of constraints D has been discussed and demonstrated on a series of molecules [14]. Here F is a force constant matrix, Λ represents the set of known experimental data (frequencies of isotopomeres available, Coriolis constants etc.), and A is an operator which puts the real symmetric matrix F into correspondence with the frequencies matrix Λ of Eq. (3.1) (or Eq. (3.3)), the Coriolis constants and so forth. The equilibrium configuration of the molecule is considered to be given. We shall determine the matrices F and the set of data Λ (a finite set of real numbers) as elements from the finite-dimensional real vector spaces with weighted norms.

The operator A, as it is clearly seen from Eqs. (3.1)–(3.3) is nonlinear and includes some not-very-evident dependencies (for example, mean square amplitudes are related to the matrix of forms L and so are dependent on matrix F. Nevertheless it can be shown that operator A is continuous and even differentiable. Analysis of the operator equation (3.4) shows that (depending on the experimental data available) it can have finite or infinite number of solutions or even no solutions at all. The latter case results from the crudeness of the mathematical model which does not take into account some essential points, such as vibrational anharmonicity, when known experimental frequencies of molecular isotopomeres don't satisfy to Eq. (3.3). Inconsistency of Eq. (3.4) can also be caused by inevitable errors in the experimental data; for example, errors may appear in operator A because the parameters of the equilibrium configuration are usually determined from experiment. The errors in right-hand side Λ and in operator A, however small, may under certain conditions cause finite and large variations of the solution F. All the above-mentioned properties of Eq. (3.4) make it clear that the mathematically formalized problem of force field calculation is an extreme example of ill-posed problems, all three conditions of correctness being generally unsatisfied.

We have proposed [9] to formalize physical model notions and use them in the force field calculation. All the necessary model assumptions may be taken into account by the choice of *a priori* given matrix of force constants F^0 and the definition of set of some constraints satisfied chosen physical model. Then we can formulate the problem of constructing the matrix F of the force constants which would be the nearest in some given metric to the matrix F^0 on the given set of constraints. Such solution can be found based on Tikhonov's regularization theory. Let us briefly summarize the mathematical formulation of the problem: let Eq. (3.4) with the exact data (A and Λ) has the unique normal solution $\bar{F}$ (with regard to a certain *a priori* specified matrix F^0). Suppose that instead of A and Λ we are given some approximate A_h and Λ_δ such that

$$\|A_h F - AF\| \leq \varphi(h,F), \quad \|\Lambda_\delta - \Lambda\| \leq \delta,$$

where h, δ are known errors (in particular, the error ($\delta > 0$) of the right-hand-side of Eq. (2.4) is determined by the experimental errors of measurement), and $\varphi(h,\delta)$ is a continuous function satisfying the condition

$$\sup_{\|F\|<C} \varphi(h,F) \to 0 \quad \text{when} \quad h \to 0$$

for any finite $C > 0$.

We now wish to construct stable approximation $F_{h\delta}$ to the normal solution $\bar{F}_n$ such that $F_{h\delta} \to \bar{F}_n$ when $(h, \delta) \to 0$. The algorithms satisfying these conditions are determined as Tikhonov's regularizing algorithms or regularizing operators.

It should be noted that if problem (3.4) with the exactly given data has a unique solution, it essentially coincides with normal $\bar{F}_n$. If Eq. (3.4) has no solutions, it has to be formulated as the problem of finding a pseudo-solution (or quasi-solution) (that is, the matrix which minimizes $\|AF - \Lambda\|$). The regularizing algorithm in this case must provide approximations converging to the normal pseudo-solution of Eq. (3.4). The last possible case to be discussed is a relatively improbable one when the problem (3.4) has more than one normal solution (or pseudo-solution). In this case the approximations $F_{h,\delta}$ may converge to the set of such solutions (in the sense of β-convergence) [9]. There were proposed [2, 9] some regularizing algorithms which are efficiently computable. The following algorithm is based on the minimization of the Tikhonov's functional

$$M^{\alpha}[F] = \|A_h F - \Lambda_\delta\|^2 + \alpha\|F - F^0\|^2 \tag{3.5}$$

where the regularization parameter $\alpha > 0$ is determined from a variant of the GDP [2,3]. This method is valid also for the special estimate of errors of operator A_h given by

$$\varphi(h, F) = h\|A_h F\|.$$

An estimate of this kind ($h < 1$) may be derived from the most commonly used Eqs. (3.1) and (3.3). In this case a parameter α can be found from the equation

$$\rho(\alpha) \equiv \|A_h F^{\alpha} - \Lambda_\delta\| - \frac{1}{1-h}[\hat{\mu} + k(\delta + h\|\Lambda_\delta\|)] = 0 \tag{3.6}$$

where $\rho(\alpha)$ depends on the extremals of the functional (3.5) and is called the generalized discrepancy [9], F^{α} is any extremal of (3.5), $k > 1$ is a constant, and $\hat{\mu}$ is a measure of incompatibility defined by

$$\hat{\mu} = \inf_F \{\|A_h F - \Lambda_\delta\| + \delta + h\|A_h F\|\}$$

to take into account the possible incompatibility of Eq. (3.4) with exact data (otherwise it should be omitted). Since $\rho(\alpha)$ may not be continuous, the generalized solution of (3.6) should be used. The extremal of (3.5) with parameter α defined by Eq. (3.6) serves as the approximate $F_{h\delta}$.

The algorithms discussed above are the basis of a software package of programs for processing spectroscopic data [9], the latest version being especially adapted to IBM PC/AT [9]. We briefly describe some capabilities of this software package. The package has several distinct modules for:

1. solving a direct vibrational problem (calculation of frequencies and forms of vibrations according to Eqs. (3.1) and (3.3));
2. solving the inverse vibrational problem from known fundamental frequencies of a molecule (and its isotopic species) without restrictions on the elements of the force constant matrix;
3. solving the inverse vibrational problem with limitations on the values of force constants of the type $f_{ij} = const$ (for instance, $f_{ij} = 0$);

4. calculating the molecular force field on the basis of an expanded set of experimental data (including Coriolis constants, centrifugal distortion constants, mean square amplitudes);

5. jointly calculating the force fields of two (or more) related molecules [9].

The calculations of force fields for a number of compounds using the given software package have demonstrated [9] its convenience and efficiency.

During the last 30 years numerous attempts were undertaken to compute the molecular force fields directly from the Schrödinger's equation. The use of very restrictive assumptions was (and still is) necessary to make such computations technically possible. These restrictions influence very strongly the accuracy of results because an increasing number of atoms in a molecule (and correspondingly of the number of vibrational degrees of freedom for nuclear motion) complicates significantly the solution of the problem and decreases the accuracy of calculations. In relatively few cases it is feasible to carry out *ab initio* calculations which can predict frequencies within the limits of experimental error (say, about 1 percent error). Nevertheless, we expect further rapid progress of *ab initio* calculations, and we have considered some new ways of utilizing even the not-so-accurate results of *ab initio* calculations that are today routinely available.

As mentioned above the choice of the initial approximation matrix F^0 which determines the stabilizer of Tikhonov's functional (3.5) is especially important in the proposed formulation of the inverse vibrational problem because we can find a solution which is the nearest (in the chosen metric) to this given matrix F^0. Thus the matrix F^0 defines the physical meaning of solution obtained. Obviously, the most attractive variant for choosing of F^0 is that based on *ab initio* calculations, because the quantum mechanical force matrix calculated at modern level of theory (even at moderate basis sizes) can give relatively correct distributions of frequencies (on the scale of a few tens of cm^{-1}) while also reflecting features of the potential surface that are physically more significant in the framework of the model. Insofar as a regularizing algorithm for force field calculations can be related to model assumptions in a theory of molecular structure (such as transferability of force constants in series of related molecules, monotonous changing of properties in related compounds, etc.) and provides a stable solution for the chosen model within the specified limits of error, the joint treatment of *ab initio* and experimental data by means of regularization techniques [13] is an example of the consolidation of modern chemical theory with a modern level of applied mathematics, and constructing regularized force fields of polyatomic molecules. We have illustrated the effectiveness of this approach in numerous applications to different molecules.

It easy to check that all assumptions from the previous section are valid, so we can prove the Theorem of convergence of regularized solutions of the inverse vibrational problem to the exact normal pseudosolution. Numerical realization, description of computer software package, and results of numerous applications have already been published [9]. At the conclusion we would like to emphasize that it is impossible to construct stable numerical methods for solution of ill-posed problems without knowledge of experimental error levels [8].

ACKNOWLEDGMENT

The RFBR grants No 95-01-00486 and 95-03-08268 are gratefully acknowledged for financial support.

REFERENCES

1. A. N. Tikhonov, A. V. Goncharsky, V. V. Stepanov, and A. G. Yagola, *Numerical Methods for the Solution of Ill-PosedProblems,* Nauka, Moscow 1990 (in Russian); Kluwer Academic Publ., Dordrecht, 1995 (in English).
2. A. N. Tikhonov, A. S. Leonov, and A. G. Yagola, *Nonlinear Ill-Posed Problems*, Nauka, Moscow 1995 (in Russian); Chapman and Hall (in English), to appear.
3. A. S. Leonov and A. G. Yagola, *Tikhonov's approach for constructing regularizing algorithms,* in "*Ill-Posed Problems in Natural Sciences,*" VSP, Utrecht/ TVP, Moscow, 1992, 71–83.
4. A. Bakushinsky and A. Goncharsky, *Ill-Posed Problems: Theory and Applications,* Kluwer Academic Publ., Dordrecht, 1994.
5. A. V. Goncharsky, A. M. Cherepashchuk, and A. G. Yagola, *Ill-Posed Problems in Astrophysics,* Nauka, Moscow, 1985 (in Russian).
6. A. B. Bakushinsky, *Notes on the regularization parameter choice due to quasioptimal and ratio criteria,* Russian J. Numer. Math. and Math. Phys. 24 (1984), 1253–1259.
7. A. N. Tikhonov, *On the problems with approximately specified information,* in "*Ill-Posed Problems in Natural Sciences*", Mir, Moscow, 1987, 13–20.
8. A. S. Leonov and A. G. Yagola, *Can ill-posed problems be solved if the data error is unknown ?* Moscow University Physics Bulletin, 50 (1995), 25–28.
9. I. V. Kochikov, G. M. Kuramshina, Yu. A. Pentin, and A. G. Yagola, *Inverse Problems in Vibrational Spectroscopy,* Moscow University Publ., Moscow, 1993 (in Russian); VSP (in English), to appear.
10. A. N. Tikhonov, A. S. Leonov, and A. G. Yagola, *Nonlinear ill-posed problems,* In "*World Congress of Nonlinear Analysts '92*" /Ed. V. Lakshmikantham, Walter de Gruyter, Berlin, New York, 1996, 506–511.
11. A. S. Leonov, *On the choice of regularization parameter for nonlinear ill-posed problems with operator approximately defined*, USSR Comput. Maths. and Math. Phys., 19 (1979), 1363–1376.
12. I. V. Kochikov, G. M. Kuramshina, and A. G. Yagola, *The stable numerical methods of solving some inverse problems of vibrational spectroscopy*, USSR Comput. Maths. and Math. Phys., 27 (1987), 33–40.
13. G. M. Kuramshina, F. Weinhold, I. V. Kochikov, A. G. Yagola, and Yu. A. Pentim, *Joint treatment of ab initio and experimental data in molecular force field calculations with Tikhonov's method of regularization*, J. Chem. Phys., 100 (1994), 1414–1424.
14. G. M. Kuramshina and A. G. Yagola, *A priori model constraints on polyatomic molecule force field parameters,* Russian Journal of Structural Chemistry, 38, N2 (1997), 221–239 (in Russian).

14

INVERSE PROBLEM FOR DIFFERENTIAL EQUATIONS SYSTEM OF ELECTROMAGNETOELASTICITY IN LINEAR APPROXIMATION

Valery G. Yakhno*

Institute of Mathematics
Russian Academy of Sciences
Novosibirsk, Russia, 630090

1. INTRODUCTION

The recent development of the radio engineering, automation, computing and measuring technology are closely connected with the application of piezoelectric objects. The main attention of researchers to such type of materials connects with the appearance of the piezoeffect which consists in arising electrical charges inside the piezoelectric bodies as the result of their deformations. Such charges will be proportional to the deformation. Thermodynamic analysis shows the existence of the inverse effect which consists in arising of mechanical stresses in the piezoelectric bodies as a result of electric field affecting. The mathematical models of these processes inside the piezoelectric bodies are described by the special system of differential equations of electromagnetoelasticity. The deduction of this differential equations system and some initial boundary value problems for this system was described in monographs [11, 27] and other articles (see references in above mentioned monographs).

As a rule in every initial boundary value problem some functions are given. Some of them determine the differential equations system (for example, the coefficients of the differential equations), the others — initial and boundary conditions. Further the initial boundary value problems are called *direct problems*. If some functions, which are usually given in the direct problem, are unknown and instead of them an additional information about the solution of the direct problem is given, then such type of problems is called *inverse problems* for the considered differential equations system.

The interest to the inverse problems has been stimulated by the study of applied problems of geophysics, astrophysics, flaw detection, nondestructive testing and so on. These problems are the problems of the determination of unknown coefficients of differential equations which

*The work was supported by the Russian Foundation for Fundamental Research under grant 96-01-01937

are the functions depending on the point of the space. These functions from physical point of view are the characteristics of media in which the physical processes take place.

The basis of the theory of inverse problems of mathematical physics was established by A. N. Tikhonov, V. K. Ivanov, M. M. Lavrent'ev (see [41,42]). The systematic investigation of inverse problems was leaded by A. S. Alekseev, M. Akamatsu, G. Anger, Yu. Anikonov, A. S. Blagoveshchenskii, A. L. Bukhgeim, A. P. Calderón, J. R. Cannon, D. Colton, V. I. Dmitriev, H. Engl, I. M. Gel'fand, V. B. Glasko, C. W. Groetsch, M. Klibanov, A. Kirsch, R. Kress, M. M. Lavrent'ev, B. M. Levitan, A. Lorenzi, F. Natterer, G. Nakamura, A. G. Ramm, V. G. Romanov, S. I. Kabanikhin, P. Sacks, F. Santosa, W. Symes, J. Sylvester, G. Uhlmann, G. Talenti, A. G. Yagola, V. G. Yakhno, M. Yamamoto and others (see articles [1–10,12–26,28–46] and references of above-mentioned articles).

A. S. Alekseev [2] and A. S. Blagoveshchenskii [5] were first who began to study the inverse problems for differential equations of elasticity. The systematic study of the inverse problems of the elasticity system was leaded by A. S. Alekseev, V. G. Romanov, P. Sacks, F. Santosa, W. Symes, G. Nakamura, V. Yakhno and others (see works [1,6,22,32,34–37,45] and references of these articles).

The systematic study of the inverse problems for electrodynamics was done by V. I. Dmitriev, V. G. Romanov, S. I. Kabanikhin, A. G. Ramm and others (see articles [12,30,32,33] and references of these articles).

At present the study of the inverse problems for the electromagnetoelasticity systems is leaded by M. M. Lavrent'ev, A. Lorenzi, I. Z. Merazhov, V. I. Priimenko, V. G. Yakhno (see articles [20,23–25]).

The purpose of the present paper consists in the study of new direct and inverse problems for the differential equations systems of electromagnetoelasticity. The investigations of direct and inverse problems in this paper is based on the theory the t-hyperbolic symmetric system of the first order and the methods which was developed by V. G. Romanov [32], V. G. Yakhno [45] for the inverse problems of elasticity and electrodynamics. The study of the direct problems is described in such form and volume which is necessary for the formulation and the investigation of the inverse problem.

2. ELECTROMAGNETOELASTICITY SYSTEM AND ITS REDUCTION TO THE *T*-HYPERBOLIC SYMMETRIC SYSTEM OF THE FIRST ORDER

The full equations system which describes the connected processes of elastic and electromagnetic wave propagations in the inhomogeneous anisotropic media consists in the following differential equations:

$$\rho\frac{\partial^2 u_i}{\partial t^2} = \sum_{j=1}^{3}\frac{\partial T_{ij}}{\partial x_j}, \quad i = 1,2,3; \tag{2.1}$$

$$\operatorname{rot} H = \frac{\partial D}{\partial t}, \quad \operatorname{rot} E = -\mu\frac{\partial H}{\partial t}, \tag{2.2}$$

Here $x = (x_1,x_2,x_3) \in \mathbf{R}^3$, $\rho = \rho(x)$ is the density of the inhomogeneous medium, $\rho(x) > 0$, $u = (u_1,u_2,u_3)$ is the displacement vector $u_i = u_i(x,t)$, $i = 1,2,3$; $E = (E_1,E_2,E_3)$ and

$H = (H_1, H_2, H_3)$ are the vectors of electric and magnetic intensities with components: $E_i = E_i(x,t)$, $H_i = H_i(x,t)$, $i = 1,2,3$; $D = (D_1, D_2, D_3)$ is the vector of the electric induction with components: $D_i = D_i(x,t)$, $i = 1,2,3$.

For stresses $T_{ij}(x,t)$ and the components of the electric induction $D_j(x,t)$ the following representations hold

$$T_{ij} = \sum_{k,l=1}^{3} c_{ijkl}\frac{\partial u_k}{\partial x_l} - \sum_{k=1}^{3} e_{kij}E_k, \quad i = 1,2,3, \quad j = 1,2,3,$$

$$D_j = \sum_{k=1}^{3} \varepsilon_{kj}E_k + \sum_{k,l=1,}^{3} e_{jkl}\frac{\partial u_k}{\partial x_l}, \quad j = 1,2,3,$$

where $c_{ijkl} = c_{ijkl}(x)$ are the elastic moduli; $e_{kij} = e_{kij}(x)$ are the piezoelectric moduli; $\varepsilon_{ij} = \varepsilon_{ij}(x)$ are the dielectric moduli, $\mu = \mu(x)$ is the magnetic permeability, $\mu > 0$

Further we shall use the following natural assumption (see [11,28]) about the symmetry of the indexes: $c_{ijkl} = c_{jikl} = c_{ijlk} = c_{klij}$, $e_{kij} = e_{kji}$, $\varepsilon_{ij} = \varepsilon_{ji}$. System (2.1)–(2.2) describes the propagation of connected elastic and electromagnetic waves. The connection of elastic and electromagnetic processes is determined by the piezoelectric moduli. In the general case equations (2.1)–(2.2) connect three branches of "slow" elastic waves with two branches of "quick" electromagnetic waves. Symmetry of the tensor of stresses reduces the number of independent elastic moduli from 81 to 21. If we shall use the denotation $c_{\alpha\beta} = c_{ijkl}$, according to the following way: $(11) \to 1$, $(22) \to 2$, $(33) \to 3$, $(23) = (32) \to 4$, $(13) = (31) \to 5$, $(12) = (21) \to 6$, then the matrix of independent elastic moduli may be rewritten in the form of the symmetric matrix of the order 6×6.

The full set of characteristics of the electromagnetoelastic medium has the form of the following matrix (see [11,27]):

$$\begin{pmatrix} c_{\alpha\beta}(6\times 6) & e_{\alpha k}(6\times 3) \\ e_{k\alpha}(3\times 6) & \varepsilon_{ij}(3\times 3) \end{pmatrix}.$$

where $C = [c_{\alpha\beta}]$, $\Upsilon = [\varepsilon_{ij}]$ are the positive definite matrices.

We shall show that system of electromagnetoelasticity may be rewritten in the form of the t-hyperbolic symmetric Friedrichs system of the first order.

Let us introduce the notations:

$$\tau_\alpha = \tau_{ij} = \sum_{k,l=1}^{3} c_{ijkl}\frac{\partial u_l}{\partial x_k}, \quad i = 1,2,3, \quad j = 1,2,3, \tag{2.3}$$

$$U_i = \frac{\partial u_i}{\partial t}, \quad i = 1,2,3.$$

Differentiating (2.3) respect to t we obtain six equations of the following form:

$$\frac{\partial \tau_\alpha}{\partial t} = \sum_{k,l=1}^{3} c_{ijkl}\frac{\partial U_l}{\partial x_k}. \tag{2.4}$$

In the terms of the functions τ_α, U_i system (2.1), (2.2) has the following form

$$A_0 \frac{\partial U}{\partial t} + \sum_{i=1}^{3} A_i \frac{\partial U}{\partial x_i} + QU = 0, \tag{2.5}$$

where $U = [u_1, u_2, u_3, \tau_1, \tau_2, \tau_3, \tau_4, \tau_5, \tau_6, E_1, E_2, E_3, H_1, H_2, H_3]^\star$, here and further the symbol $(\star)$ is the sign of the transposition, A_0 is the block-diagonal matrix of the following form

$$A_0 = \mathrm{diag} \quad (\rho I_3, C^{-1}, \varepsilon, \mu I_3),$$

I_3 is the unit matrix of the order 3×3, C^{-1} is the inverse matrix to the matrix $C = [c_{\alpha\beta}]$, which has the order 6×6,

$$\varepsilon = \begin{pmatrix} \varepsilon_{11} & \varepsilon_{12} & \varepsilon_{13} \\ \varepsilon_{12} & \varepsilon_{22} & \varepsilon_{23} \\ \varepsilon_{13} & \varepsilon_{23} & \varepsilon_{33} \end{pmatrix}, \quad A_i = \begin{pmatrix} 0_{3,3} & A_i^1 & A_i^2 & 0_{3,3} \\ A_i^{1\star} & 0_{6,6} & 0_{6,3} & 0_{6,3} \\ A_i^{2\star} & 0_{3,6} & 0_{3,3} & A_i^3 \\ 0_{3,3} & 0_{3,6} & A_i^{3\star} & 0_{3,3} \end{pmatrix}, \quad i = 1,2,3;$$

$$A_1^1 = \begin{pmatrix} -1 & 0 & 0 & 0 & 0 & 0 \\ 0 & 0 & 0 & 0 & 0 & -1 \\ 0 & 0 & 0 & 0 & -1 & 0 \end{pmatrix}, \quad A_2^1 = \begin{pmatrix} 0 & 0 & 0 & 0 & 0 & -1 \\ 0 & -1 & 0 & 0 & 0 & 0 \\ 0 & 0 & 0 & -1 & 0 & 0 \end{pmatrix},$$

$$A_3^1 = \begin{pmatrix} 0 & 0 & 0 & 0 & -1 & 0 \\ 0 & 0 & 0 & -1 & 0 & 0 \\ 0 & 0 & -1 & 0 & 0 & 0 \end{pmatrix}, \quad A_1^2 = \begin{pmatrix} e_{11} & e_{21} & e_{31} \\ e_{16} & e_{26} & e_{36} \\ e_{15} & e_{25} & e_{35} \end{pmatrix},$$

$$A_2^2 = \begin{pmatrix} e_{16} & e_{26} & e_{36} \\ e_{12} & e_{22} & e_{32} \\ e_{14} & e_{24} & e_{34} \end{pmatrix}, \quad A_3^2 = \begin{pmatrix} e_{15} & e_{25} & e_{35} \\ e_{14} & e_{24} & e_{34} \\ e_{13} & e_{23} & e_{33} \end{pmatrix},$$

$$A_1^3 = \begin{pmatrix} 0 & 0 & 0 \\ 0 & 0 & -1 \\ 0 & 1 & 0 \end{pmatrix}, \quad A_2^3 = \begin{pmatrix} 0 & 0 & 1 \\ 0 & 0 & 0 \\ -1 & 0 & 0 \end{pmatrix}, \quad A_3^3 = \begin{pmatrix} 0 & 1 & 0 \\ -1 & 0 & -1 \\ 0 & 0 & 0 \end{pmatrix};$$

$$Q = \begin{pmatrix} 0_{3,9} & Q_1 & 0_{3,3} \\ 0_{12,9} & 0_{12,3} & 0_{12,3} \end{pmatrix}; \quad Q_1 = -\begin{pmatrix} \mathrm{div}\, q^1 & \mathrm{div}\, q^2 & \mathrm{div}\, q^3 \\ \mathrm{div} p^1 & \mathrm{div} p^2 & \mathrm{div} p^3 \\ \mathrm{div}\, l^1 & \mathrm{div}\, l^2 & \mathrm{div}\, l^3 \end{pmatrix};$$

$$q^k = (e_{k1}, e_{k6}, e_{k5}), \quad p^k = (e_{k6}, e_{k2}, e_{k4}), \quad l^k = (e_{k5}, e_{k4}, e_{k3}), \quad k = 1,2,3,$$

where $0_{m,n}$ is the zero matrix which has the order $m \times n$, here m is the number of lines, n is the number of columns.

In present paper we shall consider the anisotropic medium of the cubic structure only. In this case the matrix of characteristics has the following form (see [11])

$$\begin{pmatrix} \begin{bmatrix} c_{11} & c_{12} & c_{12} \\ c_{12} & c_{11} & c_{12} \\ c_{12} & c_{12} & c_{11} \end{bmatrix} & 0 & 0 \\ 0 & \begin{bmatrix} c_{44} & & 0 \\ & c_{44} & \\ 0 & & c_{44} \end{bmatrix} & \begin{bmatrix} e_{14} & & 0 \\ & e_{14} & \\ 0 & & e_{14} \end{bmatrix} \\ 0 & \begin{bmatrix} e_{14} & & 0 \\ & e_{14} & \\ 0 & & e_{14} \end{bmatrix} & \begin{bmatrix} \varepsilon & & 0 \\ & \varepsilon & \\ 0 & & \varepsilon \end{bmatrix} \end{pmatrix}.$$

3. LINEARIZATION PROCESS FOR THE HYPERBOLIC SYMMETRIC SYSTEM. DIRECT AND INVERSE PROBLEMS IN LINEAR APPROXIMATION

Let us consider for $x = (x_1, x_2, x_3) \in \mathbf{R}^3$, $0 \le x_3 \le H$, $t \in \mathbf{R}$ an arbitrary t-hyperbolic symmetric Friedrichs system of differential equations of the first order

$$A_0 \frac{\partial}{\partial t} U + \sum_{j=1}^{3} A_j \frac{\partial}{\partial x_j} U + QU = 0, \quad 0 \le x_3 \le H, \tag{3.1}$$

with the following conditions

$$U|_{t<0} = 0, \tag{3.2}$$

$$G_1 U|_{x_3=0} = g_1,$$

$$G_2 U|_{x_3=H} = g_2, \tag{3.3}$$

where $A_j, j = 0,1,2,3$ are the symmetric matrices. Moreover A_0 is the positive definite matrix, Q is the arbitrary fixed matrix, G_1, G_2 are given matrices which guarantee the dissipativity of boundary conditions, $g_1(x_1, x_2, t)$, $g_2(x_1, x_2, t)$ are given functions.

For given smooth matrices $Q(x), A_j(x), j = 0,1,2,3$, the problem of the determination of the function $U(x, t, x_1^0, x_2^0)$ which satisfies equations (3.1)–(3.3) is called the **direct problem**.

Let some functions which appear as elements in the matrices $A_j(x), j = 0,1,2,3$, $Q(x)$ are unknown functions then the problem of the determination of these unknown functions, if respect to the solution $U(x, t, x_1^0, x_2^0)$ of the direct problem is given the following additional information

$$G_1 U|_{x_3=H} = h_1(x_1, x_2, t),$$

$$G_2 U|_{x_3=0} = h_2(x_1, x_2, t), \tag{3.4}$$

where $h_1(x_1, x_2, t)$, $h_2(x_1, x_2, t)$ are given functions, is called *the inverse problem*.

We shall describe reasoning which leads to the formulation of direct and inverse problems in the linear approximation. We shall suppose that $A_j(x), j=0,1,2,3,\ Q(x),\ G_j(x), j=1,2$, have the following representations

$$A_j(x)=A_j^0+A_j^1(x), \quad j=0,1,2,3,$$

$$Q(x)=Q^0+Q^1(x), \quad G_j(x)=G_j^0+G_j^1(x), \quad j=1,2, \tag{3.5}$$

where $A_j^0, j=0,1,2,3;\ \ Q^0,\ \ G_j^0, j=1,2$ are given matrices and matrices $A_j^1(x), j=0,1,2,3, Q^1(x), G_j^1(x), j=1,2$, have the values which are less than the values $A_j^0, j=0,1,2,3, Q^0, G_j^0$.

Let us introduce the parameter of the smallness λ such that equations (3.5) may be rewritten as

$$A_j(x)=A_j^0+\lambda\tilde{A}_j^1(x), \quad j=0,1,2,3,$$

$$Q(x)=Q^0+\lambda\tilde{Q}^1(x) \quad G_j(x)=G_j^0+\lambda\tilde{G}_j^1(x), \quad j=1,2, \tag{3.6}$$

where $\tilde{A}_j^1(x), j=0,1,2,3, \tilde{Q}^1(x), \tilde{G}_j^1(x), j=1,2$ have the same order of the values as A_j^0, $j=0,1,2,3, Q^0, G_j^0, j=1,2$.

We represent the solution of direct problem (3.1)–(3.3) in the form

$$U(x,t)=U^0(x,t)+\lambda\tilde{U}^1(x,t)+\dots \tag{3.7}$$

Substituting (3.6), (3.7) in equalities (3.1)–(3.3) and equating the values in the same degrees of the parameter λ we obtain:

$$A_0^0\frac{\partial}{\partial t}U^0+\sum_{j=1}^{3}A_j^0\frac{\partial}{\partial x_j}U^0+Q^0=0, \quad 0\le x_3\le H, \tag{3.8}$$

$$U^0|_{t<0}=0, \tag{3.9}$$

$$G_1^0U^0|_{x_3=0}=g_1(x_1-x_1^0,x_2-x_2^0,t),$$

$$G_2^0U^0|_{x_3=H}=g_2(x_1-x_1^0,x_2-x_2^0,t), \tag{3.10}$$

$$A_0^0\frac{\partial}{\partial t}\tilde{U}^1+\sum_{j=1}^{3}A_j^0\frac{\partial}{\partial x_j}\tilde{U}^1=$$

$$=-\left[\tilde{A}_0^1\frac{\partial}{\partial t}U^0+\sum_{j=1}^{3}\tilde{A}_j^1\frac{\partial}{\partial x_j}U^0+\tilde{Q}^1U^0\right], \quad 0\le x_3\le H, \tag{3.11}$$

$$\tilde{U}^1|_{t<0} = 0, \tag{3.12}$$

$$G_1^0 \tilde{U}^1|_{x_3=0} = -G_1^1(x_1,x_2,0)U^0|_{x_3=0},$$

$$G_2^0 \tilde{U}^1|_{x_3=H} = -G_2^1(x_1,x_2,H)U^0|_{x_3=H}. \tag{3.13}$$

The transfer from (3.1)–(3.3) to correlations (3.8)–(3.13) is justified if it is known a priori that in the right hand side of correlation (3.7) the values of the terms with factors λ^s, $s = 2,3,\ldots$ are small.

Neglecting of terms of the order of the smallness λ^2 and higher we obtain

$$U(x,t,x_1^0,x_2^0) \cong U^0(x,t,x_1^0,x_2^0) + U^1(x,t,x_1^0,x_2^0), \tag{3.14}$$

where $U^1 = \lambda \tilde{U}^1$.

Multiplying the right and left hand sides of equations (3.11)–(3.13) on the number λ we come to the correlations:

$$A_0^0 \frac{\partial}{\partial t} U^1 + \sum_{j=1}^{3} A_j^0 \frac{\partial}{\partial x_j} U^1 + Q^0 U^1 =$$

$$= -\left[A_0^1 \frac{\partial}{\partial t} U^0 + \sum_{j=1}^{3} A_j^1 \frac{\partial}{\partial x_j} U^0 + Q^1 U^0 \right], \quad 0 \le x_3 \le H, \tag{3.15}$$

$$U^1|_{t<0} = 0, \tag{3.16}$$

$$G_1^0 U^1|_{x_3=0} = 0,$$

$$G_2^0 U^1|_{x_3=H} = 0. \tag{3.17}$$

From equalities (3.14), (3.4) we hold:

$$G_1^0 U^1|_{x_3=H} = H_1(x,t,x_1^0,x_2^0),$$

$$G_2^0 U^1|_{x_3=0} = H_2(x,t,x_1^0,x_2^0), \tag{3.18}$$

where

$$H_1(x,t,x_1^0,x_2^0) = h_1(x,t,x_1^0,x_2^0) - U^0|_{x_3=H},$$

$$H_2(x,t,x_1^0,x_2^0) = h_2(x,t,x_1^0,x_2^0) - U^0|_{x_3=0}.$$

The problem of the determination of the function U having representation (3.14), where U^0 is the solution of problem (3.8)–(3.10) and U^1 is the solution of problem (3.11)–(3.13) in which A_j^0, $A_j^1(x), j = 0,1,2,3$, $Q^1(x)$ G_j^0, $G_j^1(x), j = 1,2$ are known matrices $g_j(x_1,x_2,t), j = 1,2$ are given functions, we shall call **the direct multidimensional linearized problem.**

The problem of the determination of unknown functions which appear in differential equations system (3.15) as the elements of the matrices $A_j^1(x), j = 0,1,2,3$, $Q^1(x)$, if we know the additional information of form (3.18), we shall call *the inverse multidimensional linearized problem*. In this connection $A_j^0, j = 0,1,2,3$, Q^0, $G_j^0, j = 1,2$, $H_j(x,t,x_1^0,x_2^0), j = 1,2$ are given matrices and vector-functions, U^0 is given solution of problem (3.8)–(3.10).

4. MULTIDIMENSIONAL DIRECT AND INVERSE PROBLEMS FOR EMES

Electromagnetoelasticity system (EMES) (2.5) for the medium of the cubic structure may be represented for $x=(x_1,x_2,x_3)\in\mathbf{R}^3$, $0\le x_3\le H$, $t\in\mathbf{R}$ in the form:

$$A_0\frac{\partial}{\partial t}U+\sum_{j=1}^{3}A_j\frac{\partial}{\partial x_j}U+QU=0,\quad 0\le x_3\le H, \tag{4.1}$$

where A_0 is the block diagonal matrix of the form

$$A_0=\text{diag}\quad(\rho I_3, S, \varepsilon I_3, \mu I_3),$$

I_3 is the unit matrix of the order 3×3, S is the inverse matrix to the matrix $C=[c_{\alpha\beta}]$ and has the form:

$$S=\begin{pmatrix} s_{11} & s_{12} & s_{12} & 0 & 0 & 0\\ s_{12} & s_{11} & s_{12} & 0 & 0 & 0\\ s_{12} & s_{12} & s_{11} & 0 & 0 & 0\\ 0 & 0 & 0 & s_{44} & 0 & 0\\ 0 & 0 & 0 & 0 & s_{44} & 0\\ 0 & 0 & 0 & 0 & 0 & s_{44} \end{pmatrix},$$

$$s_{11}=-\frac{c_{11}+c_{12}}{\Delta},\quad s_{12}=\frac{c_{12}}{\Delta},\quad s_{44}=\frac{1}{c_{44}},\quad \Delta=(c_{12}-c_{11})(c_{11}+2c_{12}),$$

$$A_i=\begin{pmatrix} 0_{3,3} & A_i^1 & A_i^2 & 0_{3,3}\\ A_i^{1\star} & 0_{6,6} & 0_{6,3} & 0_{6,3}\\ A_i^{2\star} & 0_{3,6} & 0_{3,3} & A_i^3\\ 0_{3,3} & 0_{3,6} & A_i^{3\star} & 0_{3,3} \end{pmatrix},\quad i=1,2,3;$$

$$A_1^1=\begin{pmatrix} -1 & 0 & 0 & 0 & 0 & 0\\ 0 & 0 & 0 & 0 & 0 & -1\\ 0 & 0 & 0 & 0 & -1 & 0 \end{pmatrix},\quad A_2^1=\begin{pmatrix} 0 & 0 & 0 & 0 & 0 & -1\\ 0 & -1 & 0 & 0 & 0 & 0\\ 0 & 0 & 0 & -1 & 0 & 0 \end{pmatrix},$$

$$A_3^1=\begin{pmatrix} 0 & 0 & 0 & 0 & -1 & 0\\ 0 & 0 & 0 & -1 & 0 & 0\\ 0 & 0 & -1 & 0 & 0 & 0 \end{pmatrix},\quad A_1^2=\begin{pmatrix} 0 & 0 & 0\\ 0 & 0 & e_{14}\\ 0 & e_{14} & 0 \end{pmatrix},$$

$$A_2^2=\begin{pmatrix} 0 & 0 & e_{14}\\ 0 & 0 & 0\\ e_{14} & 0 & 0 \end{pmatrix},\quad A_3^2=\begin{pmatrix} 0 & e_{14} & 0\\ e_{14} & 0 & 0\\ 0 & 0 & 0 \end{pmatrix},$$

$$A_1^3=\begin{pmatrix} 0 & 0 & 0\\ 0 & 0 & -1\\ 0 & 1 & 0 \end{pmatrix},\quad A_2^3=\begin{pmatrix} 0 & 0 & 1\\ 0 & 0 & 0\\ -1 & 0 & 0 \end{pmatrix},\quad A_3^3=\begin{pmatrix} 0 & 1 & 0\\ -1 & 0 & -1\\ 0 & 0 & 0 \end{pmatrix},$$

$$Q=\begin{pmatrix} 0_{3,9} & Q_1 & 0_{3,3} \\ 0_{12,9} & 0_{12,3} & 0_{12,3} \end{pmatrix}, \quad Q_1=\begin{pmatrix} 0 & -\frac{\partial}{\partial x_3}e_{14} & -\frac{\partial}{\partial x_2}e_{14} \\ -\frac{\partial}{\partial x_3}e_{14} & 0 & -\frac{\partial}{\partial x_1}e_{14} \\ 0 & -\frac{\partial}{\partial x_1}e_{14} & -\frac{\partial}{\partial x_1}e_{14} \end{pmatrix},$$

where $0_{m,n}$ is the zero matrix of the order $m \times n$, where m is the number of lines, n is the number of columns.

Further we shall suppose that the functions: $\rho(x)$, $s_{11}(x)$, $s_{12}(x)$, $s_{44}(x)$, $\varepsilon(x)$, $\mu(x)$, $e_{14}(x)$ may be represented in the domain D in the form:

$$\rho(x)=\rho^0+\rho^1(x), \quad s_{11}(x)=s_{11}^0+s_{11}^1(x), \quad s_{12}(x)=s_{12}^0+s_{12}^1(x),$$

$$s_{44}(x)=s_{44}^0+s_{44}^1(x), \quad \varepsilon(x)=\varepsilon^0+\varepsilon^1(x), \quad \mu(x)=\mu^0+\mu^1(x), \tag{4.2}$$

$$e_{14}(x)=e_{14}^1(x), \quad e_{14}^0=0,$$

where ρ^0, s_{11}^0, s_{12}^0, s_{44}^0, ε^0, μ^0 are given constants, $\rho^1(x)$, $s_{11}^1(x)$, $s_{12}^1(x)$, $s_{44}^1(x)$, $\varepsilon^1(x)$, $\mu^1(x)$, $e_{14}^1(x)$ are the functions having the small values.

Further we shall suppose that

$$\rho^0>0, \quad s_{44}^0>0, \quad s_{11}^0>0, \quad \varepsilon^0>0, \quad \mu^0>0,$$

$$s_{11}^0+2s_{12}^0>0, \quad s_{11}^0+s_{12}^0>0, \quad \varepsilon^0\mu^0<s_{44}^0\rho^0, \tag{4.3}$$

$$\rho^1(x),s_{11}^1(x),s_{12}^1(x),s_{44}^1(x),\varepsilon^1(x),\mu^1(x),e_{14}^1(x)\in C_0^1(\mathbf{R}^2\times[0,H]), \tag{4.4}$$

where $C_0^1(\mathbf{R}^2\times[0,H])$ is the class of functions which are continuously differentiable and compactly supported on $\mathbf{R}^2\times[0,H]$.

Let us consider differential equations system (4.1) for $x=(x_1,x_2,x_3)\in\mathbf{R}^3$, $0\le x_3\le H$, $t\in\mathbf{R}$ with the following data

$$U|_{t<0}=0, \tag{4.5}$$

$$G^1U|_{x_3=0}=g_1(x_1-x_1^0,x_2-x_2^0,t),$$

$$G^2U|_{x_3=H}=g_2(x_1-x_1^0,x_2-x_2^0,t), \tag{4.6}$$

where the functions $g_1(x_1,x_2,t)$, $g_2(x_1,x_2,t)$ are given and the matrices G^1, G^2 have the order 5×15. The elements of the matrices $G^1=[G_{ij}^1]$, $G^2=[G_{ij}^2]$ have the forms:

$$G_{11}^1=G_{22}^1=G_{33}^1=G_{11}^2=G_{22}^2=G_{33}^2=\sqrt{\frac{\rho^0}{2}},$$

$$G_{18}^1=G_{27}^1=-G_{18}^2=-G_{27}^2=-\sqrt{\frac{s_{44}^0}{2}},$$

$$G^1_{34} = G^1_{35} = -G^2_{34} = -G^2_{35} = -s^0_{12}\sqrt{\frac{s^0_{11}+s^0_{12}}{(s^0_{11}-s^0_{12})(s^0_{11}+2s^0_{12})}},$$

$$G^1_{36} = -G^2_{36} = -\frac{s^{02}_{11}+s^0_{11}s^0_{12}+2s^{02}_{11}}{2\sqrt{(s^0_{11}-s^0_{12})(s^0_{11}+2s^0_{12})}},$$

$$G^1_{4.10} = G^1_{5.11} = G^2_{4.10} = G^2_{5.11} = \sqrt{\frac{\varepsilon^0}{2}},$$

$$G^1_{4.14} = -G^1_{5.13} = -G^2_{4.14} = G^2_{5.13} = -\sqrt{\frac{\mu^0}{2}},$$

and all other elements G^k_{ij} are equal to zero.

We shall suppose that the parameter $x^0 = (x^0_1, x^0_2, 0)$ belongs to the set of points of the boundary D and we shall consider the following multidimensional direct and inverse linearized problems.

Multidimensional direct linearized problem 1. Find the function $U(x,t)$ having the form:

$$U(x,t) = U^0(x,t,x^0_1,x^0_2) + U^1(x,t,x^0_1,x^0_2), \tag{4.7}$$

where $U^0(x,t,x^0_1,x^0_2)$, $U^1(x,t,x^0_1,x^0_2)$ are the solutions of the following initial boundary value problems respectively:

$$A^0_0\frac{\partial}{\partial t}U^0 + \sum_{j=1}^{3} A^0_j \frac{\partial}{\partial x_j}U^0 = 0, \quad 0 \le x_3 \le H, \tag{4.8}$$

$$U^0|_{t<0} = 0, \tag{4.9}$$

$$G^1U^0|_{x_3=0} = g_1(x_1 - x^0_1, x_2 - x^0_2, t),$$

$$G^2U^0|_{x_3=H} = g_2(x_1 - x^0_1, x_2 - x^0_2, t), \tag{4.10}$$

$$A^0_0\frac{\partial}{\partial t}U^1 + \sum_{j=1}^{3} A^0_j \frac{\partial}{\partial x_j}U^1 =$$

$$= -\left[A^1_0\frac{\partial}{\partial t}U^0 + \sum_{j=1}^{3} A^1_j \frac{\partial}{\partial x_j}U^0 + Q^1U^0\right], \quad 0 \le x_3 \le H, \tag{4.11}$$

$$U^1|_{t<0} = 0, \tag{4.12}$$

$$G^1U^1|_{x_3=0} = 0,$$

$$G^2U^1|_{x_3=H} = 0. \tag{4.13}$$

Here A^0_j, $A^1_j(x), j = 0,1,2,3$, $Q^1(x)$ are given matrices.

Multidimensional inverse linearized problem 1. We shall suppose that the functions $\rho^1(x), s^1_{11}(x), s^1_{12}(x), s^1_{44}(x), \varepsilon^1(x), \mu^1(x), e^1_{14}(x)$ which appear in differential equations system (4.11) are unknown. It is necessary to find these functions if we know the additional information about the solution of direct linearized problem 1 in the following form:

$$G^1\tilde{U}^1|_{x_3=H} = h_1(x_1,x_2,t,x_1^0,x_2^0),$$

$$G^2\tilde{U}^1|_{x_3=0} = h_2(x_1,x_2,t,x_1^0,x_2^0), \tag{4.14}$$

where $h_1(x_1,x_2,t)$, $h_2(x_1,x_2,t)$ are given vector-functions for $(x_1,x_2) \in \mathbf{R}^2$, $(x_1^0,x_2^0) \in \mathbf{R}^2$, $t \in [0,T]$.

5. INITIAL BOUNDARY VALUE PROBLEM (4.8)–(4.10)

Let us consider for $x = (x_1,x_2,x_3)$, $x_1,x_2,x_1^0,x_2^0 \in \mathbf{R}$, $0 \le x_3 \le H$, $t \in \mathbf{R}$ initial boundary value problem (4.8)–(4.10) in which ρ^0, s^0_{11}, s^0_{12}, s^0_{44}, ε^0, μ^0 are given constants and the functions $g_j(x_1,x_2,t), j = 1,2$ have the forms

$$g_k(x_1,x_2,t) = e^k\delta(x_1,x_2)\theta(t), \qquad k = 1,2, \tag{5.1}$$

where e^k, $k = 1,2$ are vectors of the space $\mathbf{R}^5$.

Let us introduce the class of vector-functions

$$\mathcal{U} = \Bigg\{ U(x,t) | U(x,t) = \frac{\partial}{\partial t}w(x,t), w|_{t<0} = 0,$$

$$w(x,t) \in C^{1,1}_{t,x_3}(\mathbf{R}_+ \times (0,H); \mathcal{E}'(\mathbf{R}^2)), w(x,+0) = 0, \Bigg\},$$

where $\mathcal{E}'(\mathbf{R}^2)$ is the space of generalized functions with the compact supports; $C^{1,1}_{t,x_3}(\mathbf{R}_+ \times (0,H))$ is the class of continuously differentiable mappings in $(t,x_3) \in \mathbf{R}_+ \times (0,H)$ and of the form $(t,x_3) \to w(x,t) \in \mathcal{E}'(\mathbf{R}^2)$. Further

$$w_j^\varepsilon(x,t) = w_j * \omega_\varepsilon(x_1,x_2), \quad j = \overline{1,15},$$

where $\omega_\varepsilon(x_1,x_2)$ is the infinitely differentiable function for which the weak limit for $\varepsilon \to +0$ is the Dirac delta function $\delta(x_1,x_2)$; $*$ is the operation of the convolution product respect to x_1,x_2.

Rewriting equations (4.8)–(4.10) in the term of the vector-function $w(x,t)$ which is connected with $U(x,t)$ by the correlation $U(x,t) = \frac{\partial}{\partial t}w(x,t)$ and then applying the operation of the convolution product respect to x_1,x_2 with the function $\omega_\varepsilon(x_1,x_2)$ to the right and left hand sides of obtained equations then we obtain:

$$\left[A_0^0\frac{\partial}{\partial t} + \sum_{j=1}^{3} A_j^0\frac{\partial}{\partial x_j}\right] w^\varepsilon = 0, \quad 0 \le x_3 \le H, \tag{5.2}$$

$$w^{\varepsilon}(x,+0)=0, \tag{5.3}$$

$$G^1 w^{\varepsilon}|_{x_3=0}=e^1\omega^{\varepsilon}\theta_1(t),$$

$$G^2 w^{\varepsilon}|_{x_3=H}=e^2\omega^{\varepsilon}\theta_1(t), \tag{5.4}$$

where $\theta_1(t)=t\theta(t)$.

Here $\omega^{\varepsilon}(x_1,x_2)\theta_1(t)$ is the differentiable function. Therefore for every $\varepsilon>0$ problem (5.2)–(5.4) has an unique solution which is determined on $\mathbf{R}^2\times[0,H]\times\mathbf{R}_+$ and for every fixed values x_1,x_2,t this solution has the finite support. For arbitrary $(x_1,x_2)\in\mathbf{R}^2$, $(x_3,t)\in[0,H]\times\mathbf{R}_+$ let us consider the limit $\lim_{\varepsilon\to+0}w^{\varepsilon}(x,t)$ in the sense of the convergence of the space $\mathcal{D}'(0,H)$. By the virtue of the fullness of the space $\mathcal{D}'(0,H)$ this limit exists and the function which is this limit belongs to the space

$$C^{\infty,\infty,2,2}_{x_1,x_2,x_3,t}(\mathbf{R}^2\times\mathbf{R}_+;\mathcal{E}'(0,H)).$$

Therefore the solution of problem (4.8)–(4.10) exists in the class $\mathcal{U}$. We can apply the Fourier transformation respect to x_1,x_2 to functions from the class $\mathcal{U}$ for fixed $t\in R$, $x_3\in[0,H]$. Moreover by the virtue of the Wiener theorem the image of the Fourier transformation is the analytic function. Consequently if we apply the Fourier transformation respect to x_1,x_2 to the right and left sides of equations (4.8)–(4.10) then we obtain the problem which we can consider as the classical initial boundary value problem with the fixed Fourier parameters:

$$\left(A_0^0\frac{\partial}{\partial t}+A_3^0\frac{\partial}{\partial x_3}-i\sum_{k=1}^{2}\nu_k A_k^0\right)\tilde{U}^0(\nu,x_3,t)=0,\quad 0\le x_3\le H, \tag{5.5}$$

$$\tilde{U}^0\big|_{t<0}=0, \tag{5.6}$$

$$G^1\tilde{U}^0\big|_{x_3=0}=e^1\theta(t),$$

$$G^2\tilde{U}^0\big|_{x_3=H}=e^2\theta(t), \tag{5.7}$$

where

$$\tilde{U}^0(\nu_1,\nu_2,x_3,t)=F_{x_1,x_2}[U^0](\nu_1,\nu_2,x_3,t).$$

Problem (5.5)–(5.7) for the fixed Fourier parameters $\nu_1,\nu_2\in\mathbf{R}^2$ has a unique solution only. This fact proves the uniqueness of the solution of original problem (4.8)–(4.10).

Conducted arguments proved the following theorem.

Theorem 5.1. *Let ρ^0, s^0_{11}, s^0_{12}, s^0_{44}, ε^0, μ^0 be the known constants satisfying conditions (4.3). Then it exists the unique solution of problem (4.8)–(4.10) $U^0(x_1-x_1^0,x_2-x_2^0,t)$, such that $U^0(x,t)\in\mathcal{U}$.*

Remark 5.1. The Fourier transformation respect to x_1,x_2 may be used to the functions of the class $\mathcal{U}$. Moreover it follows from Wiener theorem that Fourier image

$$\tilde{U}^0(\nu_1,\nu_2,x_3,t)=F_{x_1,x_2}[U^0](\nu_1,\nu_2,x_3,t).$$

of the function $U^0(x,t)\in\mathcal{U}$ satisfies the following condition: it exists such positive constants N,C that for every $\nu=(\nu_1,\nu_2)\in\mathbf{R}^2$

$$|\tilde{U}^0(\nu,x_3,t)|\le C(1+|\nu|)^N, \tag{5.8}$$

6. INITIAL BOUNDARY VALUE PROBLEM (4.11)–(4.13)

Further we shall consider problem (4.11)–(4.13). The following theorem holds.

Theorem 6.1. *Let ρ^0, s^0_{11}, s^0_{12}, s^0_{44}, ε^0, μ^0 be known constants and $\rho^1(x)$, $s^1_{11}(x)$, $s^1_{12}(x)$, $s^1_{44}(x)$, $\varepsilon^1(x)$, $\mu^1(x)$, $e^1_{14}(x)$ be the known functions satisfying conditions (4.3), (4.4) respectively; $U^0(x_1-x^0_1,x_2-x^0_2,x_3,t)$ be the solution of problem (4.8)–(4.10), where $U^0(x,t)\in\mathfrak{U}$; $(x^0_1,x^0_2)\in\mathbf{R}^2$ be a parameter. Then it exists the unique solution $U^1(x,t,x^0_1,x^0_2)$ of problem (4.11)–(4.13) such that*

$$U^1(x,t,x^0_1,x^0_2)\in C([0,T];S'(\mathbf{R}^4\times(0,H))),$$

$$\tilde U^1(\nu_1,\nu_2,x_3,t,\kappa_1,\kappa_2)\in C_{\nu_1,\nu_2,x_3}(\mathbf{R}^2\times\mathbf{R}^+;S'(\mathbf{R}^3)).$$

Proof of Theorem 6.1: Applying the Fourier transformation respect to x_1, x_2, x^0_1, x^0_2 to the left and right sides of equalities (4.11)–(4.13) (while formally) we obtain:

$$\left(A^0_0\frac{\partial}{\partial t}+A^0_3\frac{\partial}{\partial x_3}-i\sum_{k=1}^{2}\nu_kA^0_k\right)\tilde U^1(\nu,x_3,t,\kappa)=\tilde f(t,x_3,\nu,\kappa),\quad 0\le x_3\le H,\qquad(6.1)$$

$$\tilde U^1\big|_{t<0}=0,\qquad(6.2)$$

$$G^1\tilde U^1\big|_{x_3=0}=0,$$

$$G^2\tilde U^1\big|_{x_3=H}=0,\qquad(6.3)$$

where

$$\tilde U^1(\nu,x_3,t,\kappa)=F_{x_1,x_2,x^0_1,x^0_2}[U^1(x,t,x^0)](\nu_1,\nu_2,x_3,t,\kappa_1,\kappa_2)=$$

$$=\int_{\mathbf{R}^4}U^1(x,t,x^0)\exp\left\{i\sum_{k=1}^{2}\left[(\kappa_k-\nu_k)x^0_k+\nu_kx_k\right]\right\}dx_1dx_2dx^0_1dx^0_2,\qquad(6.4)$$

$\nu=(\nu_1,\nu_2)$ $\quad\kappa=(\kappa_1,\kappa_2)$ are parameters from $\mathbf{R}^2$,

$$\tilde f(t,x_3,\nu,\kappa)=-\left[\tilde A^1_0(\kappa,x_3)\frac{\partial}{\partial t}+\tilde A^1_3(\kappa,x_3)\frac{\partial}{\partial x_3}-\right.$$

$$\left.-i\sum_{k=1}^{2}\nu_k\tilde A^1_k(\kappa,x_3)+\tilde Q^1(\kappa,x_3)\right]\tilde U^0(\nu-\kappa,x_3,t),$$

$$\tilde A^1_j(\kappa,x_3)=F_{x_1,x_2}[A^j(x)](\nu_1,\nu_2,x_3)\equiv$$

$$=\int_{\mathbf{R}^2}A^j(x)\exp\left\{i\sum_{k=1}^{2}[(\nu_kx_k]\right\}dx_1dx_2,\quad j=0,1,2,3.$$

Here we used the following lemma.

Lemma 6.2. *Let $A_j^0, j = 0,1,2,3$ be given constant matrices; $A_j^1(x), j = 0,1,2,3$ be given matrices having the elements from the class $C_0^1(\mathbf{R}^2 \times [0,H])$; $(x_1^0, x_2^0) \in \mathbf{R}^2$ be a parameter; $U^0(x_1 - x_1^0, x_2 - x_2^0, t)$ be the solution of problem (4.11)–(4.13) such that $U^0(x,t) \in \mathfrak{U}$. Then the following equality holds:*

$$F_{x_1,x_2,x_1^0,x_2^0}[A^1(x)\frac{\partial^{s^1+s^2}}{\partial x_1^{s^1}\partial x_1^{s^1}}U^0(x_1 - x_1^0, x_2 - x_2^0, x_3, t)](\nu_1, \nu_2, x_3, t, \kappa_1, \kappa_2) =$$

$$= (-i\nu_1)^{s_1}(-i\nu_2)^{s_2}\tilde{A}^1(\kappa_1, \kappa_2, x_3, t)\tilde{U}^0(\nu_1 - \kappa_1, \nu_2 - \kappa_2, x_3, t).$$

Proof of Lemma 6.2: is conducted by immediate calculation with the use of properties of the Fourier transformation.

The following lemma is necessary for the further proof of Theorem 6.1.

Lemma 6.3. *Let the conditions of Theorem 6.1 hold. Then the function $\tilde{f}(t, x_3, \nu, \kappa)$ belongs to the class $C_{t,x_3}(\mathbf{R}_+ \times [0,T]; S'(\mathbf{R}^4))$, and for fixed $(t, x_3) \in \mathbf{R}_+ \times [0,T]$ it exists the positive number m such that:*

$$\int_{\mathbf{R}^4} |\tilde{f}(t, x_3, \nu, \kappa)|(1 + |\nu| + |\kappa|)^{-m} d\nu d\kappa < \infty.$$

Proof of Lemma 6.3: Without loss of generality it is sufficient to prove the confirmation of Lemma 6.3 for the case when

$$\tilde{f}(t, x_3, \nu, \kappa) = i\sum_{k=1}^{2} \nu_k \tilde{A}_k^1(\kappa, x_3)\tilde{U}^0(\nu - \kappa, x_3, t).$$

Using inequality (5.8) and the Cauchy–Schwartz–Bunyakovskii inequality we obtain:

$$\int_{\mathbf{R}^4} |\sum_{k=1}^{2} \nu_k \tilde{A}_k^1(\kappa, x_3)\tilde{U}^0(\nu - \kappa, x_3, t)|(1 + |\nu| + |\kappa|)^{-m} d\nu d\kappa$$

$$\leq \left[\int_{\mathbf{R}^2} \sum_{k=1}^{2} |\tilde{A}_k^1(\kappa, x_3)|^2 d\kappa\right]^{\frac{1}{2}} \left[\int_{\mathbf{R}^2} \frac{d\nu}{1 + |\nu|^2}\right]^{\frac{1}{2}}$$

$$\left[\int_{\mathbf{R}^4} |\tilde{U}^0(\nu - \kappa, x_3, t)|^2 (1 + |\nu| + |\kappa|)^{-2m+2} d\nu d\kappa\right]^{\frac{1}{2}}.$$

It follows the confirmation of Lemma 6.3 from last inequality for $m = N + 3$ and the condition: $\tilde{A}_j^1(\kappa, x_3), j = 0,1,2,3$, $\tilde{Q}(\kappa, x_3) \in C([0,H], L_2(\mathbf{R}^2))$.

Let us continue the proof of Theorem 6.1. It is known from linear algebra that it exists the nonsingular matrix T such that $T^* A_0^0 T = I$, where I is the unit matrix and $T^* A_3^0 T = D_0$ is the diagonal matrix.

The elements of the matrices $T = (\tau_{ij})$, $T^* = (\tau_{ij}^*)$ are determined by means of the following formulas:

$$\tau_{11} = \tau_{18} = \tau_{22} = \tau_{27} = \tau_{11}^* = \tau_{81}^* = \tau_{22}^* = \tau_{72}^* = \frac{1}{\sqrt{2\rho^0}},$$

$$\tau_{81} = -\tau_{88} = \tau_{72} = -\tau_{77} = \tau^*_{18} = -\tau^*_{88} = \tau^*_{27} = -\tau^*_{77} = -\frac{1}{\sqrt{2s^0_{44}}},$$

$$\tau_{10,10} = \tau_{10,14} = \tau_{11,11} = \tau_{11,13} = \tau^*_{10,10} = \tau^*_{14,10} = \tau^*_{11,11} = \tau^*_{13,11} = \frac{1}{\sqrt{2\varepsilon^0}},$$

$$\tau_{14,10} = -\tau_{14,14} = \tau_{13,11} = -\tau_{13,13} = \tau^*_{14,10} = -\tau^*_{14,14} = \tau^*_{11,13} = -\tau^*_{13,13} = \frac{1}{\sqrt{2\mu^0}},$$

$$\tau_{35} = \tau_{36} = \frac{1}{\sqrt{\rho^0}}, \qquad \tau_{43} = \tau_{53} = \frac{3}{\sqrt{2(s^0_{11} + 2s^0_{12})}},$$

$$\tau_{44} = \frac{\sqrt{2(s^0_{11} + 2s^0_{12})} + \sqrt{3(s^0_{11} - s^0_{12})}}{2\sqrt{(s^0_{11} - s^0_{12})(s^0_{11} + 2s^0_{12})}},$$

$$\tau_{45} = -\tau_{46} = \tau_{55} = -\tau_{56} = -\frac{s^0_{12}}{3\sqrt{(s^0_{11} - s^0_{12})(s^0_{11} + 2s^0_{12})}},$$

$$\tau_{54} = -\frac{\sqrt{2(s^0_{11} + 2s^0_{12})} - \sqrt{3(s^0_{11} - s^0_{12})}}{2\sqrt{(s^0_{11} - s^0_{12})(s^0_{11} + 2s^0_{12})}},$$

$$\tau_{65} = -\tau_{66} = \sqrt{\frac{s^0_{11} + s^0_{12}}{(s^0_{11} - s^0_{12})(s^0_{11} + 2s^0_{12})}},$$

$$\tau^*_{34} = \frac{\sqrt{2(s^0_{11} + 2s^0_{12})(s^0_{11} - s^0_{12})} - \sqrt{3}(s^0_{11} + s^0_{12})}{6\sqrt{(s^0_{11} - s^0_{12})(s^0_{11} + s^0_{12})}},$$

$$\tau^*_{35} = \frac{\sqrt{2(s^0_{11} + 2s^0_{12})(s^0_{11} - s^0_{12})} + \sqrt{3}(s^0_{11} + s^0_{12})}{6\sqrt{(s^0_{11} - s^0_{12})(s^0_{11} + s^0_{12})}},$$

$$\tau^*_{44} = -\tau^*_{45} = -\frac{1}{\sqrt{2(s^0_{11} - s^0_{12})}}, \qquad \tau^*_{53} = -\tau^*_{63} = \frac{1}{2\sqrt{\rho^0}},$$

$$\tau_{54}^* = \tau_{55}^* = -\tau_{64}^* = -\tau_{65}^* = \frac{s_{12}^0}{2\sqrt{(s_{11}^0 - s_{12}^0)(s_{11}^0 + 2s_{12}^0)}},$$

$$\tau_{56}^* = -\tau_{66}^* = \frac{1}{2}\sqrt{\frac{s_{11}^0 + s_{12}^0}{(s_{11}^0 - s_{12}^0)(s_{11}^0 + 2s_{12}^0)}},$$

all different elements are equal to zero. The matrix D_0 has the following representation:

$$D_0 = \mathrm{diag}(\lambda_j^0, \quad j = \overline{1,15}),$$

where

$$\lambda_1^0 = \lambda_2^0 = -\lambda_7^0 = -\lambda_8^0 = \frac{1}{\sqrt{s_{44}^0 \rho^0}},$$

$$\lambda_5^0 = -\lambda_6^0 = -\sqrt{\frac{s_{11}^0 + s_{12}^0}{\rho^0 (s_{11}^0 - s_{12}^0)(s_{11}^0 + 2s_{12}^0)}},$$

$$\lambda_{10}^0 = -\lambda_{11}^0 = \lambda_{13}^0 = -\lambda_{14}^0 = \frac{1}{\sqrt{\varepsilon^0 \mu^0}},$$

$$\lambda_j^0 = 0, \quad j = 3,4,9,12,15.$$

Let us introduce the function

$$\tilde{V}^1(\nu, x_3, t, \kappa) = T\tilde{U}^1(\nu, x_3, t, \kappa). \tag{6.5}$$

Equalities (6.1)–(6.3) have the following forms in the term of the function $\tilde{V}^1(\nu, x_3, t, \kappa)$:

$$\left[I\frac{\partial}{\partial t} + D_0 \frac{\partial}{\partial x_3}\right] \tilde{V}^1(t, x_3, \nu, \kappa) - i\nu B\tilde{V}^1(t, x_3, \nu, \kappa) = \tilde{f}^1(t, x_3, \nu, \kappa), \quad 0 \le x_3 \le H, \tag{6.6}$$

$$\tilde{V}^1\big|_{t<0} = 0, \tag{6.7}$$

$$\tilde{V}_j^1\big|_{x_3=0} = 0, \quad j = 1,2,6,10,13,$$

$$\tilde{V}_j^1\big|_{x_3=H} = 0, \quad j = 5,7,8,11,14. \tag{6.8}$$

where

$$\nu B = \sum_{k=1}^{2} \nu_k T^* A_k^0, \tag{6.9}$$

$$\tilde{f}^1(\nu,x_3,t,\kappa) = T^*\tilde{f}(t,x_3,\nu,\kappa). \tag{6.10}$$

Equality (6.6) may be rewritten along of the every characteristic

$$(\xi - x_3) - \lambda_j(\tau - t) = 0$$

as

$$\frac{d}{d\tau}\left[\tilde{V}^1\right](x_3,t,\nu,\kappa,\tau) - i\nu B[\tilde{V}^1](x_3,t,\nu,\kappa,\tau) = [\tilde{f}^1](x_3,t,\nu,\kappa,\tau),$$

where

$$\frac{d}{d\tau}\left[\tilde{V}^1\right](x_3,t,\nu,\kappa,\tau) = \left(\frac{d}{d\tau}\left(\tilde{V}_j^1(\nu,x_3+\lambda_j(t-\tau),\tau,\kappa)\right),\quad j=\overline{1,15}\right),$$

$$\left[\tilde{V}^1\right](x_3,t,\nu,\kappa,\tau) = \left(\tilde{V}_j^1(\nu,x_3+\lambda_j(t-\tau),\tau,\kappa),\quad j=\overline{1,15}\right),$$

$$\left[\tilde{f}^1\right](x_3,t,\nu,\kappa,\tau) = \left(\tilde{f}_j^1(\tau,x_3+\lambda_j(t-\tau),\nu,\kappa),\quad j=\overline{1,15}\right).$$

Therefore the solution of problem (6.6)–(6.8) may be found by the following formula:

$$\tilde{V}^1(\nu,x_3,t,\kappa) = \exp(i\nu tB)\int_0^t K(x_3,t,\tau)\exp(-i\nu\tau B)[\tilde{f}^1](\tau,x_3+\lambda_j\tau,\nu,\kappa)d\tau, \tag{6.11}$$

where

$$K(x_3,t,\tau) = \left(\theta(\tau - t_j^*(x_3,t)),\quad j=\overline{1,15}\right),$$

the value of the function $t_j^*(x_3,t)$ in the fixed point (x_3,t) is determined as the value of the variable $\tau \in [0,t]$ for which the characteristic $(\xi - x_3) - \lambda_j(\tau - t) = 0$ intersects the axis $\xi = 0$ or the direct line $\xi = H$ or the axis $\tau = 0$. The confirmation of Theorem 6.1 follows from Lemma 6.3, formulas (6.9)–(6.11) and the theory of integral equations of the Volterra type.

7. INVERSE LINEARIZED PROBLEM

In this section we describe the inverse problem to determine unknown functions $\varepsilon^1(x)$, $s_{11}^1(x)$, $s_{44}^1(x)$, $e_{14}^1(x)$ which appear in differential equations (4.11)–(4.13). Moreover we suppose that vector-function U^0, which appearing in system (4.11), is the solution of initial boundary value problem (4.8)–(4.10) for

$$g^1 = e^1\delta(x_1)\delta(x_2)\theta(t),$$

$$g^2 = e^2\delta(x_1)\delta(x_2)\theta(t),$$

where $e^1 = 0, \quad e^2 = (1,0,1,0,1)$.

This inverse problem solving is the part of inverse linearized problem 1 solving. The main object of our investigation in this section is the following inverse problem.

Inverse linearized problem 2. Let ρ^0, s_{11}^0, s_{12}^0, s_{44}^0, ε^0, μ^0 be given constants satisfying conditions (4.3); $s_{12}^1(x)$, $\rho^1(x)$, $\mu^1(x)$ be given functions from the class $C_0^1(R^2 \times [0,H])$; $s_{44}^1(x)$, $\varepsilon^1(x)$, $s_{11}^1(x)$, $e_{14}^1(x)$ be unknown functions from the class $C_0^1(R^2 \times [0,H])$.

Find unknown functions $s_{44}^1(x)$, $\varepsilon^1(x)$, $e_{14}^1(x)$, $s_{11}^1(x)$ if it is given the additional information about the solution $U^1(x,t,x_1^0,x_2^0)$ of problem (4.11)–(4.13):

$$\tilde{V}_j^1(\nu_1,\nu_2,x_3,t,\kappa)\big|_{\nu_1=\nu_2=0,x_3=H} = h_j(\kappa_1,\kappa_2,t), \quad j=1,6,10,13, \tag{7.1}$$

where the vector-function $\tilde{V}^1(\nu_1,\nu_2,x_3,t,\kappa)$ is determined by means of formulas (6.4), (6.5); $h_j(\kappa_1,\kappa_2,t)$, $\quad j=1,6,10,13$ are given functions.

Let us introduce the numbers:

$$a_{33} = \frac{3(s_{11}^0+s_{12}^0)-2(s_{12}^0)^2}{6\Delta}, \quad \Delta = (s_{11}^0-s_{12}^0)(s_{11}^0+2s_{12}^0).$$

The main result of this section consists in the following uniqueness theorem of the inverse linearized problem 2 solution.

Theorem 7.1. *Let H be a fixed positive number; ρ^0, s_{11}^0, s_{12}^0, s_{44}^0, ε^0, μ^0 be given constants satisfying conditions (4.3), and $a_{33} \neq 0$. Then the solution of inverse linearized problem 2 is uniquely determined in the class $C_0^1(\mathbf{R}^2 \times [0,H])$ by means of additional information (7.1).*

Proof: Using given conditions we find that the Fourier images of the functions $\rho^1(x)$, $\varepsilon^1(x)$, $s_{11}^1(x)$, $s_{12}^1(x)$, $s_{44}^1(x)$, $\mu^1(x)$, $e_{14}^1(x)$ respect to the variables x_1, x_2 are the analytic functions respect to the parameters of the Fourier transformation. Therefore these Fourier images $\tilde{\rho}^1(\kappa_1,\kappa_2,x_3)$, $\tilde{\varepsilon}^1(\kappa_1,\kappa_2,x_3)$, $\tilde{s}_{11}^1(\kappa_1,\kappa_2,x_3)$, $\tilde{s}_{12}^1(\kappa_1,\kappa_2,x_3)$, $\tilde{s}_{44}^1(\kappa_1,\kappa_2,x_3)$, $\tilde{\mu}^1(\kappa_1,\kappa_2,x_3)$, $\tilde{e}_{14}^1(\kappa_1,\kappa_2,x_3)$ may be represented by means of the power Taylor series respect to the powers of the parameters κ_1,κ_2. The coefficients of these series depend on one variable x_3 only. Further we shall describe the process of successive determination of the coefficients of the power series of unknown functions $\tilde{\varepsilon}^1(\kappa_1,\kappa_2,x_3)$, $\tilde{s}_{11}^1(\kappa_1,\kappa_2,x_3)$, $\tilde{s}_{12}^1(\kappa_1,\kappa_2,x_3)$, $\tilde{s}_{44}^1(\kappa_1,\kappa_2,x_3)$, $\tilde{e}_{14}^1(\kappa_1,\kappa_2,x_3)$. For this case it is necessary to study in detail the structure of the traces $\tilde{U}^0(\nu,x_3,t)\big|_{\nu_1=0,\nu_2=0}$, and $\tilde{U}^1(\nu,x_3,t,\kappa_1,\kappa_2)\big|_{\nu_1=0,\nu_2=0}$.

First, we consider problem (5.5)–(5.7) and the following denotation:

$$U^{01} = \text{column} \quad (\tilde{U}_1^0,\tilde{U}_8^0), \qquad U^{02} = \text{column} \quad (\tilde{U}_2^0,\tilde{U}_7^0),$$

$$U^{03} = \text{column} \quad (\tilde{U}_3^0,\tilde{U}_4^0,\tilde{U}_5^0,\tilde{U}_6^0),$$

$$U^{04} = \text{column} \quad (\tilde{U}_{10}^0,\tilde{U}_{14}^0), \qquad U^{05} = \text{column} \quad (\tilde{U}_{11}^0,\tilde{U}_{13}^0),$$

$$U^{06} = \tilde{U}_9^0, \quad U^{07} = \tilde{U}_{12}^0, \quad U^{08} = \tilde{U}_{15}^0,$$

$$g^{k1} = \text{column} \quad (g_1^k,g_8^k), \qquad g^{k2} = \text{column} \quad (g_2^k,g_7^k),$$

$$g^{k3} = \text{column} \quad (g_3^k,g_4^k,g_5^k,g_6^k),$$

$$g^{k4} = \text{column} \quad (g_{10}^k,g_{14}^k), \qquad g^{k5} = \text{column} \quad (g_{11}^k,g_{13}^k),$$

$$g^{k6} = g_9^k, \quad g^{k7} = g_{12}^k, \quad g^{k8} = g_{15}^k.$$

Equations system (4.8) is decomposed on several equations systems for $\nu_1 = \nu_2 = 0$ and therefore problem (4.8)–(4.10) may be rewritten in the block form:

$$\left(A_0^{0J} \frac{\partial}{\partial t} + A_3^{0J} \frac{\partial}{\partial x_3} \right) U^{0J} = 0, \quad 0 \le x_3 \le H, \tag{7.2}$$

$$U^{0J}|_{t<0} = 0, \tag{7.3}$$

$$G^{1J} U^{0J}|_{x_3=0} = g_1^{1J}(t),$$

$$G^{2J} U^{0J}|_{x_3=H} = g_2^{2J}(t), \tag{7.4}$$

where $J = \overline{1,8}$,

$$A_0^{0J} = \operatorname{diag} \quad (\rho^0, s_{44}^0), \quad J = 1,2$$

$$A_0^{03} = \begin{pmatrix} \rho^0 & 0 & 0 & 0 \\ 0 & s_{11}^0 & s_{12}^0 & s_{12}^0 \\ 0 & s_{12}^0 & s_{11}^0 & s_{12}^0 \\ 0 & s_{12}^0 & s_{12}^0 & s_{11}^0 \end{pmatrix},$$

$$A_0^{0J} = \operatorname{diag} \quad (\varepsilon^0, \mu^0), \quad J = 4,5,$$

$$A_0^{06} = s_{44}^0, \quad A_0^{07} = \varepsilon^0, \quad A_0^{08} = \mu^0,$$

$$A_3^{0J} = \begin{pmatrix} 0 & -1 \\ -1 & 0 \end{pmatrix}, \quad J = 1,2,4, \qquad A_3^{03} = \begin{pmatrix} 0 & 0 & 0 & -1 \\ 0 & 0 & 0 & 0 \\ 0 & 0 & 0 & 0 \\ -1 & 0 & 0 & 0 \end{pmatrix},$$

$$A_3^{05} = \begin{pmatrix} 0 & 1 \\ 1 & 0 \end{pmatrix}, \qquad A_3^{0J} = 0, \quad J = 6,7,8,$$

$$G^{i1} = \begin{pmatrix} G_{11}^i & G_{18}^i \end{pmatrix}, \quad i = 1,2,$$

$$G^{i2} = \begin{pmatrix} G_{22}^i & G_{27}^i \end{pmatrix}, \quad i = 1,2,$$

$$G^{i3} = \begin{pmatrix} G_{33}^i & G_{34}^i & G_{35}^i & G_{36}^i \end{pmatrix}, \quad i = 1,2,$$

$$G^{i4} = \begin{pmatrix} G^i_{4.10} & G^i_{4.14} \end{pmatrix}, \quad i = 1,2,$$

$$G^{i5} = \begin{pmatrix} G^i_{5.11} & G^i_{5.13} \end{pmatrix}, \quad i = 1,2.$$

We reduce differential equations system (7.2) to the canonical form. For this case we consider such matrices T_0^J, T_0^{*J} that $T_0^{*J}A_0^{0J}T_0^J = I$, $T_0^{*J}A_3^{0J}T_0^J = D_0^J$, $J = \overline{1,8}$, where D_0^J is the diagonal matrix, I is the unit matrix. The matrices T_0^J, T_0^{*J}, $J = \overline{1,8}$ have the following form:

$$T_0^j = \begin{pmatrix} \frac{1}{\sqrt{2\rho^0}} & \frac{1}{\sqrt{2\rho^0}} \\ -\frac{1}{\sqrt{2s_{44}^0}} & \frac{1}{\sqrt{2s_{44}^0}} \end{pmatrix}, \qquad T_0^{*j} = \begin{pmatrix} \frac{1}{\sqrt{2\rho^0}} & -\frac{1}{\sqrt{2s_{44}^0}} \\ \frac{1}{\sqrt{2\rho^0}} & \frac{1}{\sqrt{2s_{44}^0}} \end{pmatrix}, \quad j = 1,2,$$

$$T_0^j = \begin{pmatrix} \frac{1}{\sqrt{\varepsilon^0}} & \frac{1}{\sqrt{\varepsilon^0}} \\ -\frac{1}{\sqrt{\mu^0}} & \frac{1}{\sqrt{\mu^0}} \end{pmatrix}, \qquad T_0^{*j} = \begin{pmatrix} \frac{1}{\sqrt{\varepsilon^0}} & -\frac{1}{\sqrt{\mu^0}} \\ \frac{1}{\sqrt{\varepsilon^0}} & \frac{1}{\sqrt{\mu^0}} \end{pmatrix}, \quad j = 4,5,$$

$$T_0^3 = \begin{pmatrix} 0 & 0 & t_{13} & t_{13} \\ t_{21} & t_{22} & t_{23} & -t_{23} \\ t_{21} & t_{32} & t_{23} & -t_{23} \\ 0 & 0 & t_{43} & -t_{43} \end{pmatrix},$$

$$t_{13} = \frac{1}{\sqrt{\rho^0}}, \quad t_{21} = \frac{3}{\sqrt{2(s_{11}^0 + 2s_{12}^0)}}, \qquad t_{22} = \frac{\sqrt{2(s_{11}^0 + 2s_{12}^0)} + \sqrt{3(s_{11}^0 - s_{12}^0)}}{2\sqrt{(s_{11}^0 - s_{12}^0)(s_{11}^0 + 2s_{12}^0)}},$$

$$t_{23} = -\frac{s_{12}^0}{3\sqrt{(s_{11}^0 - s_{12}^0)(s_{11}^0 + 2s_{12}^0)}}, \qquad t_{32} = -\frac{\sqrt{2(s_{11}^0 + 2s_{12}^0)} - \sqrt{3(s_{11}^0 - s_{12}^0)}}{2\sqrt{(s_{11}^0 - s_{12}^0)(s_{11}^0 + 2s_{12}^0)}},$$

$$t_{43} = \sqrt{\frac{s_{11}^0 + s_{12}^0}{(s_{11}^0 - s_{12}^0)(s_{11}^0 + 2s_{12}^0)}},$$

$$T_0^{3*} = \begin{pmatrix} 0 & t_{12}^* & t_{13}^* & 0 \\ 0 & t_{22}^* & -t_{22}^* & 0 \\ t_{31}^* & t_{32}^* & t_{32}^* & t_{34}^* \\ t_{31}^* & -t_{32}^* & -t_{32}^* & -t_{34}^* \end{pmatrix},$$

$$t_{12}^* = \frac{\sqrt{2(s_{11}^0 + 2s_{12}^0)(s_{11}^0 - s_{12}^0)} - \sqrt{3}(s_{11}^0 + s_{12}^0)}{6\sqrt{(s_{11}^0 - s_{12}^0)(s_{11}^0 + s_{12}^0)}},$$

$$t_{13}^* = \frac{\sqrt{2(s_{11}^0 + 2s_{12}^0)(s_{11}^0 - s_{12}^0)} + \sqrt{3}(s_{11}^0 + s_{12}^0)}{6\sqrt{(s_{11}^0 - s_{12}^0)(s_{11}^0 + s_{12}^0)}},$$

$$t_{22}^* = -\frac{1}{\sqrt{2(s_{11}^0 - s_{12}^0)}}, \quad t_{31}^* = \frac{1}{2\sqrt{\rho^0}}, \quad t_{32}^* = \frac{s_{12}^0}{2\sqrt{(s_{11}^0 - s_{12}^0)(s_{11}^0 + 2s_{12}^0)}},$$

$$t_{34}^* = \frac{1}{2}\sqrt{\frac{s_{11}^0 + s_{12}^0}{(s_{11}^0 - s_{12}^0)(s_{11}^0 + 2s_{12}^0)}},$$

$$T_0^6 = T_0^{*6} = \frac{1}{\sqrt{s_{44}^0}}, \quad T_0^7 = T_0^{*7} = \frac{1}{\sqrt{\varepsilon^0}}, \quad T_0^8 = T_0^{*8} = \frac{1}{\sqrt{\mu^0}}.$$

Further we use the following notations

$$V^{0j} = T_0^j U^{0j}, \quad j = \overline{1,8}, \quad V^0 = (V_j^0, \quad j = \overline{1,15}),$$

$$V^{01} = \text{column} \quad (V_1^0, V_8^0), \qquad V^{02} = \text{column} \quad (V_2^0, V_7^0),$$

$$V^{03} = \text{column} \quad (V_3^0, V_4^0, V_5^0, V_6^0),$$

$$V^{04} = \text{column} \quad (V_{10}^0, V_{14}^0), \qquad V^{05} = \text{column} \quad (V_{11}^0, V_{13}^0),$$

$$V^{06} = V_9^0, \quad V^{07} = V_{12}^0, \quad V^{08} = V_{15}^0.$$

Equations (7.2)–(7.4) in the terms of the vector functions V^{0J}, $J = \overline{1,8}$, V_i^0, $i = \overline{1,15}$ have the form:

$$\left(I\frac{\partial}{\partial t} + D_0^J \frac{\partial}{\partial x_3}\right) V^{0J} = 0, \quad 0 \le x_3 \le H, \tag{7.5}$$

$$V^{0J}|_{t<0} = 0, \tag{7.6}$$

$$V_i^0|_{x_3=0} = g_i^1(t), \qquad i = 1,2,6,10,13,$$

$$V_i^0|_{x_3=H} = g_i^2(t), \qquad i = 5,7,8,11,14, \tag{7.7}$$

where $J = \overline{1,8}$,

$$D_0^j = \text{diag}(\lambda_1^0, -\lambda_1^0), \quad j = 1,2, \lambda_1^0 = \frac{1}{\sqrt{s_{44}^0 \rho^0}},$$

$$D_0^3 = \mathrm{diag}(0,0,-\lambda_2^0,\lambda_2^0), \quad \lambda_2^0 = \sqrt{\frac{s_{11}^0 + s_{12}^0}{\rho^0 (s_{11}^0 - s_{12}^0)(s_{11}^0 + 2s_{12}^0)}},$$

$$D_0^4 = \mathrm{diag}(\lambda_3^0, -\lambda_3^0), \quad \lambda_3^0 = \frac{1}{\sqrt{\varepsilon^0 \mu^0}},$$

$$D_0^5 = \mathrm{diag}(-\lambda_3^0, \lambda_3^0), \qquad D_0^j = 0, \quad j = 6,7,8.$$

The solution of problem (7.5)–(7.7) is determined by the following explicit formulas:

$$V_j^0 = \theta(t) \qquad g_j^1\left(t - \frac{x_3}{\lambda_1^0}\right), \quad j = 1,2,$$

$$V_5^0 = \theta(t) \qquad g_5^2\left(t - \frac{x_3 - H}{\lambda_2^0}\right), \qquad V_6^0 = \theta(t) \qquad g_6^1\left(t - \frac{x_3}{\lambda_2^0}\right),$$

$$V_j^0 = \theta(t) \qquad g_j^2\left(t - \frac{x_3 - H}{\lambda_1^0}\right), \quad j = 7,8, \tag{7.8}$$

$$V_j^0 = \theta(t) \qquad g_j^1\left(t - \frac{x_3}{\lambda_3^0}\right), \quad j = 10,13,$$

$$V_j^0 = \theta(t) \qquad g_j^2\left(t - \frac{x_3 - H}{\lambda_3^0}\right), \quad j = 11,14,$$

$$V_j^0 = 0, \quad j = 3,4,9,12,15.$$

Let us consider problem (4.11)–(4.13). These equations may be rewritten for $\nu_1 = \nu_2 = 0$ in the form:

$$\left(\mathcal{A}_0^{0J}\frac{\partial}{\partial t} + \mathcal{A}_3^{0J}\frac{\partial}{\partial x_3}\right)\mathcal{U}^{1J} =$$

$$= -\left[\tilde{\mathcal{A}}_0^{1J}(\kappa,x_3)\frac{\partial}{\partial t} + \tilde{\mathcal{A}}_3^{1J}(\kappa,x_3)\frac{\partial}{\partial x_3} + \tilde{\mathfrak{Q}}^{1J}(\kappa,x_3)\right]\mathcal{U}^{0J}(-\kappa,x_3,t), \quad 0 \le x_3 \le H, \tag{7.9}$$

$$\mathcal{U}^{1J}|_{t<0} = 0, \tag{7.10}$$

$$G^{1J}U^{1I}|_{x_3=0} = 0,$$

$$G^{2J}U^{1I}|_{x_3=H} = 0, \quad I = \overline{1,8}, \tag{7.11}$$

where $J = \overline{1,6}$,

$$\mathcal{A}_0^{01} = \text{diag} \quad (A_0^{01}, A_0^{04}), \qquad \mathcal{A}_3^{01} = \text{diag} \quad (A_3^{01}, A_3^{05}), \qquad \mathcal{A}_0^{02} = \mathcal{A}_0^{03},$$

$$\mathcal{A}_3^{02} = \mathcal{A}_3^{03}, \qquad \mathcal{A}_0^{03} = \text{diag} \quad (A_0^{02}, A_0^{04}), \qquad \mathcal{A}_3^{03} = \text{diag} \quad (A_3^{02}, A_3^{04}),$$

$$\mathcal{A}_0^{04} = A_0^{06}, \qquad \mathcal{A}_0^{05} = A_0^{07}, \qquad \mathcal{A}_0^{06} = A_0^{08}, \qquad \mathcal{A}_0^{0j} = 0, \quad j = 4,5,6;$$

$$\mathcal{A}_0^{1j} = \text{diag} \quad (\tilde{\rho}^1(\kappa_1,\kappa_2,x_3), \tilde{s}_{44}^1(\kappa_1,\kappa_2,x_3), \tilde{\varepsilon}^1(\kappa_1,\kappa_2,x_3), \tilde{\mu}^1(\kappa_1,\kappa_2,x_3)), \quad j = 1,3;$$

$$\mathcal{A}_3^{1J} = \begin{pmatrix} 0 & 0 & \tilde{e}_{14}^1 & 0 \\ 0 & 0 & 0 & 0 \\ \tilde{e}_{14}^1 & 0 & 0 & 1 \\ 0 & 0 & 1 & 0 \end{pmatrix}, \quad \mathcal{Q}^{1J} = \begin{pmatrix} 0 & 0 & \tilde{e}_{14}^{1\prime} & 0 \\ 0 & 0 & 0 & 0 \\ 0 & 0 & 0 & 0 \\ 0 & 0 & 0 & 0 \end{pmatrix} \quad J = 1,3,$$

$$\mathcal{A}_0^{12} = \begin{pmatrix} \tilde{\rho}^1 & 0 & 0 & 0 \\ 0 & \tilde{s}_{11}^1 & \tilde{s}_{12}^1 & \tilde{s}_{12}^1 \\ 0 & \tilde{s}_{12}^1 & \tilde{s}_{11}^1 & \tilde{s}_{12}^1 \\ 0 & \tilde{s}_{12}^1 & \tilde{s}_{12}^1 & \tilde{s}_{11}^1 \end{pmatrix}, \qquad \mathcal{A}_3^{12} = 0, \qquad \mathcal{Q}^{1J} = 0, \quad J = 2,4,5,6;$$

$$\mathcal{A}_3^{14} = \tilde{s}_{44}^1, \qquad \mathcal{A}_3^{15} = \tilde{\varepsilon}^1, \qquad \mathcal{A}_3^{16} = \tilde{\mu}^1,$$

$$\mathcal{U}^{11} = \text{column} \quad (\tilde{U}_1^1, \tilde{U}_8^1, \tilde{U}_{11}^1, \tilde{U}_{13}^1), \quad \mathcal{U}^{12} = \text{column} \quad (\tilde{U}_3^1, \tilde{U}_4^1, \tilde{U}_5^1, \tilde{U}_6^1),$$

$$\mathcal{U}^{13} = \text{column} \quad (\tilde{U}_2^1, \tilde{U}_7^1, \tilde{U}_{10}^1, \tilde{U}_{14}^1), \quad \mathcal{U}^{14} = \tilde{U}_9^1, \quad \mathcal{U}^{15} = \tilde{U}_{12}^1, \quad \mathcal{U}^{16} = \tilde{U}_{15}^1,$$

$$\mathcal{U}^{01} = \text{column} \quad (\tilde{U}_1^0, \tilde{U}_8^0, \tilde{U}_{11}^0, \tilde{U}_{13}^0), \quad \mathcal{U}^{02} = \text{column} \quad (\tilde{U}_3^0, \tilde{U}_4^0, \tilde{U}_5^0, \tilde{U}_6^0),$$

$$\mathcal{U}^{03} = \text{column} \quad (\tilde{U}_2^0, \tilde{U}_7^0, \tilde{U}_{10}^0, \tilde{U}_{14}^0), \quad \mathcal{U}^{04} = \tilde{U}_9^0, \quad \mathcal{U}^{05} = \tilde{U}_{12}^0, \quad \mathcal{U}^{06} = \tilde{U}_{15}^0.$$

We rewrite differential equations system (7.9)–(7.11) in the canonical form. For this case we consider such matrices T_1^j, T_1^{*j} that $T_1^{*j}\mathcal{A}_0^{0j}T_1^j = I$, $T_1^{*j}\mathcal{A}_3^{0j}T_1^j = \mathcal{D}_1^j, j = \overline{1,6}$, where I is the unit matrix, $\mathcal{D}$ is the diagonal matrix. The matrices T_1^j, T_1^{*j} have the following structure:

$$T_1^1 = \begin{pmatrix} T_0^1 & 0 \\ 0 & T_0^5 \end{pmatrix}, \qquad T_1^3 = \begin{pmatrix} T_0^2 & 0 \\ 0 & T_0^4 \end{pmatrix},$$

$$T_1^2 = T_0^3, \quad T_1^4 = T_0^6, \quad T_1^5 = T_0^7, \quad T_1^6 = T_0^8.$$

We use the following notations:

$$\mathcal{V}^{1j} = T_1^j \mathcal{U}^{1j}, \quad j = \overline{1,6}, \quad V^1 = (V_i^1, \quad i = \overline{1,15}).$$

We remark that the following correlations take place:

$$\mathcal{V}^{11} = \text{column} \quad (V_1^1, V_8^1, V_{11}^1, V_{13}^1), \quad \mathcal{V}^{12} = \text{column} \quad (V_3^1, V_4^1, V_5^1, V_6^1),$$

$$\mathcal{V}^{13} = \text{column} \quad (V_2^1, V_7^1, V_{10}^1, V_{14}^1), \quad \mathcal{V}^{14} = V_9^1, \quad \mathcal{V}^{15} = V_{12}^1, \quad \mathcal{V}^{16} = V_{15}^1.$$

Equations system (7.9)–(7.11) has the following form in the term of $\mathcal{V}^{1j}$, $j = \overline{1,6}$:

$$\left(I\frac{\partial}{\partial t} + \mathcal{D}_1^J \frac{\partial}{\partial x_3} \right) \mathcal{V}^{1J} =$$

$$= - \left[\hat{\mathcal{A}}_0^J \frac{\partial}{\partial t} + \hat{\mathcal{A}}_3^J \frac{\partial}{\partial x_3} + \hat{\mathcal{Q}}^J \right] \mathcal{V}^{0J}(-\kappa, x_3, t), \quad 0 \le x_3 \le H, \tag{7.12}$$

$$\mathcal{V}^{1J}|_{t<0} = 0, \tag{7.13}$$

$$\mathcal{V}_i^1|_{x_3=0} = 0, \qquad i = 1, 2, 6, 10, 13,$$

$$\mathcal{V}_i^1|_{x_3=H} = 0, \qquad i = 5, 7, 8, 11, 14, \tag{7.14}$$

where $J = \overline{1,6}$,

$$\mathcal{D}_1^1 = \text{diag}(\lambda_1^0, -\lambda_1^0, -\lambda_3^0, \lambda_3^0),$$

$$\mathcal{D}_1^2 = D_0^2, \quad \mathcal{D}_1^3 = \text{diag}(\lambda_1^0, -\lambda_1^0, \lambda_3^0, -\lambda_3^0), \qquad \mathcal{D}_0^j = 0, \quad j = 4, 5, 6,$$

$$\hat{\mathcal{A}}_0^J = T_1^{*j} \tilde{\mathcal{A}}_0^{1J} T_1^j, \quad \hat{\mathcal{A}}_3^J = T_1^{*j} \tilde{\mathcal{A}}_3^{1J} T_1^j, \quad \hat{\mathcal{Q}}^J = T_1^{*j} \tilde{\mathcal{Q}}_3^{1J} T_1^j,$$

$$\hat{\mathcal{A}}_0^J = \begin{pmatrix} R^1 & 0 \\ 0 & R^2 \end{pmatrix}, \quad \hat{\mathcal{A}}_3^J = \begin{pmatrix} D_0^1 & R^3 \\ R^3 & D_0^4 \end{pmatrix}, \quad \hat{\mathcal{Q}}^J = \begin{pmatrix} 0 & R^4 \\ 0 & 0 \end{pmatrix}, \quad J = 1, 3,$$

$$R^1 = \begin{pmatrix} \frac{1}{2\rho^0}\tilde{\rho}^1 + \frac{1}{2s_{44}^0}\tilde{s}_{44}^1 & \frac{1}{2\rho^0}\tilde{\rho}^1 - \frac{1}{2s_{44}^0}\tilde{s}_{44}^1 \\ \frac{1}{2\rho^0}\tilde{\rho}^1 - \frac{1}{2s_{44}^0}\tilde{s}_{44}^1 & \frac{1}{2\rho^0}\tilde{\rho}^1 + \frac{1}{2s_{44}^0}\tilde{s}_{44}^1 \end{pmatrix},$$

$$R^2 = \begin{pmatrix} \frac{1}{2\varepsilon^0}\tilde{\varepsilon}^1 + \frac{1}{2\mu^0}\tilde{\mu}^1 & \frac{1}{2\varepsilon^0}\tilde{\varepsilon}^1 - \frac{1}{2\mu^0}\tilde{\mu}^1 \\ \frac{1}{2\varepsilon^0}\tilde{\varepsilon}^1 - \frac{1}{2\mu^0}\tilde{\mu}^1 & \frac{1}{2\varepsilon^0}\tilde{\varepsilon}^1 + \frac{1}{2\mu^0}\tilde{\mu}^1 \end{pmatrix},$$

$$R^3 = \begin{pmatrix} -\frac{1}{2\varepsilon^0\rho^0}\tilde{e}_{14}^1 & -\frac{1}{2\varepsilon^0\rho^0}\tilde{e}_{14}^1 \\ -\frac{1}{2\varepsilon^0\rho^0}\tilde{e}_{14}^1 & -\frac{1}{2\varepsilon^0\rho^0}\tilde{e}_{14}^1 \end{pmatrix}, \quad R^4 = \begin{pmatrix} \frac{1}{2\varepsilon^0\rho^0}\tilde{e}_{14}^{1\prime} & \frac{1}{2\varepsilon^0\rho^0}\tilde{e}_{14}^{1\prime} \\ \frac{1}{2\varepsilon^0\rho^0}\tilde{e}_{14}^{1\prime} & \frac{1}{2\varepsilon^0\rho^0}\tilde{e}_{14}^{1\prime} \end{pmatrix},$$

$$\hat{\mathcal{A}}_0^2$$

$$\begin{pmatrix} a_{11}\tilde{s}_{11}^1 + a_{11}\tilde{s}_{12}^1 & a_{12}\tilde{s}_{11}^1 + b_{12}\tilde{s}_{12}^1 & a_{13}\tilde{s}_{11}^1 + b_{13}\tilde{s}_{12}^1 & -a_{13}\tilde{s}_{11}^1 - b_{13}\tilde{s}_{12}^1 \\ 0 & a_{22}\tilde{s}_{11}^1 + a_{22}\tilde{s}_{12}^1 & 0 & 0 \\ a_{31}\tilde{s}_{11}^1 + b_{31}\tilde{s}_{12}^1 & a_{32}\tilde{s}_{11}^1 + a_{32}\tilde{s}_{12}^1 & r\tilde{\rho}^1 + a_{33}\tilde{s}_{11}^1 + b_{33}\tilde{s}_{12}^1 & r\tilde{\rho}^1 - a_{33}\tilde{s}_{11}^1 - b_{33}\tilde{s}_{12}^1 \\ -a_{31}\tilde{s}_{11}^1 - b_{31}\tilde{s}_{12}^1 & -a_{32}\tilde{s}_{11}^1 + b_{42}\tilde{s}_{12}^1 & r\tilde{\rho}^1 - a_{33}\tilde{s}_{11}^1 - b_{33}\tilde{s}_{12}^1 & r\tilde{\rho}^1 + a_{33}\tilde{s}_{11}^1 + b_{33}\tilde{s}_{12}^1 \end{pmatrix},$$

$$a_{11} = t_{21}(t_{12}^* + t_{13}^*), \qquad a_{12} = t_{12}^* t_{22} + t_{13}^* t_{32},$$

$$b_{12} = t_{12}^* t_{32} + t_{13}^* t_{22}, \qquad a_{13} = t_{12}^* t_{23} + t_{13}^* t_{23},$$

$$b_{13} = (t_{12}^* + t_{13}^*)(t_{23} + t_{43}), \qquad a_{22} = t_{22}^*(t_{22} - t_{32}),$$

$$a_{31} = 2t_{32}^* t_{21}, \qquad b_{31} = 2t_{21}(t_{32}^* + t_{34}^*),$$

$$a_{32} = t_{32}^*(t_{22} + t_{32}), \qquad r = \frac{1}{2\rho^0}, \qquad a_{33} = 2t_{32}^* t_{23} + t_{34}^* t_{43},$$

$$b_{34} = t_{32}^*(t_{23} + t_{22}) + t_{34}^* t_{23}, \qquad b_{42} = -(t_{32} + t_{22})(t_{34}^* + t_{34}^*),$$

$$\hat{A}_3^2 = \begin{pmatrix} 0 & 0 \\ 0 & R^5 \end{pmatrix}, \quad R^5 = \begin{pmatrix} r_{11} & r_{12} \\ -r_{12} & -r_{11} \end{pmatrix}, \quad b_{33} = 2[t_{32}^*(t_{23} + t_{43}) + t_{34}^* t_{23}],$$

$$r_{11} = -t_{34}^* \frac{1}{\rho^0} - t_{31}^* t_{43}, \qquad r_{12} = -t_{34}^* \frac{1}{\rho^0} + t_{31}^* t_{43},$$

$$\mathcal{V}^{01} = \text{column} \quad (V_1^0, V_8^0, V_{11}^0, V_{13}^0), \qquad \mathcal{V}^{12} = \text{column} \quad (V_3^0, V_4^0, V_5^0, V_6^0),$$

$$\mathcal{V}^{03} = \text{column} \quad (V_2^0, V_7^0, V_{10}^0, V_{14}^0),$$

$$\mathcal{V}^{04} = V_9^0, \quad \mathcal{V}^{05} = V_{12}^0, \quad \mathcal{V}^{06} = V_{15}^0.$$

We find the following equalities from equations (7.9)–(7.11) and (7.8):

$$V_1^1(0, x_3, t, 0) = -\frac{1}{2}\theta(t)\theta(t + \frac{x_3 - H}{\lambda_1^0})\theta(\frac{x_3 + H}{\lambda_1^0} - t) \times$$

$$\times \left[\frac{1}{2\rho^0}\tilde{\rho}^1(0, \frac{1}{2}(x_3 + H - \lambda_1^0 t)) - \frac{1}{2s_{44}^0}\tilde{s}_{44}^1(0, \frac{1}{2}(x_3 + H - \lambda_1^0 t)\right], \tag{7.15}$$

$$V_{10}^1(0,x_3,t,0) = -\frac{1}{2}\theta(t)\theta(t+\frac{x_3-H}{\lambda_3^0})\theta(\frac{x_3+H}{\lambda_3^0}-t)\times$$

$$\times\left[\frac{1}{2\varepsilon^0}\tilde{\varepsilon}^1(0,\frac{1}{2}(x_3+H-\lambda_3^0 t)) - \frac{1}{2\mu^0}\tilde{\mu}^1(0,\frac{1}{2}(x_3+H-\lambda_3^0 t)\right], \tag{7.16}$$

$$V_{13}^1(0,x_3,t,0) = \frac{1}{2\varepsilon^0\rho^0}\frac{1}{\lambda_3^0-\lambda_1^0}\theta(t)\theta(t-\frac{x_3}{\lambda_3^0})\theta(\frac{x_3}{\lambda_1^0}-t)$$

$$\tilde{e}_{14}^1(0,\frac{\lambda_1^0\lambda_3^0}{\lambda_3^0-\lambda_1^0}\left(t-\frac{x_3}{\lambda_3^0}\right)), \tag{7.17}$$

$$V_6^1(0,x_3,t,0) = -\frac{1}{2}\theta(t)\theta(t+\frac{x_3-H}{\lambda_2^0})\theta(\frac{x_3+H}{\lambda_2^0}-t)\times$$

$$\times\left[r\tilde{\rho}^1(0,\frac{1}{2}(x_3+H-\lambda_2^0 t)) + a_{33}\tilde{s}_{11}^1(0,\frac{1}{2}(x_3+H-\lambda_2^0 t)+\right.$$

$$\left.+b_{33}\tilde{s}_{12}^1(0,\frac{1}{2}(x_3+H-\lambda_2^0 t)\right], \tag{7.18}$$

where r, and the constants a_{33}, b_{33} are determined by the formulas which located above the formulation of Theorem 7.1.

Using additional information (7.8) for inverse problem 2 solving we obtain from equation (7.15)–(7.18):

$$h_1(0,t) = -\frac{1}{2}\theta(t)\theta(\frac{2H}{\lambda_1^0}-t)\left[\frac{1}{2\rho^0}\tilde{\rho}^1(0,H-\frac{\lambda_1^0}{2}t) - \frac{1}{2s_{44}^0}\tilde{s}_{44}^1(0,H-\frac{\lambda_1^0}{2}t)\right], \tag{7.19}$$

$$h_{10}(0,t) = -\frac{1}{2}\theta(t)\theta(\frac{2H}{\lambda_3^0}-t)\left[\frac{1}{2\varepsilon^0}\tilde{\varepsilon}^1(0,H-\frac{\lambda_3^0}{2}t) + \frac{1}{2\mu^0}\tilde{\mu}^1(0,H-\frac{\lambda_3^0}{2}t)\right], \tag{7.20}$$

$$h_{13}(0,t) = \frac{1}{2\varepsilon^0\rho^0}\frac{1}{\lambda_3^0-\lambda_1^0}\theta(t)\theta(t-\frac{H}{\lambda_3^0})\theta(\frac{H}{\lambda_1^0}-t)\tilde{e}_{14}^1(0,\frac{\lambda_1^0\lambda_3^0}{\lambda_3^0-\lambda_1^0}\left(t-\frac{H}{\lambda_3^0}\right)), \tag{7.21}$$

$$h_6(0,t) = -\frac{1}{2}\theta(t)\theta(\frac{2H}{\lambda_2^0}-t)\left[r\tilde{\rho}^1(0,H-\frac{\lambda_2^0}{2}t)+\right.$$

$$\left.+a_{33}\tilde{s}_{11}^1(0,H-\frac{\lambda_2^0}{2}t) + b_{33}\tilde{s}_{12}^1(0,H-\frac{\lambda_2^0}{2}t)\right], \tag{7.22}$$

Using equalities (7.19)–(7.22) we obtain the explicit formulas for determination of the functions $\tilde{s}^1_{44}(0,x_3)$, $\tilde{\varepsilon}^1(0,x_3)$, $\tilde{e}^1_{14}(0,x_3)$, $\tilde{s}^1_{11}(0,x_3)$ for $x_3 \in [0,H]$:

$$\tilde{s}^1_{44}(0,x_3) = s^0_{44}\left[\frac{1}{\rho^0}\tilde{\rho}^1(0,x_3) + 4h_1(0,\frac{2}{\lambda^0_1}(H-x_3))\right],$$

$$\tilde{\varepsilon}^1(0,x_3) = -\varepsilon^0\left[\frac{1}{\mu^0}\tilde{\mu}^1(0,x_3) + 4h_{10}(0,\frac{2}{\lambda^0_3}(H-x_3))\right],$$

$$\tilde{e}^1_{14}(0,x_3) = 2\rho^0\varepsilon^0 h_{13}(0,\frac{\lambda^0_3-\lambda^0_1}{\lambda^0_1\lambda^0_3}x_3 + \frac{H}{\lambda^0_3}),$$

$$\tilde{s}^1_{11}(0,x_3) = -\frac{1}{a_{33}}\left[r\tilde{\rho}^1(0,x_3) + b_{33}\tilde{s}^1_{12}(0,x_3) - h_6(0,\frac{2}{\lambda^0_2}(H-x_3))\right].$$

Let us suppose that all derivatives of the orders less then $k+m$ of the functions $\tilde{\varepsilon}^1(\kappa_1,\kappa_2,x_3)$, $\tilde{s}^1_{11}(\kappa_1,\kappa_2,x_3)$, $\tilde{s}^1_{44}(\kappa_1,\kappa_2,x_3)$, $\tilde{e}^1_{14}(\kappa_1,\kappa_2,x_3)$ are known for $\kappa_1 = 0$, $\kappa_2 = 0$. Now we describe the process of the determination of the derivative $\frac{\partial^{k+m}}{\partial\kappa_1\partial\kappa_2}$ of the functions $\tilde{\varepsilon}^1(\kappa_1,\kappa_2,x_3)$, $\tilde{s}^1_{11}(\kappa_1,\kappa_2,x_3)$, $\tilde{s}^1_{44}(\kappa_1,\kappa_2,x_3)$, $\tilde{e}^1_{14}(\kappa_1,\kappa_2,x_3)$ for $\kappa_1 = 0$, $\kappa_2 = 0$. For this case we apply the differential operator $\frac{\partial^{k+m}}{\partial\kappa_1\partial\kappa_2}$ to the right and left sides of equations (7.9)–(7.11) and use the Leibnitz classical formula, then we obtain:

$$\left(I\frac{\partial}{\partial t} + \mathcal{D}^J_1\frac{\partial}{\partial x_3}\right)\frac{\partial^{k+m}}{\partial\kappa_1^k\partial\kappa_2^m}\mathcal{V}^{1J} =$$

$$= -\frac{\partial^{k+m}}{\partial\kappa_1^k\partial\kappa_2^m}\left[\hat{\mathcal{A}}^J_0\frac{\partial}{\partial t} + \hat{\mathcal{A}}^J_3\frac{\partial}{\partial x_3} + \hat{\mathcal{Q}}^J\right]\mathcal{V}^{0J}(-\kappa,x_3,t) +$$

$$\mathcal{F}[\mathcal{P}^J,\mathcal{V}^{0J}](\kappa,x_3,t)), \quad 0 \le x_3 \le H, \tag{7.23}$$

$$\frac{\partial^{k+m}}{\partial\kappa_1^k\partial\kappa_2^m}V^{1J}|_{t<0} = 0, \tag{7.24}$$

$$\frac{\partial^{k+m}}{\partial\kappa_1^k\partial\kappa_2^m}V^1_i|_{x_3=0} = 0, \qquad i = 1,2,6,10,13,$$

$$\frac{\partial^{k+m}}{\partial\kappa_1^k\partial\kappa_2^m}V^1_i|_{x_3=H} = 0, \qquad i = 5,7,8,11,14, \tag{7.25}$$

where $J = \overline{1,6}$,

$$\mathcal{F}[\mathcal{P}^J,\mathcal{V}^{0J}](\kappa,x_3,t)) = \sum_{i=0}^{m-1} C^i_m\frac{\partial^{k+i}\mathcal{P}^J}{\partial\kappa_1^k\partial\kappa_2^i}\frac{\partial^{m-i}\mathcal{V}^{0J}}{\partial\kappa_2^{m-i}} +$$

$$\sum_{i=0}^{m}\sum_{j=0}^{k-1} C_k^j C_m^i \frac{\partial^{j+i} \mathcal{L}^J}{\partial \kappa_1^j \partial \kappa_2^i} \frac{\partial^{k+m-j-i} \mathcal{V}^{0J}}{\partial \kappa_1^{m-i} \partial \kappa_2^{k-j}},$$

$$\mathcal{L}^J = -\left[\hat{\mathcal{A}}_0^J \frac{\partial}{\partial t} + \hat{\mathcal{A}}_3^J \frac{\partial}{\partial x_3} + \hat{\mathcal{Q}}^J\right].$$

Let $\mathcal{V}^{*J}(x_3,t)$, $J = \overline{1,6}$ be the solution of the following problem:

$$\left(I\frac{\partial}{\partial t} + \mathcal{D}_1^J \frac{\partial}{\partial x_3}\right)\mathcal{V}^{*J}(x_3,t) = \mathcal{F}[\mathcal{L}^J, \mathcal{V}^{0J}](\kappa, x_3, t)|_{\kappa=0}, \tag{7.26}$$

$$V^{*J}(x_3,t)|_{t<0} = 0, \tag{7.27}$$

$$V_i^*(x_3,t)|_{x_3=0} = 0, \qquad i = 1,2,6,10,13,$$

$$V_i^*(x_3,t)|_{x_3=H} = 0, \qquad i = 5,7,8,11,14. \tag{7.28}$$

Remark 7.1. The functions $\mathcal{V}^{*J}(x_3,t)$, $J = \overline{1,6}$ are the known functions because the functions $\mathcal{F}[\mathcal{L}^J, \mathcal{V}^{0J}](\kappa, x_3, t)|_{\kappa=0}$, $J = \overline{1,6}$ are known.

Let further

$$W^J(x_3,t) = \frac{\partial^{k+m}}{\partial \kappa_1^k \partial \kappa_2^m} \mathcal{V}^{1J}|_{\kappa=0} - \mathcal{V}^{*J}(x_3,t).$$

Using formulas (7.23)–(7.25), (7.26)–(7.28) we obtain:

$$\left(I\frac{\partial}{\partial t} + \mathcal{D}_1^J \frac{\partial}{\partial x_3}\right) W^J =$$

$$= -\frac{\partial^{k+m}}{\partial \kappa_1^k \partial \kappa_2^m}\left[\hat{\mathcal{A}}_0^J \frac{\partial}{\partial t} + \hat{\mathcal{A}}_3^J \frac{\partial}{\partial x_3} + \hat{\mathcal{Q}}^J\right]|_{\kappa=0} \mathcal{V}^{0J}(0,x_3,t), \quad 0 \le x_3 \le H, \tag{7.29}$$

$$W^J|_{t<0} = 0, \tag{7.30}$$

$$W_i|_{x_3=0} = 0, \qquad i = 1,2,6,10,13,$$

$$W_i|_{x_3=H} = 0, \qquad i = 5,7,8,11,14, \tag{7.31}$$

where $J = \overline{1,6}$.

Moreover we obtain from (7.1) that

$$W_j(x_3,t)\big|_{x_3=H} = h_j^{km}(t), \quad j = 1,6,10,13, \tag{7.32}$$

where

$$h_j^{km}(t) = \frac{\partial^{k+m}}{\partial \kappa_1^k \partial \kappa_2^m} h_j(\kappa_1, \kappa_2, t)|_{\kappa_1=0,\kappa_2=0} - V_i^*(x_3, t)|_{x_3=0}, \quad j = 1, 6, 10, 13.$$

We obtained the equations which are analogous to equations (7.9)–(7.11). Using equations (7.29)–(7.31) and reasoning which we used for the determination of the functions $\tilde{\varepsilon}^1(0,x_3)$, $\tilde{s}_{11}^1(0,x_3)$, $\tilde{s}_{44}^1(0,x_3)$, $\tilde{e}_{14}^1(0,x_3)$ for $x_3 \in [0,H]$ we can find the values of the functions

$$\frac{\partial^{k+m}}{\partial \kappa_1 \partial \kappa_2} \tilde{\varepsilon}^1(\kappa_1, \kappa_2, x_3), \qquad \frac{\partial^{k+m}}{\partial \kappa_1 \partial \kappa_2} \tilde{s}_{11}^1(\kappa_1, \kappa_2, x_3),$$

$$\frac{\partial^{k+m}}{\partial \kappa_1 \partial \kappa_2} \tilde{s}_{44}^1(\kappa_1, \kappa_2, x_3), \qquad \frac{\partial^{k+m}}{\partial \kappa_1 \partial \kappa_2} \tilde{e}_{14}^1(\kappa_1, \kappa_2, x_3), \qquad for \quad \kappa_1 = 0, \quad \kappa_2 = 0.$$

Hence we described the process of successive determinations for $x_3 \in [0,H]$, $\kappa_1 = 0$, $\kappa_2 = 0$ of all derivatives of the functions $\tilde{\varepsilon}^1(\kappa_1,\kappa_2,x_3)$, $\tilde{s}_{11}^1(\kappa_1,\kappa_2,x_3)$, $\tilde{s}_{44}^1(\kappa_1,\kappa_2,x_3)$, $\tilde{e}_{14}^1(\kappa_1,\kappa_2,x_3)$ analytic respect to κ_1, κ_2.

Therefore Theorem 7.1 is proved.

REFERENCES

1. M. Akamatsu, G. Nakamura, and S. Steinberg. Identification of Lamé coefficients from boundary observations. *Inverse Problems*, 7:335–354, 1991.
2. A. S. Alekseev. Some inverse problems in wave propagation theory. *Izvestiya Academy Sciences of USSR*, 1962. Geophysics.
3. G. Anger. *Inverse and Improperly Posed Problems in Differential Equations*. Akademie Verlag, Berlin, 1979.
4. Y. Anikonov. *Some Methods of the Study of Multidimensional Inverse Problems for Differential Equations*. Nauka, Novosibirsk, 1978. Russian.
5. A. Blagoveshchenskii. The inverse problem in the theory of seismic–wave propagation. In *In Topics in Mathematical Physics*, number 1. Plenum Press, New York, 1967.
6. K. Bube, P. Lailly, P. Sacks, F. Santosa, and W. Symes. Simultaneous determination of source wavelet and velocity profile using impulsive point–source reflections from a layered fluid. *Geophysical Journal*, 95:449–462, 1988.
7. A. L. Bukhgeim. *Volterra Equations and Inverse Problems*. Nauka, Novosibirsk, 1983. Russian.
8. A. Calderón. On an inverse boundary value problem. In *Seminar on Numerical Analysis and its Applications to Continuum Mechanics*, pages 65–73, Rio de Janeiro, 1980. Society Brasileira de Mathematica.
9. J. Cannon and U. Hornung. *Inverse Problems*. Birkhäuser-Verlag, Basel, 1986.
10. D. Colton and R. Kress. *Inverse Acoustic and Electromagnetic Scattering Theory*. Springer-Verlag, New York, 1992.
11. E. Dieulesaint and D. Royer. *Ondes Elastiques Dans les Solides. Application au Tratement du Signal*. Masson et Cie, Paris, 1974.
12. V. I. Dmitriev. Inverse problems electromagnetic sounding. In *Ill-Posed Problems of Mathematical Physics and Analysis*, pages 85–97. Nauka, Novosibirsk, 1992.
13. H. Engl and C. W. Groetshc. *Inverse and Ill-posed Problems*. Academic Press, Boston, 1987.
14. I. M. Gel'fand and B. M. Levitan. On the determination of a differential operator from its spectral function. *American Mathematical Society Translation*, 1:253–304, 1951.
15. V. Glasko. *Inverse Problems of Mathematical Physics*. American Institute of Physics, New York, 1984.
16. C. Groetsch. *Inverse Problems in the Mathematical Sciences*. Vieweg-Verlag, Wiesbaden, 1993.
17. S. Gutman and M. Klibanov. Iterative method for multidimensional inverse scattering problems at fixed frequencies. *Inverse Problems*, 10:573–599, 1994.
18. A. Kirsch. *An Introduction to Mathematical Theory of Inverse Problems*. Springer-Verlag, New York, 1996.
19. M. M. Lavrent'ev. *Some Improperly Posed Problems of Mathematical Physics*. Springer-Verlag, Berlin, 1967.
20. M. M. Lavrent'ev and V. I. Priimenko. Simultaneous determination of elastic and electromagnetic medium parameters. In *Computerized Tomography*, pages 302–308. TVP/VSP Utrecht, The Netherlands, 1995.

21. M. M. Lavrent'ev, K. G. Reznitskaya, and V. G. Yakhno. *One-Dimensional Inverse Problems of Mathematical Physics*. American Mathematical Society Translations, Providence Rhode Island, 1986.
22. M. M. Lavrent'ev, V. G. Romanov, and V. G. Vasil'ev. *Multidimensional Inverse Problems for Differential Equations*. Springer-Verlag, Berlin, 1970.
23. A. Lorenzi and V. I. Priimenko. Identification problems related to electromagnetoelastic interactions. *Inverse and Ill-Posed Problems*, 4(2):115–144, 1996.
24. I. Z. Merazhov and V. G. Yakhno. Direct and inverse problems for electroelastic equations. In *Computerized Tomography*, pages 332–338. TVP/VSP Utrecht, The Netherlands, 1995.
25. I. Z. Merazhov and V. G. Yakhno. Direct and inverse problems for differential equations of electromagnetoelasticity. In *Inverse Geophysics Problems*, pages 134–138. Computer Center of Siberian Division of Russian Academy of Sciences, Novosibirsk, 1996.
26. G. Nakamura and G. Uhlmann. Identification of Lame parameters by boundary measurements. *American Journal of Mathematics*, (115):1161–1187, 1993.
27. F. Natterer. *The Mathematics of Computerized Tomography*. Teubner-Verlag, Stuttgart, 1986.
28. V. Z. Parton and B. A. Kudryavzev. *Electromagnetoelasticity of Piezoelectric and Electrically Conducting Bodies*. Nauka, Moscow, 1988. Russian.
29. A. Ramm. *Multidimensional Inverse Scattering Problems*. Longman Scientific and Wiley, New York, 1992. Expanded Russian edition Mir Moscow 1994.
30. A. G. Ramm. An inverse problem for Maxwell's equations. *Physical Letters*, 138A:459–462, 1989.
31. A. G. Ramm and A. Katsevich. *The Radon Transform and Local Tomography*. CRC Press, Boca Raton, 1996.
32. V. Romanov. *Inverse Problems of Mathematical Physics*. VNU Science Press BV, Utrecht, 1987.
33. V. G. Romanov and S. I. Kabanikhin. *Inverse Problems of Geoelectricity*. Nauka, Moscow, 1991. Russian.
34. P. Sacks. A velocity inversion problem involving an unknown source. *SIAM Journal of Applied Mathematics*, 50(3):931–941, 1990.
35. P. Sacks. Reconstruction of steplike potentials. *Wave Motion*, (18):21–30, 1993.
36. P. Sacks and W. Symes. Recovery of the elastic parameters of a layered half–space. *Geophysical Journal R. astr. Society*, (88):593–620, 1987.
37. P. Sacks and W. Symes. The inverse problem for a fluid over a layered elastic. *Inverse Problems*, (6):1031–1054, 1990.
38. J. Sylvester and G. Uhlmann. A uniqueness theorem for an inverse boundary problem in electrical prospection. *Communication Pure Applied Mathematics*, (39):91–112, 1986.
39. J. Sylvester and G. Uhlmann. A global uniqueness theorem for an inverse boundary value problem. *Ann. Mathematics*, (125):153–169, 1987.
40. J. Sylvester and G. Uhlmann. The Dirichlet to Neumann map and applications. In *Inverse Problems in Partial Differential Equations*, pages 101–139. SIAM Publications, Philadelphia, 1990.
41. G. Talenti. *Inverse Problems*. Springer-Verlag, Berlin, 1986.
42. A. Tikhonov. On the stability of inverse problems. *Doklady Academy of Sciences of URSS*, (39):176–179, 1943.
43. A. N. Tikhonov, A. V. Goncharskii, V. V. Stepanov, and A. G. Yagola. *Numerical Methods for the Solution of Ill-Posed Problems*. Kluwer, Dordrecht, 1995.
44. A. N. Tikhonov, V. K. Ivanov, and M. M. Lavrent'ev. Ill-posed problems. In *Partial Differential Equations*, volume 2. American Mathematical Society Translation, 1976.
45. V. Yakhno. *Inverse Problems for Differential Equations of Elasticity*. Nauka, Novosibirsk, 1990. Russian.
46. M. Yamamoto. Well-posedness of an inverse hyperbolic problem by the Hilbert uniqueness method. *Journal of Inverse and Ill-Posed Problems*, (2):349–368, 1994.

15

ON AN INVERSE PROBLEM OF DETERMINING SOURCE TERMS IN MAXWELL'S EQUATIONS WITH A SINGLE MEASUREMENT

Masahiro Yamamoto

Department of Mathematical Sciences
The University of Tokyo
3-8-1 Komaba Meguro 153 Tokyo Japan
E-mail: myama@ms.u-tokyo.ac.jp

ABSTRACT

In Maxwell's equations, we consider an inverse problem of determining electric source terms by a single measurement of electric and magnetic fields on lateral boundary and establish the uniqueness in the inverse problem. Our method is based on the Carleman estimate.

1. INTRODUCTION

We consider Maxwell's equations for a non-dispersive and isotropic medium in a bounded domain $\Omega \subset \mathbb{R}^3$ surrounded by a perfectly conducting C^2-boundary $\partial\Omega$ (e.g. Duvaut and Lions [3]):

$$D'(x,t) = \nabla \times \left(\frac{1}{\mu(x)} B(x,t) \right) - J(x,t), \quad x \in \Omega, \ -T < t < T \tag{1.1}$$

$$B'(x,t) = -\nabla \times \left(\frac{1}{\epsilon(x)} D(x,t) \right), \quad x \in \Omega, \ -T < t < T \tag{1.2}$$

$$\nabla \cdot B(x,t) = 0, \qquad x \in \Omega, \ -T < t < T \tag{1.3}$$

$$D(x,0) = B(x,0) = 0, \qquad x \in \Omega \tag{1.4}$$

Inverse Problems, Tomography, and Image Processing, edited by Ramm,
Plenum Press, New York, 1998

$$\nu(x) \times D(x,t) = 0, \qquad x \in \partial\Omega, \ -T < t < T, \tag{1.5}$$

where $x = (x_1, x_2, x_3) \in \mathbb{R}^3$ and $\nu = \nu(x)$ denotes the outward unit normal vector to $\partial\Omega$ at x. Here $J(x,t)$ is an electric current injected from the exterior and, throughout this paper, we assume

$$\begin{aligned} J(x,t) &= f(x)q(x,t) \\ &= f(x)(q_1(x,t), q_2(x,t), q_3(x,t))^T, \quad x \in \Omega, \ -T < t < T. \end{aligned} \tag{1.6}$$

Here and henceforth $\cdot^T$ denotes the transpose of vectors under consideration.

In a system of Maxwell's equations, an electric charge density $\rho = \rho(x,t)$ satisfies

$$\nabla \cdot D(x,t) = \rho(x,t), \qquad x \in \Omega, \ -T < t < T, \tag{1.7}$$

and in our inverse problem, ρ is regarded as an unknown function, and so we do not consider (1.7) in the governing system for our inverse problem. Here we notice that a magnetic current $J^*(x,t)$ injected from the exterior does not exist physically, that is, for determination of source terms in Maxwell's equations, we need not consider

$$B'(x,t) = -\nabla \times \left(\frac{1}{\epsilon(x)} D(x,t) \right) - J^*(x,t), \quad x \in \Omega, \ -T < t < T$$

in place of (1.2).

In this paper, we discuss

1.1. Inverse Source Problem

Let $q(x,t)$ be prescribed and $T > 0$ be given. Does

$$D(x,t), \quad B(x,t), \qquad x \in \partial\Omega, \ -T < t < T$$

determine $f(x)$, $x \in \Omega$ uniquely?

This is one of inverse problems for Maxwell's equations and we can refer to Ola, Päivärinta and Somersalo [7], Ramm [8], Section 10 of III in Ramm [9], Ramm and Somersalo [10], Sun and Uhlmann [12] for a formulation with many measurements, and a monograph by Romanov and Kabanikhin [11] for a formulation with impulsive inputs. We can refer also to Yamamoto [13]. For inverse scattering problems for Maxwell's equations, see Colton and Kress [2]. In this paper, we apply the argument on the basis of Carleman estimate (Bukhgeim and Klibanov [1], Isakov [4, 5] and Klibanov [6]) and prove the uniqueness under some "non-degenerate" assumption on $q(\cdot, 0)$, ϵ and μ on $\overline{\Omega}$.

2. MAIN RESULT

We assume that $\epsilon, \mu \in C^2(\overline{\Omega})$, $\epsilon(x), \mu(x) > 0$, $x \in \overline{\Omega}$ and

$$0 \in \Omega \tag{2.1}$$

$$1 + \frac{(x, \nabla(\epsilon\mu)(x))}{2(\epsilon\mu)(x)} > 0, \quad x \in \overline{\Omega}. \tag{2.2}$$

Here and henceforth, $(\cdot, \cdot)$ denotes the scalar product in $\mathbb{R}^3$.

Remark 2.1. The condition (2.2) is necessary for application of the Carleman estimate. More precisely, under (2.2) we can construct a weight function which is good for a Carleman estimate. The condition (2.2) requires that $\nabla(\epsilon\mu)$ is small along the x-direction in comparison with Ω or that $\nabla(\epsilon\mu)$ is monotonically increasing along the x-direction. In particular, if the medium is homogeneous, i.e., ϵ and μ are constant, then (2.2) is satisfied. However, (2.2) is not satisfied in the following physically interesting case: ϵ and μ depend only on x_3 (i.e. the depth), not in a monotone way. To the author's knowledge, without extra conditions such as (2.2), it is open whether we can construct a suitable weight function for the Carleman estimate which is globally true over Ω.

We set

$$\omega = \inf_{\xi\in\Omega}\sup_{x\in\Omega}|x-\xi|.$$

Henceforth we may assume that in the definition of ω, the infimum is attained at $\xi = 0$, that is,

$$\omega = \sup_{x\in\Omega}|x|, \tag{2.3}$$

without loss of generality. We choose $\theta > 0$ such that

$$0 < \theta < \inf_{x\in\Omega}\left[\left\{\sqrt{\omega^2\frac{|\nabla(\epsilon\mu)(x)|^2}{(\epsilon\mu)(x)} + 4(\epsilon\mu)(x)\left(1+\frac{(x,\nabla(\epsilon\mu)(x))}{2(\epsilon\mu)(x)}\right)} - \omega\frac{|\nabla(\epsilon\mu)(x)|}{\sqrt{(\epsilon\mu)(x)}}\right\}^2 \times \frac{1}{4}(\epsilon\mu)(x)^{-2}\right] \tag{2.4}$$

and

$$0 < \theta \le \inf_{x\in\Omega}\frac{1}{(\epsilon\mu)(x)}. \tag{2.5}$$

Moreover we set

$$\nabla \times \left(\frac{q(x,t)}{\epsilon(x)}\right) = (r_1(x,t), r_2(x,t), r_3(x,t))^T \tag{2.6}$$

$$A_1(x,t) = \begin{pmatrix} r_1(x,t) & 0 & \frac{q_3(x,t)}{\epsilon(x)} \\ r_2(x,t) & -\frac{q_3(x,t)}{\epsilon(x)} & 0 \\ r_3(x,t) & \frac{q_2(x,t)}{\epsilon(x)} & -\frac{q_1(x,t)}{\epsilon(x)} \end{pmatrix} \tag{2.7}$$

and

$$A_2(x,t) = \begin{pmatrix} -\frac{q_2(x,t)}{\epsilon(x)} & 0 & 0 \\ 0 & \frac{q_1(x,t)}{\epsilon(x)} & 0 \\ 0 & 0 & 1 \end{pmatrix}, \qquad x\in\Omega,\ -T<t<T. \tag{2.8}$$

Now we are ready to state our main result on uniqueness in determining a source term of (1.1) in the form (1.6):

Theorem 2.1. *Let us assume*

$$T > \frac{\sup_{x\in\Omega}|x|}{\sqrt{\theta}} \tag{2.9}$$

and

$$\left|\det\begin{pmatrix} A_1(x,0) & A_2(x,0) \\ A_1'(x,0) & A_2'(x,0)\end{pmatrix}\right| \ge q_0 > 0, \quad x\in\overline{\Omega} \tag{2.10}$$

where a constant $q_0 > 0$ *is independent of* $x\in\overline{\Omega}$. *Let*

$$B, D, q \in C^4([-T,T]; C^2(\overline{\Omega})^3), \qquad f\in C^1(\overline{\Omega}) \tag{2.11}$$

satisfy (1.1)–(1.5). If

$$D(x,t) = B(x,t) = 0, \quad x\in\partial\Omega,\ -T<t<T, \tag{2.12}$$

then $f(x) = 0$, $x\in\Omega$ *and* $B(x,t) = D(x,t) = 0$, $x\in\Omega$, $-T<t<T$.

Remark 2.2. Let ϵ and μ be constants. Then (2.4) and (2.5) are equivalent to $0<\theta<\frac{1}{\epsilon\mu}$, and so the condition (2.9) for the observation time length is

$$T > \sqrt{\epsilon\mu}\sup_{x\in\Omega}|x|.$$

Since $\frac{1}{\sqrt{\epsilon\mu}}$ is the speed of the electromagnetic wave, this condition is reasonable from the physical point of view.

Remark 2.3. The condition (2.10) is restrictive. For example, we set $\epsilon(x) = 1, x\in\Omega, q_1(x,t) = e^{\alpha t}a(x), q_2(x,t) = e^{\beta t}b(x), q_3(x,t) = 1, x\in\Omega, -T<t<T$ where $\alpha\ne 0$ and $\beta\ne 0$ are constants, and

$$a(x)\ne 0, \quad b(x)\ne 0, \quad \beta\frac{\partial b}{\partial x_1}(x) \ne \alpha\frac{\partial a}{\partial x_2}(x), \quad x = (x_1,x_2,x_3)\in\overline{\Omega}.$$

Then (2.10) is verified by direct calculations.

3. PROOF OF THEOREM

The proof is based on

1. reduction of the system (1.1)–(1.5) with (2.12) to an overdetermining system for a hyperbolic system
2. application of the Carleman estimate to an inverse hyperbolic problem by Bukhgeim and Klibanov [1], Isakov [4,5] and Klibanov [6].

3.1. First Step

By (2.9) we may assume

$$T = \frac{\omega}{\sqrt{\theta}} + \xi \quad \text{with sufficiently small } \xi > 0. \tag{3.1}$$

By (1.1), (1.3) and a formula: $\nabla \times (\nabla \times A) = -\Delta A + \nabla(\nabla \cdot A)$, we have

$$\begin{aligned}
\nabla \times D' &= \nabla \times \left(\nabla \times \left(\frac{1}{\mu}B\right)\right) - \nabla \times (fq)\\
&= -\Delta\left(\frac{1}{\mu}B\right) + \nabla\left(\nabla \cdot \left(\frac{1}{\mu}B\right)\right) - \nabla \times (fq)\\
&= -\Delta\left(\frac{1}{\mu}B\right) + \nabla\left(\frac{1}{\mu}(\nabla \cdot B) + \nabla\left(\frac{1}{\mu}\right) \cdot B\right) - \nabla \times (fq)\\
&= -\frac{1}{\mu}\Delta B - 2\nabla\left(\frac{1}{\mu}\right) \cdot \nabla B - B\Delta\left(\frac{1}{\mu}\right) + \nabla\left(\nabla\left(\frac{1}{\mu}\right) \cdot B\right) - \nabla \times (fq).
\end{aligned}$$

Therefore we can write $\nabla \times D'$ as

$$\frac{1}{\epsilon}\nabla \times D' = -\frac{1}{\epsilon\mu}\Delta B + P_1 B - \frac{1}{\epsilon}\nabla \times (fq) \tag{3.2}$$

where P_1 is a differential operator in x whose order is 1. We note by $\epsilon, \mu \in C^2(\overline{\Omega})$ that all the coefficients in P_1 are in $C(\overline{\Omega})$.

On the other hand, noting a formula $\nabla \times (fA) = \nabla f \times A + f(\nabla \times A)$ for a scalar function f and a $\mathbb{R}^3$-valued function A, from (1.2) we have

$$-B'' = \nabla \times \left(\frac{1}{\epsilon}D'\right) = \frac{1}{\epsilon}\nabla \times D' + \nabla\left(\frac{1}{\epsilon}\right) \times D'.$$

Therefore again by (1.1), we obtain

$$\begin{aligned}
-B'' &= \frac{1}{\epsilon}\nabla \times D' + \nabla\left(\frac{1}{\epsilon}\right) \times \left(\nabla \times \left(\frac{1}{\mu}B\right)\right) - \nabla\left(\frac{1}{\epsilon}\right) \times (fq)\\
&= \frac{1}{\epsilon}\nabla \times D' + P_2 B - \nabla\left(\frac{1}{\epsilon}\right) \times (fq)
\end{aligned} \tag{3.3}$$

where P_2 is a differential operator of order 1 in x whose coefficients are all in $C(\overline{\Omega})$. Therefore (3.2) and (3.3) yield

$$B'' = \frac{1}{\epsilon\mu}\Delta B - (P_1 + P_2)B + \frac{1}{\epsilon}\nabla \times (fq) + \nabla\left(\frac{1}{\epsilon}\right) \times (fq)$$

in $\Omega \times (-T, T)$, namely,

$$B'' = \frac{1}{\epsilon\mu}\Delta B - (P_1 + P_2)B + \frac{1}{\epsilon}(\nabla f) \times q + \begin{pmatrix} r_1 \\ r_2 \\ r_3 \end{pmatrix} f \tag{3.4}$$

in $\Omega \times (-T, T)$, by

$$\frac{1}{\epsilon}\nabla \times (fq) + \nabla\left(\frac{1}{\epsilon}\right) \times (fq) = \frac{1}{\epsilon}(\nabla f) \times q + \left(\frac{1}{\epsilon}(\nabla \times q)\right)f + \left(\nabla\left(\frac{1}{\epsilon}\right) \times q\right)f$$
$$= \frac{1}{\epsilon}(\nabla f) \times q + \left(\nabla \times \left(\frac{q}{\epsilon}\right)\right)f.$$

Here we recall (2.6). Moreover we set $P_3 = -P_1 - P_2$ and

$$F(x) = \begin{pmatrix} F_1(x) \\ F_2(x) \end{pmatrix}, \quad F_1(x) = \begin{pmatrix} f(x) \\ \frac{\partial f}{\partial x_1}(x) \\ \frac{\partial f}{\partial x_2}(x) \end{pmatrix}, \quad F_2(x) = \frac{\partial f}{\partial x_3}(x)\begin{pmatrix} 1 \\ 1 \\ 0 \end{pmatrix}. \tag{3.5}$$

Then we rewrite (3.4) as

$$(PB)(x,t) \equiv B'' - \frac{1}{\epsilon\mu}\Delta B - P_3 B$$
$$= A_1(x,t)F_1(x) + A_2(x,t)F_2(x), \qquad x \in \Omega,\ -T < t < T \tag{3.6}$$

where A_1 and A_2 are given by (2.7) and (2.8). By (3.6) we have

$$(PB')(x,t) = A_1'(x,t)F_1(x) + A_2'(x,t)F_2(x), \qquad x \in \Omega,\ -T < t < T,$$

so that

$$(PV)(x,t) = Q(x,t)F(x), \qquad x \in \Omega,\ -T < t < T, \tag{3.7}$$

where

$$V(x,t) = (B(x,t), B'(x,t))^T, \qquad x \in \Omega,\ -T < t < T \tag{3.8}$$

$$Q(x,t) = \begin{pmatrix} A_1(x,t) & A_2(x,t) \\ A_1'(x,t) & A_2'(x,t) \end{pmatrix} = (q_{ij}(x,t))_{1\le i,j\le 6}. \tag{3.9}$$

For fixed $0 < \eta < \delta$, we define a function $\kappa = \kappa_{\delta,\eta}(t)$ such that $\kappa \in C_0^\infty(\mathbb{R})$, $0 \le \kappa(t) \le 1$, $t \in \mathbb{R}$,

$$\kappa(t) = \begin{cases} 1, & |t| \le \sqrt{\delta^2 - \eta^2} \\ 0, & |t| > \delta. \end{cases} \tag{3.10}$$

Moreover we define $\widetilde{q_{ij}}(x,t)$, $x \in \Omega$, $-T < t < T$, $1 \le i,j \le 6$ by

$$\widetilde{q_{ij}}(x,t) = q_{ij}(x,0) + \kappa(t)(q_{ij}(x,t) - q_{ij}(x,0))$$
$$x \in \Omega,\ -T < t < T,\ 1 \le i,j \le 6. \tag{3.11}$$

We set

$$\widetilde{Q}(x,t) = (\widetilde{q_{ij}}(x,t))_{1\le i,j\le 6}, \quad x \in \Omega,\ -T < t < T.$$

Then by (3.11) we see

$$|\widetilde{q_{ij}}(x,t) - q_{ij}(x,0)| = |\kappa(t)(q_{ij}(x,t) - q_{ij}(x,0))|$$
$$\le C\delta\|q_{ij}\|_{C^1(\overline{\Omega}\times[-T,T])}, \quad x \in \overline{\Omega},\ |t| \le \delta,\ 1 \le i,j \le 6.$$

Therefore by the assumption (2.10), we can choose sufficiently small $\delta > 0$ and $\eta > 0$ with $0 < \eta < \delta$ such that

$$\det \widetilde{Q}(x,t) \neq 0, \qquad x \in \overline{\Omega},\ |t| \leq \delta \tag{3.12}$$

and

$$\det Q(x,t) \neq 0, \qquad x \in \overline{\Omega},\ |t| \leq \delta. \tag{3.13}$$

Moreover by (3.10) and (3.11), we obtain

$$\widetilde{Q}(x,t) = \begin{cases} Q(x,t), & x \in \overline{\Omega},\ |t| \leq \sqrt{\delta^2 - \eta^2} \\ Q(x,0), & x \in \overline{\Omega},\ |t| > \delta. \end{cases} \tag{3.14}$$

Therefore $Q^{-1}PV = F$ in $\overline{\Omega} \times (-\delta, \delta)$, and the time differentiation yields

$$Q^{-1}(PV)' - Q^{-1}Q'Q^{-1}PV = 0,$$

namely, $(PV)' - Q'Q^{-1}PV = 0$ in $\overline{\Omega} \times (-\delta, \delta)$. Defining an ordinary differential operator N in t by

$$(NU)(x,t) = U'(x,t) - Q'(x,t)Q^{-1}(x,t)U(x,t), \quad x \in \Omega,\ |t| < \delta \tag{3.15}$$

for $U = (U_1, U_2, U_3, U_4, U_5, U_6)^T$, we obtain

$$(NPV)(x,t) = 0, \qquad x \in \Omega,\ |t| < \delta. \tag{3.16}$$

3.2. Second Step

We derive boundary conditions of $V = \begin{pmatrix} B \\ B' \end{pmatrix}$ and NV from (2.12). Since $\partial\Omega$ is of C^2-class, for any $x^0 = (x_1^0, x_2^0, x_3^0) \in \partial\Omega$, we can take neighborhoods $\mathcal{V}$ in $\mathbb{R}^3$ of x^0 and $\mathcal{U}$ in $\mathbb{R}^2$ of (x_1^0, x_2^0), a function $h = h(x_1, x_2) \in C^2(\mathcal{U})$ such that

$$(x_1, x_2, x_3) \in \mathcal{V} \cap \partial\Omega \text{ if and only if } x_3 = h(x_1, x_2). \tag{3.17}$$

We introduce a new coordinate $y = (y_1, y_2, y_3)$ by

$$y_1 = x_1, \quad y_2 = x_2, \quad y_3 = x_3 - h(x_1, x_2) \tag{3.18}$$

for $(x_1, x_2) \in \mathcal{U}$. We set

$$\phi(y,t) = D(x,t), \qquad \psi(y,t) = B(x,t), \quad x \in \mathcal{V} \cap \overline{\Omega},\ -T < t < T.$$

Then the boundary condition (2.12) implies

$$\phi(y_1, y_2, 0, t) = \psi(y_1, y_2, 0, t) = 0, \qquad (y_1, y_2) \in \mathcal{U},\ -T < t < T. \tag{3.19}$$

Therefore by the regularity condition (2.11), from (1.1), (1.4) and (3.19), we can derive

$$\begin{aligned} 0 = &\phi'(y_1, y_2, 0, 0) = \nabla_x \times \left(\frac{1}{\mu(x)} B(x,0) \right) - f(x)q(x,0) \\ &= -f(x)q(x,0), \qquad x \in \partial\Omega. \end{aligned}$$

On the other hand, the assumption (2.10) implies

$$\left|\det\begin{pmatrix} A_1(x,0) & A_1'(x,0) \\ A_2(x,t) & A_2'(x,0)\end{pmatrix}\right|$$
$$=\left|\det\frac{1}{\epsilon(x)}\begin{pmatrix} r_1(x,0) & 0 & \dots \\ r_2(x,0) & -q_3(x,0) & \dots \\ r_3(x,0) & q_2(x,0) & \dots \\ -\frac{q_2}{\epsilon}(x,0) & 0 & \dots \\ 0 & q_1(x,0) & \dots \\ 0 & 0 & \dots \end{pmatrix}\right| \ne 0, \quad x\in\overline{\Omega}.$$

Therefore, noting $q(x,0)=(q_1(x,0),q_2(x,0),q_3(x,0))^T$, we have $q(x,0)\ne 0$, $x\in\overline{\Omega}$. Hence

$$f(x)=0, \qquad x\in\partial\Omega. \tag{3.20}$$

Consequently by (3.20), the equation (1.1) and (2.12) yield

$$\nabla_x\times\left(\frac{1}{\mu(x)}B(x,t)\right)=0, \qquad x\in\partial\Omega,\ -T<t<T,$$

so that

$$\nabla_x\times B(x,t)=0, \qquad x\in\partial\Omega,\ -T<t<T, \tag{3.21}$$

by (2.12) and $\nabla_x\times\left(\frac{1}{\mu(x)}B(x,t)\right)=\nabla_x\left(\frac{1}{\mu(x)}\right)\times B(x,t)+\frac{1}{\mu(x)}(\nabla_x\times B(x,t))$. In the (y_1,y_2,y_3)-coordinate, the equality (3.21) is

$$\begin{aligned}&\frac{\partial\psi_1}{\partial y_3}(y_1,y_2,0,t)=\frac{\partial\psi_3}{\partial y_1}(y_1,y_2,0,t)-\frac{\partial h}{\partial x_1}\frac{\partial\psi_3}{\partial y_3}(y_1,y_2,0,t)\\ &\frac{\partial\psi_2}{\partial y_3}(y_1,y_2,0,t)=\frac{\partial\psi_3}{\partial y_2}(y_1,y_2,0,t)-\frac{\partial h}{\partial x_2}\frac{\partial\psi_3}{\partial y_3}(y_1,y_2,0,t),\\ &(y_1,y_2)\in\mathfrak{U},\ -T<t<T,\end{aligned} \tag{3.22}$$

by noting that $\frac{\partial}{\partial x_1}=\frac{\partial}{\partial y_1}-\frac{\partial h}{\partial x_1}\frac{\partial}{\partial y_3}$, $\frac{\partial}{\partial x_2}=\frac{\partial}{\partial y_2}-\frac{\partial h}{\partial x_2}\frac{\partial}{\partial y_3}$ and $\frac{\partial}{\partial x_3}=\frac{\partial}{\partial y_3}$. The relation (3.19) means that

$$\begin{aligned}&\frac{\partial\psi_i}{\partial y_1}(y_1,y_2,0,t)=\frac{\partial\psi_i}{\partial y_2}(y_1,y_2,0,t)=0,\\ &\qquad (y_1,y_2)\in\mathfrak{U},\ -T<t<T,\ 1\le i\le 3,\end{aligned} \tag{3.23}$$

so that

$$\begin{aligned}&\frac{\partial\psi_1}{\partial y_3}(y_1,y_2,0,t)=-\frac{\partial h}{\partial x_1}\frac{\partial\psi_3}{\partial y_3}(y_1,y_2,0,t)\\ &\frac{\partial\psi_2}{\partial y_3}(y_1,y_2,0,t)=-\frac{\partial h}{\partial x_2}\frac{\partial\psi_3}{\partial y_3}(y_1,y_2,0,t),\\ &(y_1,y_2)\in\mathfrak{U},\ -T<t<T.\end{aligned} \tag{3.24}$$

On the other hand, (1.3) and (2.11) yield

$$\left(\frac{\partial\psi_1}{\partial y_1}+\frac{\partial\psi_2}{\partial y_2}+\frac{\partial\psi_3}{\partial y_3}-\frac{\partial h}{\partial x_1}\frac{\partial\psi_1}{\partial y_3}-\frac{\partial h}{\partial x_2}\frac{\partial\psi_2}{\partial y_3}\right)(y_1,y_2,0,t)=0$$

for $(y_1,y_2)\in\mathcal{U}$ and $-T<t<T$, with which (3.23) and (3.24) imply

$$\frac{\partial\psi_3}{\partial y_3}(y_1,y_2,0,t)=0,\qquad (y_1,y_2)\in\mathcal{U},\ -T<t<T.$$

Therefore again (3.24) yields

$$\frac{\partial\psi_i}{\partial y_3}(y_1,y_2,0,t)=0,\qquad (y_1,y_2)\in\mathcal{U},\ -T<t<T,\ 1\le i\le 3, \tag{3.25}$$

With (2.12), the equalities (3.23) and (3.25) imply

$$B(x,t)=\frac{\partial B}{\partial\nu}(x,t)=0,\quad x\in\mathcal{V}\cap\partial\Omega,\ -T<t<T.$$

Since $x^0\in\mathcal{V}$ is an arbitrary point of $\partial\Omega$, we obtain

$$B(x,t)=\frac{\partial B}{\partial\nu}(x,t)=0,\quad x\in\partial\Omega,\ -T<t<T. \tag{3.26}$$

Then we obtain

$$\begin{aligned}V(x,t)&=\frac{\partial V}{\partial\nu}(x,t)=(NV)(x,t)\\&=\frac{\partial(NV)}{\partial\nu}(x,t)=0,\quad x\in\partial\Omega,\ -T<t<T.\end{aligned} \tag{3.27}$$

3.3. Third Step

In this step, we apply the argument by the Carleman estimate in view of (3.16), (3.27) and (1.4). Our argument is based on Isakov [4, 5] and Klibanov [6] with modifications like an extension $\widetilde{Q}$ defined by (3.14).

For $\theta>0$ given by (2.4)–(2.5) and any $c>0$, we set

$$\phi=\phi(x,t)=|x|^2-\theta t^2, \tag{3.28}$$

and

$$\phi_c=\{(x,t)\in\Omega\times(-T,T);\phi(x,t)>c^2\}. \tag{3.29}$$

Then from Corollary 1.2.5 in Isakov [5], we can derive the following estimate called a Carleman estimate:

Lemma 3.1. *Let us assume (2.1) and (2.2), and let $\eta > 0$ be given. Then there exists constants $\tau = \tau(\eta) > 0$, $M = M(\eta) > 0$ and $\Lambda = \Lambda(\eta) > 0$ such that if $\lambda > \Lambda$, then*

$$\begin{aligned}&\lambda\|V\exp(\lambda e^{\tau\phi})\|^2_{L^2(\phi_\eta)} + \lambda\|V'\exp(\lambda e^{\tau\phi})\|^2_{L^2(\phi_\eta)}\\ &+\lambda\sum_{k=1}^{3}\left\|\frac{\partial V}{\partial x_k}\exp(\lambda e^{\tau\phi})\right\|^2_{L^2(\phi_\eta)}\\ &\le M\|(PV)\exp(\lambda e^{\tau\phi})\|^2_{L^2(\phi_\eta)}\end{aligned}$$

for any $V \in H_0^2(\phi_\eta)^6$.

Here we recall that P is defined in (3.6). For convenience, we will give a sketch of the derivation of the lemma in Appendix.

Now we fix a sufficiently small $\eta > 0$ and we set

$$c(\eta) = (\omega^2 - \theta\delta^2 + \theta\eta^2)^{\frac{1}{2}}. \tag{3.30}$$

Let $\chi \in C^\infty(\phi_{c(\eta)})$ such that $0 \le \chi(x,t) \le 1$ in $\overline{\Omega}\times[-\delta,\delta]$, and

$$\chi(x,t) = \begin{cases} 1, & (x,t)\in\phi_{c(3\eta)} \\ 0, & (x,t)\notin\phi_{c(\eta)\setminus c(2\eta)}. \end{cases} \tag{3.31}$$

Let

$$W(x,t) = \chi(x,t)V(x,t), \qquad (x,t)\in\phi_{c(\eta)}. \tag{3.32}$$

First direct calculations show that $\phi_{c(\eta)} \subset \overline{\Omega}\times[-\delta,\delta]$, so that in $\phi_{c(\eta)}$, the operator N is well-defined (see (3.15)).

By (3.26), (3.31) and the definition (3.15) of N, we easily see that

$$NW = N(\chi V) \in H_0^2(\phi_{c(\eta)})^6. \tag{3.33}$$

Therefore by Lemma 3.1 we obtain

$$\begin{aligned}&\lambda\|(NW)\exp(\lambda e^{\tau\phi})\|^2_{L^2(\phi_{c(\eta)})} + \lambda\|(NW)'\exp(\lambda e^{\tau\phi})\|^2_{L^2(\phi_{c(\eta)})}\\ &+\lambda\sum_{k=1}^{3}\left\|\frac{\partial}{\partial x_k}(NW)\exp(\lambda e^{\tau\phi})\right\|^2_{L^2(\phi_{c(\eta)})}\\ &\le M\|(PNW)\exp(\lambda e^{\tau\phi})\|^2_{L^2(\phi_{c(\eta)})}\end{aligned}$$

for large $\lambda > 0$. On the other hand, by (3.16) we have

$$\begin{aligned}PNW &= NPW + [P,N]W = [NP,\chi]V + \chi NPV + [P,N]W\\ &=[NP,\chi]V + [P,N]W \qquad \text{in } \phi_{c(\eta)}.\end{aligned}$$

Here and henceforth $[P,N]$ denotes the commutator: $[P,N] = PN - NP$. Consequently

$$\begin{aligned}&\lambda\|(NW)\exp(\lambda e^{\tau\phi})\|^2_{L^2(\phi_{c(\eta)})} + \lambda\|(NW)'\exp(\lambda e^{\tau\phi})\|^2_{L^2(\phi_{c(\eta)})}\\ &+\lambda\sum_{k=1}^{3}\left\|\frac{\partial}{\partial x_k}(NW)\exp(\lambda e^{\tau\phi})\right\|^2_{L^2(\phi_{c(\eta)})}\\ &\le M\|[NP,\chi]V\exp(\lambda e^{\tau\phi})\|^2_{L^2(\phi_{c(\eta)})} + M\|[P,N]W\exp(\lambda e^{\tau\phi})\|^2_{L^2(\phi_{c(\eta)})}\end{aligned} \tag{3.34}$$

for large $\lambda > 0$. Direct calculations yield

$$[P,N]W(x,t) = \sum_{k=1}^{3} a_k(x,t)\frac{\partial W}{\partial x_k}(x,t)$$
$$+a_0(x,t)W'(x,t) + b_0(x,t)W(x,t), \quad (x,t) \in \phi_{c(\eta)} \tag{3.35}$$

with some $a_k,\ b_0 \in C^0(\overline{\phi_{c(\eta)}})^{6\times 6}$, $0 \le k \le 3$. Substitution of (1.4) into (1.2) gives $B'(x,0) = 0$, $x \in \overline{\Omega}$, and so

$$W(x,0) = 0, \qquad x \in \overline{\Omega} \tag{3.36}$$

by (3.8) and (3.32). Therefore from the definition (3.15) of N, we can construct a 6×6 matrix $K(x,t,s) \in C^2(\overline{\Omega}\times[-\delta,\delta]^2)$ such that

$$W(x,t) = \int_0^t K(x,t,s)(NW)(x,s)ds, \quad (x,t) \in \phi_{c(\eta)}. \tag{3.37}$$

On the other hand, the following lemma holds (e.g. Klibanov [6]):

Lemma 3.2. *Let $\eta > 0$. Then*

$$\int_{\phi_\eta} \exp(2\lambda e^{\tau\phi}) \left(\int_0^t |p(x,s)|ds\right)^2 dxdt \le \sup_{(x,t)\in\phi_\eta} |t| \int_{\phi_\eta} \exp(2\lambda e^{\tau\phi})|p(x,t)|^2 dxdt$$

for $p \in L^2(\phi_\eta)$.

Since

$$\frac{\partial W}{\partial x_k}(x,t) = \int_0^t \frac{\partial K}{\partial x_k}(x,t,s)(NW)(x,s)ds$$
$$+\int_0^t K(x,t,s)\frac{\partial (NW)}{\partial x_k}(x,s)ds,$$

and

$$W'(x,t) = K(x,t,t)(NW)(x,t) + \int_0^t \frac{\partial K}{\partial t}(x,t,s)(NW)(x,s)ds,$$

we apply Lemma 3.2 and by (3.35) we see

$$\|[P,N]W\exp(\lambda e^{\tau\phi})\|^2_{L^2(\phi_{c(\eta)})}$$
$$\le M\left(\sum_{k=1}^{3}\left\|\frac{\partial W}{\partial x_k}\exp(\lambda e^{\tau\phi})\right\|^2_{L^2(\phi_{c(\eta)})} + \|W'\exp(\lambda e^{\tau\phi})\|^2_{L^2(\phi_{c(\eta)})}\right.$$
$$\left. + \|W\exp(\lambda e^{\tau\phi})\|^2_{L^2(\phi_{c(\eta)})}\right)$$
$$\le M\left(\|(NW)\exp(\lambda e^{\tau\phi})\|^2_{L^2(\phi_{c(\eta)})} + \|(NW)'\exp(\lambda e^{\tau\phi})\|^2_{L^2(\phi_{c(\eta)})}\right.$$
$$\left. + \sum_{k=1}^{3}\left\|\frac{\partial}{\partial x_k}(NW)\exp(\lambda e^{\tau\phi})\right\|^2_{L^2(\phi_{c(\eta)})}\right).$$

Hence (3.34) implies

$$\lambda\|(NW)\exp(\lambda e^{\tau\phi})\|^2_{L^2(\phi_{c(\eta)})} + \lambda\|(NW)'\exp(\lambda e^{\tau\phi})\|^2_{L^2(\phi_{c(\eta)})}$$
$$+\lambda\sum_{k=1}^{3}\left\|\frac{\partial}{\partial x_k}(NW)\exp(\lambda e^{\tau\phi})\right\|^2_{L^2(\phi_\eta)}$$
$$\le M\|[NP,\chi]V\exp(\lambda e^{\tau\phi})\|^2_{L^2(\phi_{c(\eta)})}$$

and, in particular, we obtain

$$\lambda\|(NW)\exp(\lambda e^{\tau\phi})\|^2_{L^2(\phi_{c(\eta)})} \le M\|[NP,\chi]V\exp(\lambda e^{\tau\phi})\|^2_{L^2(\phi_{c(\eta)})} \tag{3.38}$$

for large $\lambda > 0$. Since $[NP,1]V = 0$, we see that

$$[\text{the right hand side of (3.38)}] = M\|[NP,\chi]V\exp(\lambda e^{\tau\phi})\|^2_{L^2(\phi_{c(\eta)}\setminus\phi_{c(3\eta)})}$$
$$\le M\exp(2\lambda e^{\tau c(3\eta)^2})\|[NP,\chi]V\|^2_{L^2(\phi_{c(\eta)}\setminus\phi_{c(3\eta)})}$$

by (3.31). On the other hand, we have

$$[\text{the left hand side of (3.38)}] \ge \lambda\|(NW)\exp(\lambda e^{\tau\phi})\|^2_{L^2(\phi_{c(3\eta)})}$$
$$\ge \lambda\exp(2\lambda e^{\tau c(3\eta)^2})\|NW\|^2_{L^2(\phi_{c(3\eta)})}.$$

Therefore we see

$$\|NW\|^2_{L^2(\phi_{c(3\eta)})} \le \frac{M}{\lambda}\|[NP,\chi]V\|^2_{L^2(\phi_{c(\eta)}\setminus\phi_{c(3\eta)})}$$

for sufficiently large $\lambda > 0$. Letting λ tend to ∞, we obtain $NW = 0$ in $\phi_{c(3\eta)}$, and $W = \chi V = 0$ in $\phi_{c(3\eta)}$ by (3.37). That is, $V = 0$ in $\phi_{c(3\eta)}$ by (3.31). Since Q^{-1} exists in $\phi_{c(3\eta)}$, it follows from (3.7) that

$$F(x) = 0, \qquad x \in \phi_{c(3\eta)} \cap \{t = 0\},$$

namely,

$$F(x) = 0 \quad \text{in } \{x \in \Omega; \sqrt{\omega^2 - \theta\delta^2 + 9\theta\eta^2} < |x| < \omega\}.$$

Since $\eta > 0$ is arbitrary, we see

$$V(x,t) = 0, \qquad (x,t) \in \phi_{c(0)}$$
$$F(x) = 0 \quad \text{in } \{x \in \Omega; \sqrt{\omega^2 - \theta\delta^2} < |x| < \omega\}. \tag{3.39}$$

3.4. Fourth Step

By (3.7), (3.27) and (3.39), we have

$$(PV)(x,t) = 0, \qquad x \in \Omega,\ \sqrt{\omega^2 - \theta\delta^2} < |x| < \omega,\ -T < t < T, \tag{3.40}$$

$$V(x,0) = 0, \qquad x \in \Omega \tag{3.41}$$

and

$$V(x,t) = \frac{\partial V}{\partial \nu}(x,t) = 0, \quad x \in \partial\Omega, \ -T < t < T. \tag{3.42}$$

In this step, we will first prove

$$F(x) = 0, \quad x \in \Omega, \ \sqrt{\omega^2 - 2\theta\delta^2} < |x| < \omega \tag{3.43}$$

and

$$V(x,t) = 0, \qquad (x,t) \in \phi_{c_1(\eta)} \tag{3.44}$$

for sufficiently small $\eta > 0$. Here and henceforth we set

$$c_1(\eta) = \sqrt{\omega^2 - 2\theta\delta^2 + \theta\eta^2}. \tag{3.45}$$

By (3.14), (3.39), (3.40) and the property of the level set determined by $\phi_{c_1(\eta)}$, we see

$$(PV)(x,t) = \widetilde{Q}(x,t)F(x), \qquad (x,t) \in \phi_{c_1(\eta)}. \tag{3.46}$$

In fact, since $\phi_{c_1(\eta)} \subset \{(x,t); \sqrt{\omega^2 - 2\theta\delta^2 + \theta\eta^2} < |x| < \omega, \ x \in \Omega, \ -T < t < T\}$, we will verify (3.46) by dividing $\phi_{c_1(\eta)}$ into $\phi^+_{c_1(\eta)} = \phi_{c_1(\eta)} \cap \{(x,t); \sqrt{\omega^2 - \theta\delta^2} \le |x| \le \omega, \ -T < t < T\}$ and $\phi^-_{c_1(\eta)} = \phi_{c_1(\eta)} \cap \{(x,t); \sqrt{\omega^2 - 2\theta\delta^2 + \theta\eta^2} < |x| < \sqrt{\omega^2 - \theta\delta^2}, \ -T < t < T\}$. In $\phi^+_{c_1(\eta)}$, the equation (3.39) and (3.40) imply (3.46). On the other hand, let $(x,t) \in \phi^-_{c_1(\eta)}$. Direct computations show that $\phi^-_{c_1(\eta)} \subset \{(x,t); x \in \Omega, \ |t| < \sqrt{\delta^2 - \eta^2}\}$, and $\widetilde{Q}(x,t) = Q(x,t)$ in $\phi^-_{c_1(\eta)}$ by (3.14). Hence (3.46) follows from (3.7). Thus the verification of (3.46) is complete.

Therefore we can apply the argument in Third Step to (3.46) with (3.41) and (3.42), and we see that $V(x,t) = 0$, $(x,t) \in \phi_{c_1(\eta)}$. Since $\eta > 0$ is arbitrary, we have $V(x,t) = 0$, $(x,t) \in \phi_{c_1(0)}$ and $F(x) = 0$ in $\{(x,t); \sqrt{\omega^2 - 2\theta\delta^2} < |x| < \omega, \ x \in \Omega\}$. Now repeating $(n-1)$-times the above argument, we obtain $F(x) = 0$ in $\{(x,t); \sqrt{\omega^2 - n\theta\delta^2} < |x| < \omega, \ x \in \Omega\}$ and $V(x,t) = 0$ in $\phi_{\sqrt{\omega^2 - n\theta\delta^2}}$. Here by (3.29) we recall that $\phi_{\sqrt{\omega^2 - n\theta\delta^2}} = \{(x,t) \in \Omega \times (-T,T); |x|^2 - \theta t^2 > \omega^2 - n\theta\delta^2\}$. Moreover, $\partial\phi_{\sqrt{\omega^2 - n\theta\delta^2}} \cap \{(x,t) \in \Omega \times (-T,T); |x| = \omega\} \subset \Omega \times \{t; |t| < \sqrt{n}\delta\}$, so that we can continue the argument until $n \in \mathbb{N}$ satisfies $\sqrt{n}\delta \le T < \sqrt{n+1}\delta$, namely, $\sqrt{\omega^2 - (n+1)\theta\delta^2} < \sqrt{\omega^2 - \theta T^2} \le \sqrt{\omega^2 - n\theta\delta^2}$. The condition (2.9) implies that $\omega^2 - \theta T^2 < 0$. Therefore our process can be repeated until $\omega^2 - n\theta\delta^2 = 0$. Hence we see that $F(x) = 0$, $x \in \Omega$, that is,

$$f(x) = 0, \qquad x \in \Omega. \tag{3.47}$$

Consequently returning to (3.6), by (1.2), (1.4) and (2.12) we obtain

$$\left\{ \begin{array}{ll} B''(x,t) = \frac{1}{\epsilon(x)\mu(x)}\Delta B(x,t) + P_3 B(x,t), & x \in \Omega, \ -T < t < T \\ B(x,t) = 0, \quad x \in \partial\Omega, \ -T < t < T & \\ B(x,0) = B'(x,0) = 0, \quad x \in \Omega. & \end{array} \right\} \tag{3.48}$$

Therefore

$$B(x,t) = 0, \qquad x \in \Omega, \ -T < t < T \tag{3.49}$$

follows from the uniqueness of solutions to a mixed problem (3.48). Substitution of (3.49) into (1.1) with (3.47) yields $D'(x,t) = 0$, $x \in \Omega$, $-T < t < T$. The initial condition (1.4) implies $D(x,t) = 0$, $x \in \Omega$, $-T < t < T$. Thus the proof of Theorem 2.1 is complete.

4. CONCLUDING REMARKS

I. For our uniqueness, we assume that the electric charge density ρ is also unknown, in other words, we do not use $\nabla \cdot D = \rho$ for the determination of f. If we assume that ρ is known, then for D we can similarly obtain a hyperbolic system whose principal part is

$$D''(x,t) - \frac{1}{\epsilon(x)\mu(x)}\Delta D(x,t).$$

Otherwise the principal part is

$$D''(x,t) - \frac{1}{\epsilon(x)\mu(x)}\Delta D(x,t) + \frac{1}{\epsilon(x)\mu(x)}\nabla(\nabla \cdot D(x,t)),$$

which is not diagonalized and the application of a usual Carleman estimate is quite difficult.

II. Let the electric charge density ρ be known, say $\rho = 0$. Then we can obtain the uniqueness in determining $(f_1(x), f_2(x))$ from boundary measurements of B and D on $\partial\Omega \times (-T, T)$ for the system:

$$D'(x,t) = \nabla \times \left(\frac{1}{\mu(x)}B(x,t)\right) - f_1(x)q(x,t), \quad x \in \Omega,\ -T < t < T \tag{4.1}$$

$$B'(x,t) = -\nabla \times \left(\frac{1}{\epsilon(x)}D(x,t)\right) + f_2(x)r(x,t), \quad x \in \Omega,\ -T < t < T \tag{4.2}$$

$$\nabla \cdot B(x,t) = \nabla \cdot D(x,t) = 0, \qquad x \in \Omega,\ -T < t < T \tag{4.3}$$

$$D(x,0) = B(x,0) = 0, \qquad x \in \Omega \tag{4.4}$$

$$\nu(x) \times D(x,t) = 0, \qquad x \in \partial\Omega,\ -T < t < T, \tag{4.5}$$

where q and r are suitably given vector-valued functions. This discussion can be done because we can derive two hyperbolic systems in B and D from (4.1)–(4.3) and the principal parts of the respective systems are diagonal, which enables us to apply the Carleman estimate.

Moreover the uniqueness of (f_1, f_2) in the system (4.1)–(4.5) can give the uniqueness of (ϵ, μ) from the boundary measurements of B and D. Our point of this paper is, however, determination of source terms and so we do not further treat the determination of ϵ and μ. In a forthcoming paper, we will give its details.

APPENDIX. DERIVATION OF LEMMA 3.1

The Carleman estimate by Isakov (e.g. Corollary 1.2.5 in [5]) reads as follows: Let

$$\theta\left((\epsilon\mu)(x) + |t||\nabla(\epsilon\mu)(x)|(\epsilon\mu)(x)^{-\frac{1}{2}}\right) < 1 + \frac{(x, \nabla(\epsilon\mu)(x))}{2(\epsilon\mu)(x)}, \quad x \in \overline{\Omega},\ -T < t < T \tag{A.1}$$

$$0 < (\epsilon\mu)(x) \le \frac{1}{\theta}, \qquad x \in \overline{\Omega} \tag{A.2}$$

and

$$\omega^2 < \theta T^2. \tag{A.3}$$

Then the conclusion of Lemma 3.1 holds.

For the proof of Lemma 3.1, it is sufficient to verify that if θ satisfies (2.4) and (2.5), and T satisfies (3.1), then (A.1)–(A.3) hold. First (A.2) and (A.3) follows from (2.5) and (3.1). Now we have to verify (A.1). We set

$$d(x) = |\nabla(\epsilon\mu)(x)|(\epsilon\mu)(x)^{-\frac{1}{2}}$$

and

$$e(x) = 1 + \frac{(x, \nabla(\epsilon\mu)(x))}{2(\epsilon\mu)(x)}, \quad x \in \Omega$$

for simplicity. We define a function $\Psi = \Psi(x, \xi)$ by

$$\Psi(x, \xi) = \frac{-\omega d(x) + \sqrt{\omega^2 d^2(x) + 4(\epsilon\mu)(x)e(x) + 4\xi d(x)e(x)}}{2(\epsilon\mu)(x) + 2\xi d(x)}$$

for $x \in \overline{\Omega}$ and $\xi \ge 0$. By direct calculations, (2.4) implies that $\min_{x\in\overline{\Omega}} \Psi(x,0) > \sqrt{\theta}$. Since $\Psi(x, \xi)$ is continuous in $x \in \overline{\Omega}$ and $\xi \ge 0$, we see that

$$\Psi(x, \xi) > \sqrt{\theta}, \quad x \in \overline{\Omega} \tag{A.4}$$

for sufficiently small $\xi > 0$. By (3.1) we can set $T = \frac{\omega}{\sqrt{\theta}} + \xi$, where $\xi > 0$ makes (A.4) valid. That is,

$$\Psi\left(x, T - \frac{\omega}{\sqrt{\theta}}\right) > \sqrt{\theta}, \quad x \in \overline{\Omega}.$$

Direct computations show that this inequality means

$$\theta\left((\epsilon\mu)(x) + \left(T - \frac{\omega}{\sqrt{\theta}}\right)d(x)\right) + \omega d(x)\sqrt{\theta} - e(x) < 0,$$

namely,

$$\theta((\epsilon\mu)(x) + Td(x)) < e(x), \quad x \in \overline{\Omega}.$$

Recalling the definition d and e, by $|t| \le T$, we can see (A.1). Thus the derivation of Lemma 3.1 from Corollary 1.2.5 in [5] is complete.

ACKNOWLEDGMENT

This work is partially supported by the Grant-in-Aid for Cooperative Researches (No. 06305005) from the Ministry of Education, Culture and Science (Japan), Sanwa Systems Development Co., Ltd. (Tokyo, Japan). The author thanks Professor A. G. Ramm and the referee for valuable comments.

REFERENCES

1. Bukhgeim, A. L. and Klibanov, M. V., "Global uniqueness of a class of multidimensional inverse problems," *Soviet Math. Dokl.*, **24**, 244–247 (1981).
2. Colton, D. and Kress, R., *Inverse Acoustic and Electromagnetic Scattering Theory*, Springer-Verlag, Berlin, (1992).
3. Duvaut, G. and Lions, J.-L., *Inequalities in Mechanics and Physics*, Springer-Verlag, Berlin, (1976).
4. Isakov, V., "A nonhyperbolic Cauchy problem for $\square_b \square_c$ and its applications to elasticity theory," *Commun. Pure. Appl. Math.*, **39**, 747–767 (1986).
5. Isakov, V., *Inverse Source Problems*, American Mathematical Society, Providence, Rhode Island, (1990).
6. Klibanov, M. V., "Inverse problems and Carleman estimates," *Inverse Problems*, **8**, 575–596 (1992).
7. Ola, P., Päivärinta, L. and Somersalo, E., "An inverse boundary value problem in electrodynamics," *Duke Math. J.*, **70**, 617–653 (1993).
8. Ramm, A. G., "An inverse problem for Maxwell's equation," *Physics Letters A*, **138**, 459–462 (1989).
9. Ramm, A. G., *Multidimensional Inverse Scattering Problems*, Longman, Essex, (1992).
10. Ramm, A. G. and Somersalo, E., "Electromagnetic inverse problem with surface measurements at low frequencies," *Inverse Problems*, **5**, 1107–1116 (1989).
11. Romanov, V. G. and Kabanikhin, S. I., *Inverse Problems for Maxwell's Equations*, VSP, Utrecht, (1994).
12. Sun, Z. and Uhlmann, G., "An inverse boundary problem for Maxwell's equations," *Arch. Rational Mech. Anal.*, 119, 71–93 (1992).
13. Yamamoto, M., "A mathematical aspect of inverse problems for non-stationary Maxwell's equations," *Int. J. of Applied Electromagnetics and Mechanics*, **9**, 1–22 (1997).

INDEX